WORKING DISASTERS
The Politics of
Recognition and Response

Edited by
Eric Tucker
Osgoode Hall Law School, York University

Work, Health, and Environment Series
Series Editors: Charles Levenstein and John Wooding

Baywood Publishing Company, Inc.
AMITYVILLE, NEW YORK

Baywood Publishing Company, Inc.
26 Austin Avenue
PO Box 337
Amityville, NY 11701
(800) 638-7819
E-mail: baywood@baywood.com
Web site: baywood.com

Library of Congress Catalog Number: 2005054582
ISBN: 0-89503-319-4 (cloth)

Library of Congress Cataloging-in-Publication Data

Working disasters : the politics of recognition and response / edited by Eric Tucker.
    p. cm. -- (Work, health and environment series)
    Includes bibliographical references and index.
    ISBN 0-89503-319-4 (cloth)
    1. Industrial accidents--Government policy. 2. Occupational diseases--Government policy. 3. Industrial safety--Government policy. I. Tucker, Eric. II. Series.

    HD7262.W62 2006
    363. 34--dc22

                             2005054582

*This book is dedicated to the memory
of the untold number of workers
who have lost their lives and health
in working disasters.*

Table of Contents

v

Preface

In this volume of the series, WORK, HEALTH AND ENVIRONMENT, Professor Eric Tucker and his colleagues examine an essential aspect of our times: the political economy of disasters. As in the time-honored role of canaries in the mines, the chapters of this book focus on hazards (and failures) in the work environment, ones which we should understand as important in themselves as well as having implications for society at large. The collection seems particularly appropriate at this writing, given the amazing spectacle of American refugees in Mississippi, Louisiana, and Texas, presumably the result of "natural" phenomena. Intentional and unintentional disasters—from Bhopal to the World Trade Center debacle and the devastating consequences of climate change—present front and center the inadequacy of existing social mechanisms to deal with remarkably hazardous modern technologies. As Karl Polanyi pointed out in *The Great Transformation,* the self-regulating market "could not exist for any length of time without annihilating the human and natural substance of society; it would have physically destroyed man and transformed his surroundings into a wilderness" (p. 3).

Disasters that attract the attention of the media and the public at large are not the only sort of problems that confront us. In this series we have been publishing works that analyze and describe the relationship between what goes on in the workplace, the consequences for the public health, and environmental degradation. We have defined health and environment broadly. Health is not limited to the absence of disease or to individual health. It must also mean a healthy and sustainable economy, a democratic and participatory politics, a workplace where the rights of workers are respected and enforced, and communities that are sustainable, crime free, and nurturing of the physical and mental health of all.

We have argued that struggles over the control of technology at the point of production were reflected in one way or another in the wider society—so that studying the micro-environment of industrial hazards could deepen our understanding of many problems in the society and general environment. We thought, for instance, that this approach was particularly useful for understanding the issues of environmental justice and "cleaner production." The relationship between inequality and health, apparently news to social epidemiologist, comes as no shock to students of work environment policy. And that there are important social dimensions to apparent "natural" disasters is also clear.

In our book series, we have tried to provide a framework for the analysis of central problems in our times—the impact of technology on work, health, and environment. But the first book in this series, a festschrift for Barry Commoner, edited by Professor David Kriebel, was called *Science and Action,* in part because the phrase captured an essential aspect of Prof. Commoner's career, but also because we did not intend our work to be dry theorizing—academic work for its own sake. We take seriously our commitment to changing the world for the better. We believe that Eric Tucker and his colleagues have made an important contribution to this effort.

Acknowledgments

Edited collections, like all academic work, are the product of a collective effort, not just of the authors of the chapters whose contributions are obvious (and greatly appreciated), but also of numerous individuals, including those who have assisted the authors with their work. Here I want to take the opportunity to acknowledge the contributions of those who aided me in putting this volume together.

My journey into the world of working disasters began with the explosion of the Westray mine on May 26, 1992. Shortly after the explosion, as reports began to emerge of widespread violations of health and safety laws that had gone uncorrected by government regulators, my friend and colleague at Osgoode Hall Law School, Harry Glasbeek, and I presented a short talk on the Westray disaster on *A Taste of Justice*, a radio show that we, along with a number of other progressive colleagues, produced for a community station. The more we investigated the events leading up to the explosion the more we became convinced that the Westray mine disaster was not the outcome of an egregious breakdown of the system of occupational health and safety regulation, but rather the predictable result of its normal operation. Over the years that followed, we wrote and spoke about this disaster and its aftermath, both together and individually.

I first conceived of the idea of an edited volume on working disasters several years after the Westray disaster. At the time, another friend and colleague Robert Storey, a professor of sociology and labour studies at McMaster University, had recently co-authored (with Professor Wayne Lewchuk) an article on the exposure of workers at the Bendix automotive plant in Windsor, Ontario to asbestos. I talked to Robert about my idea and he enthusiastically agreed to join me in putting together a proposal and approaching potential contributors and publishers. Although other commitments eventually kept him from continuing his participation in the project, Robert's early contributions played a vital role in shaping its themes.

As chapters began to arrive, I was fortunate enough to be able to engage the services of Brent Arnold, then a first-year law student at Osgoode Hall Law School with a background in publishing and copy-editing. I think I can speak for all the contributors to this volume in thanking Brent for his meticulous copy-editing of the draft chapters.

I would also like to thank Chuck Levenstein and John Wooding, the editors of this series, for their enthusiastic support for this volume, Juniee Oneida for the outstanding job of creating the index, and Julie Krempa and Bobbi Olszewski from Baywood for their assistance in bringing the volume to publication.

Most of the work on this collection was undertaken at Osgoode Hall Law School, York University, where the administration, staff, and colleagues have contributed to the creation of a supportive research environment. I completed the volume while spending a sabbatical year as a visiting scholar at Cleveland-Marshall College of Law, Cleveland State University, and would like to thank the faculty and staff for their warm welcome and support.

My children, Myka and Zak, are now too old to be offered up as excuses for delays in bringing this project to fruition. For the same reason, I no longer need to apologize to them for occasional bouts of distraction. I do, however, want to thank them for their love and understanding, over the last few years. My parents, Selma and William, have also been a constant source of support.

Finally, I owe my greatest debt to Lisa Brand, my phoenix, on whose wings I rose from the ashes.

Eric Tucker

CHAPTER 1

Introduction:
The Politics of Recognition
and Response

Eric Tucker

On the morning of February 1, 2003 seven astronauts died when the space shuttle Columbia broke up in the sky high over Texas and Louisiana while reentering the earth's atmosphere. The event was immediately characterized as a disaster and the media interrupted its normal broadcasts to focus on the developing story. Within hours an independent review board was convened, headed by retired Admiral Harold W. Gehman Jr. (Broder with Oppel Jr. 2003). Almost unnoted in the ensuing discussions, and certainly of no great significance to commentators, was that these seven astronauts were also workers killed in the course of performing their jobs: six were members of the military (five American and one Israeli) and one a civilian employee of NASA (Shuttle Victims 2003).

At first glance, this characterization of the event and the reaction to it seems quite natural. Public attention is focused on manned-space missions, which are presented as and perceived to be dramatic instances of heroic risk-taking in the name of advancing the boundaries of human knowledge. Thus when missions fail so spectacularly and publicly, killing all those aboard, it seems intuitively obvious that we have witnessed a disaster. A noble pursuit has ended tragically in the loss of life. In that context, the status of the astronauts as workers, either military or civilian, is of no obvious public consequence because we are given to understand that they were voluntary risk takers: that is why they are celebrated as heroes, not mourned as victims. Thus, according to the *New York Times'* editorial writers, "They accepted the risks, the ones they knew and perhaps even the ones they couldn't have imagined. Their acceptance was unsentimental, just part of the job" (Remembering the Columbia Crew 2003). Moreover, we are also assured that the exposure of these workers to the risk of death and their voluntary acceptance of that risk is consistent with NASA's overarching commitment to safety. On the one hand, NASA proclaims that "[e]xploration involves risk, including the

1

risk of failure" but, on the other that, "[b]eing an Agency workforce willing to accept risk, but only in an informed manner, is consistent with our unwillingness to compromise the safety and health of people and property or do harm to the environment" (NASA 1999). Although we are not told exactly how NASA's willingness to accept the risk of failure that can materialize in multiple deaths is consistent with an unwillingness to compromise health and safety, such statements seem to be sufficient to satisfy the government and the public. Perhaps for this reason, there was almost no public outrage over the deaths at the moment they occurred: everything humanly possible had been done to ensure the safety of the astronauts, but something unforeseeably went wrong. But because the commitment to safety is genuinely felt, and because it is socially unacceptable to operate a space program whose risks materialize in multiple and highly visible deaths such as these, it also seems natural that an inquiry should be conducted to determine what went wrong so that more deaths may be avoided in the future.

As much as the public perception of and reaction to this working disaster seems natural, upon closer examination competing causal stories (Stone 1989) may begin to emerge that offer different constructions of the events and their meanings. For example, NASA's critics question the scientific utility of manned missions, taking the view that their primary purpose is to generate public support for an expensive space exploration program that provides little civilian benefit (e.g., Kuttner 2003). Viewed this way, the space shuttle program is not a noble endeavor but rather a spectacle, mounted by NASA and promoted by the cheer-leading media, that diverts the public from insisting that government address pressing problems here on Earth. If that is so, are the inherent risks to human life associated with manned spaceflight worthwhile? As well, the supposed unstinting commitment of the program to safety may be more myth than reality. According to one journalistic account produced in the days following the loss of the Columbia, although there was a renewed emphasis on safety backed by increased funding immediately after the Challenger disaster of 1986, "NASA's pursuit of a safer shuttle has largely stalled. It is a story of seesawing budgets, political infighting and radical policy shifts against a backdrop of falling public interest in space exploration" (Barstow and Moss 2003). The Columbia Accident Investigation Board (2003, p. 187) adopted much the same view of NASA's safety program. "Despite periodic attempts to emphasize safety, NASA's frequent reorganizations in the drive to become more efficient reduced the budget for safety, sending employees conflicting messages and creating conditions more conducive to the development of a conventional bureaucracy than to the maintenance of a safety-conscious research-and-development organization." From this perspective, the status of the astronauts as workers may not be so insignificant. NASA, it seems, behaved much like other employers: faced with a conflict between production and safety, they stinted on safety to achieve production targets. Perhaps these astronauts did not truly accept the risks to which they were exposed, including "the risks they could not have imagined" (whatever that means) in that, like other workers, they put too much faith in the commitment and competence of the organization to which they provided service to provide them in turn with the safest possible working conditions.

It is unlikely that the above reconstruction of the story will change anyone's view that the death of the seven Columbia astronauts was a disaster—although it may be viewed as a disaster of a different kind than initially thought—but hopefully it raises questions about the naturalness of the category and the meanings attached to it. For example, if it were revealed that tens of workers were killed and thousands injured or made ill in the course of designing, building, and maintaining the shuttle, the rockets, and the rest of the infrastructure supporting a manned space program, would that be construed as a disaster? What are the social processes that lead to the attribution of some events as disasters but not others? Why, for example, do we focus on single incidents in which there are multiple worker deaths and virtually ignore the far greater toll of death, injury, and disease that workers suffer one by one on a daily basis?

The events surrounding the deaths of the Columbia astronauts and the Challenger astronauts before them also amply demonstrate that the characterization of an event as a disaster may imbue it with enormous emotional, social, and political power. A disaster may cause people to question assumptions that allowed them to accept with more or less equanimity the conduct of risky activity. It may trigger inquiries into the social utility of the objectives for which the risk is undertaken, or at least a reassessment of whether the benefits justify the risks. The social construction of an event as a disaster may also lead to an examination of the distribution of risks and benefits: for whose benefit are workers dying or being injured? It may produce inquiries into the adequacy of the systems of risk prevention and risk regulation that were supposed to protect workers: was the risk detected?; if not, why not?; if so, what was the response and why did it fail to prevent the risk from materializing in deaths and injuries?

Just as we need to interrogate the social processes of disaster recognition and the attribution of meanings to that designation, so too we need to investigate more deeply the social, political, and legal processes that determine how the state responds to such events. Will the disaster designation change the balance of social forces so that groups previously unable to effectively assert their concerns in the policy arena may now have their voices heard and even heeded? Will the processes of re-examination result in significant and meaningful changes to public or private systems of risk regulation, or will the momentum for change be dissipated through processes that lead to a restoration or relegitimation of the *status quo ante*?

The politics of recognition and response to working disasters are the subject of the essays gathered in this book. Although there are published case studies of the struggle for recognition of occupational disease (e.g., Clark 1997; Levenstein, Delaurier, with Dunn 2002; Rosner and Markowitz 1991) and of the aftermath of occupational health and safety (OHS) disasters (e.g., Cherniak 1986), the subject of working disasters as a general phenomenon has not received sustained attention. One reason for this is that the topic intersects a number of different intellectual streams that are not commonly joined, and so it will be useful at the outset to briefly identify them.

Disaster research is a relatively new field that has been dated back to a study by Prince (1920) of the Halifax Harbour explosion of 1917. It was not until the end of World War II, however, that the field began to develop a distinctive analytical or research paradigm. To a great extent, this paradigm was shaped by the professional commitments of the authors in the field who were largely concerned with the management of the aftermaths of natural disasters such as earthquakes, floods, and hurricanes. Coming from this orientation, Charles Fritz (1961) provided one of the first definitions of disaster as:

> . . . an event, concentrated in time and space, in which a society, or a relatively self-sufficient subdivision of society undergoes severe danger and incurs losses to its members and physical appurtenances that the social structure is disrupted and the fulfillment of all or some of the essential functions of the society is prevented. (p. 655)

This definition, which focuses on time, space, and severity, continues to inform much of the literature in the field (e.g., Fischer 1998, pp. 2-3) and coincided precisely with those events that governments defined as disasters justifying extraordinary interventions. The ideal-type disaster, so to speak, was a sudden, natural occurrence that severely affected a discrete community.

This definition did not exclude social factors from an analysis of disasters, but it also did not make them central.[1] Later researchers addressed this deficiency. Yet while they emphasized that the vulnerability of a community to harm from a natural event like a hurricane was a contingent social condition, not a natural state of affairs, this did not change their understanding of what constituted a disaster (Gilbert 1998).

The study of socially or technically caused (as opposed to natural) disasters developed later. Barry Turner's seminal book, *Man-made Disasters* (1978), set the tone for much of the research that followed. He focused primarily on disaster causation, arguing that disasters largely stemmed from an accumulation of errors resulting from misinterpretation, false assumptions, poor communication, cultural lag, and misplaced optimism (p. 395). While others have criticized Turner's model and advanced alternatives (e.g., Perrow 1984; Vaughan 1996) their focus remained on events that fit Fritz's definition. For example, Turner's study was based on detailed analysis of 84 official reports of inquiries into single-incident events that produced multiple deaths; Perrow's focused on nuclear accidents; and Vaughan's on the launch of the shuttle Challenger. However, the approach to disaster causation taken by these studies laid the groundwork for undercutting the definitional certainty of their object. This was because in different ways these analysts theorized disasters not as the outcome of technological failures alone, but rather as a result of the interaction between technology and organizational, political, and economic contexts. Technological or man-made disasters, then, were not caused by single incidents and the harm they produced was not necessarily experienced immediately.

While these authors were not led to problematize the object of their study, others were beginning to question the concept of disaster itself, as they recognized that at some level disasters were socially constructed phenomena (e.g., Quarantelli 1985). This approach received an additional boost in 1980s and 90s from writers in the rapidly expanding field of risk studies. Lupton (1999, ch. 2) traced three epistemological positions in the risk literature: realist, weak constructionist, and strong constructionist. Realists treat risk as objective, measurable, and independent of social and cultural processes, but recognize that these processes may distort risk perception and assessment. Weak constructionists recognize the material reality of risk, but see its perception and assessment as inevitably mediated by social processes. Finally, strong constructionists see risk itself as a social construction.

Strong constructionism has attracted few adherents among those writing in the field of disaster studies, if only because, as Oliver-Smith (2002, p. 39) notes, "the physical reality of disaster explicitly challenges theoretical currents that hold that nature is a purely social construction at the ontological level." Assuming broad agreement with the view that it is unproductive to sever the ties between disaster and material reality, however, still leaves unanswered the question of how social constructionism operates to select some set of harm-causing events as disasters while ignoring others.

Kreps (1998) attempted to reformulate Fritz's definition in a way that incorporated social constructionist perspectives. He defined disasters as:

> nonroutine events in societies or their larger subsystems (e.g., regions, communities) that involve social disruption and physical harm. Among, the key defining properties of such events are (1) length of forewarning, (2) magnitude of impact, (3) scope of impact, and (4) duration of impact. (p. 34)

While Kreps recognized that "precise thresholds of when historical happenings are socially defined as disasters have never been determined," his attempt to impose a threshold limited to "nonroutine" events seems artificial unless the goal of the exercise is to affirm the existing selection practices of state disaster relief agencies. By definitional fiat, this precludes so-called "routine" events that cause enormous harm on an ongoing basis from being constructed as disasters, thereby contributing to a process that normalizes both the occurrence of that harm and the state practices that permit it.

A more promising model that focuses on the *process* of social construction is that of Robert Gephart Jr. (1984). His political sensemaking model joins, perhaps somewhat oddly, a post-modernist sensibility with a political economy perspective. According to Gephart, social reality is constructed by individuals through the process of reflecting on and interpreting the meaning of phenomena. However, the process of sensemaking is fundamentally political because divergent social interests, motives, and knowledge generate competing descriptions of reality. As a result, those who are more powerful are better able to have their versions of reality become the dominant one. In contemporary society, capital is better organized and mobilized to make its interests appear as the general interest, leading to the widespread acceptance of its construction of reality. The logic of Gephart's analysis lends itself to radical critique of conventional understandings of disaster:

> The occurrence of a disaster is a political accomplishment. . . . Industry/ government makes claims minimizing the disruptive impact or nature of events. . . . Public critics make claims maximizing the disruptive impact or nature of events. (Gephart 1984, pp. 214, 218)

Gephart's approach, however, does not seem to have attracted much attention among disaster researchers.[2]

Although social constructionist approaches have led to a broadening of the scope of disaster research, it still has not reached into the workplace. Perhaps for this reason, occupational health and safety researchers have not drawn on the sociology of disaster literature in their studies of the processes of recognition/ non-recognition of working disasters. Indeed, to a great extent OHS researchers have not been concerned with the labeling of the harms that workers experience as disasters because the workers they are studying are confronting the logically prior problem of just getting employers and state officials to recognize that their work environment is causing harm (e.g., Levenstein et al. 2002; Markowitz and Rosner 2002). Much of the research into harm recognition is informed by a social constructionist perspective, although not in its strong forms, if only because the materiality of workplace hazards and harms seems all too apparent, even if only retrospectively. However, it is widely accepted that the recognition and assessment of risk is a social process that takes place against a backdrop of often conflicting objectives among workers and employers, and in a world in which scientific knowledge and research, and political, administrative, and legal decision-making do not escape the effect of unequal power relations. Recognition of OHS hazards is thus an intensely political process. Thus for example, Levenstein et al. (2002, pp. 4-7) theorize that workers' OHS concerns get recognized when unions are in a position to challenge the power of employers (rarely) or when progressive forces, including occupational health researchers, coalesce to form a strong alliance in support of reforms, and some employers find it in their interest to accept that existing practices need amelioration. Numerous studies (Clark 1997; Derickson 1998; Levenstein et al. 2002; Markowitz and Rosner 2002; Rosner and Markowitz 1991) have amply documented the shocking role of industry, often assisted by doctors and scientists, in suppressing available hazard information and in blocking further research.

The essays in this collection that address the politics of recognition, draw on this body of OHS research, and seek to extend it by challenging the historically narrow paradigm that has conventionalized the harm that workers routinely suffer. That is, they seek in various ways to question why the massive harms that workers endure are either not recognized as being work-related, or if work-related are not being recognized as disasters that require an extraordinary state response. Quinlan, Mayhew, and Johnstone (Chapter 2), for example, take the case of the death and injury of truck drivers, one of the most dangerous occupations, and interrogate why it does not attract the kind of recognition that is given to a coal-mine explosion that kills far fewer workers. There is, of course, the obvious point that truck drivers are killed one-by-one while coal miners are killed in groups when mines explode, but that that does not answer the question of why only clustered deaths tend to be socially constructed as disasters that require extraordinary responses. They suggest a number of reasons for this, focusing especially on the roles of ideology and of institutions. At the ideological level, Quinlan et al. point to the growing influence of neo-liberalism and the emphasis it places on individual agency, responsibility, and risk management. This facilitates a shift in the focus of attention onto the behavior of individual drivers, rather than on the underlying social causes of transport accidents that include economic pressures, work restructuring, and regulatory failures. By obscuring common themes that might be seen to link these individual events, it is less likely they will be aggregated and viewed as a common phenomenon that causes immense harm—a disaster. They also point to the role of regulatory arrangements in the politics of trucking deaths. Road transport regulation, not OHS, has primary authority over these incidents. As a result, common work arrangements that increase the risk to drivers or induce riskier driver behavior have little regulatory or social significance. Indeed, they go largely unrecognized as health and safety officials who might be more attentive to such issues are unlikely to be involved. In sum, because truck driver deaths are individualized and not viewed through the lens of work, they are unlikely to be recognized as working disasters.

The role of institutions also plays a prominent part in Hopkins' chapter, which considers the rise and fall of repetitive strain injury (RSI) in Australia during the 1980s (Chapter 3). While not suggesting that this epidemic should have been characterized as a disaster, Hopkins' discussion of the politics of RSI recognition makes an important contribution by focusing on the process through which official statistics are constructed and how that data may be used to provide evidence of a social problem. According to Hopkins, for contingent political reasons the workers' compensation system was open to RSI claims at a time when the federal public service was being restructured and work was being intensified. Because work injury statistics are derived from successful workers' compensation claims, this facilitated bureaucratic and social recognition of RSI as a real problem demanding a regulatory response.

Rennie's study of Newfoundland (Chapter 4) fluorspar miners' struggle to gain recognition that the lung diseases they suffered from were work-related also points to the important role that the workers' compensation system plays in the politics of working disasters. But in his case, its major role was to resist, not facilitate, recognition of the work-relatedness of the high incidence of lung diseases that miners suffered. Thus a major focus of Rennie's analysis is on the struggle of the miners, their union, and community to overcome this institutional and legal resistance to recognition. Rennie works from a political economy perspective that emphasizes the role of conflict in the politics of working disaster recognition. Not only did the miners have to deal with problems of scientific uncertainty, they also faced a government and an employer that seemed more concerned with the economic consequences that would ensue from acknowledging that miners were becoming sick from their work than with providing them with proper protection and fair compensation. The combination of a growing body count, medical investigations, media attention, presentations to review committees and a royal commission, industrial action, and public protests for over thirty years was necessary to gain recognition of the full extent of the harm inflicted on the miners.

By contrast, Thörnquist's discussion of silicosis in Sweden (Chapter 5) shows that recognition of an occupational disease by workers' compensation authorities does not necessarily lead political and regulatory authorities to accept that continued exposure of workers to a given danger will have disastrous consequences unless preventive measures are taken. The central question she asks in her chapter is: why was there was an extended delay between the time silicosis was recognized as an occupational disease in 1931 and the time stricter controls on dust exposure were mandated? In part, the answer lies in the authorities' limited recognition of the scope of the problem and in their misguided belief that medical supervision of exposed workers exclusively in high-risk work places was a sufficient response. Indeed, Thörnquist argues that medical supervision legitimated the continued exposure of workers to silica. Consequently, the struggle for recognition of silica exposure as a serious problem—as a disaster requiring a strong state response—needed to continue. The shape and timing of that struggle for recognition was influenced by many factors, including the development of the Swedish model of industrial relations in the 1930s (with its emphasis on cooperative union-management self-regulation), the challenges to it in the 1960s and 1970s, and the activities of committed physicians and researchers who documented the true scope and consequences of worker exposure to silica.

These chapters also demonstrate that the politics of recognition necessarily join with the politics of response, if only because the nature and extent of the recognition of harm to workers as a disaster will influence the state's response to it. Nevertheless, it is also clear that the outcome of the political struggle over recognition will not determine how the politics of response will play out.

Therefore, it is necessary to explore separately the processes that influence whether individuals or organizations will be held accountable and whether significant change to regimes of OHS regulation will follow upon disaster recognition.

Arguably one can identify three inter-related dimensions to the politics of response. First, there is likely to be a debate over causation. Victims and others who seek accountability and change will argue that the disaster was avoidable because it was the result of purposeful actions, regardless of whether the result was intended, whereas those who wish to avoid blame will claim both that the outcome was unintended and that it was the result of unguided actions (Stone 1989). Second, even if a disaster is identified as the outcome of purposeful behavior, there will still be disputes about the measures necessary to avoid similar outcomes in the future and whether they are practicable. Finally, even if a technical consensus is reached, there are likely to be political obstacles that will need to be overcome to implement the necessary changes.

Although the politics of response to occupational health and safety disasters has received relatively little consideration, the disaster literature, especially that part dealing with man-made disasters, provides some useful insights. There seems to be widespread acceptance of two points, both of which are implicit in much of the discussion so far. The first is that is that the impact of disasters on public policy is largely determined by political processes rather than by the characteristics of the disasters themselves. For example, according to Freeman (2002, p. 3), "[t]he aftermaths of disasters are influenced less by the extent of the tragedies as by the political contexts in which they occur." The second is that the response to a disaster may produce significant changes. Thus, according to Michael Reich (1991):

> Disasters provide an opportunity, and sadly may even be necessary, for realigning the mobilization of bias and for redefining the dominant symbols in ways to tip the balance of power, at least momentarily, in the direction of public interests and in favor of the relatively powerless. Crises not only provide opportunities for viewing the ordinary processes of society, they also provide the powerless with brief chances for reforming those processes, for redirecting social resources in more equitable ways. (p. 266)

The more difficult question on which there is less agreement is what factors shape the politics of disaster response and influence their outcomes. One focus of research has been on the characteristics of victims and their power resources. Ortwin Renn uses the metaphor of an arena to describe institutional settings in which policy is determined and is particularly concerned with decision-making about risk. In his view, "[t]he fundamental axiom is that resource availability determines the degree of influence for shaping policies" (Renn 1992, p. 195). Social resources include money, power, social influence, value commitment, and evidence. Renn recognizes that these resources are unequally distributed, but has little to say on the subject. Writing about the likelihood of activism in response to pain and loss events (of which disasters would be a subset), Michael Jennings (1999, p. 8) suggested a four-category typology generated from the combination of two characteristics of the affected group: their power and their social approval. The resulting categories are the advantaged (high on both dimensions), contenders (high on power, low on approval), dependents (low on power, high on approval), and deviants (low on both). OHS disasters will by definition have working-class victims and although locating them within this matrix is not entirely straightforward, in most cases they would be identified as a group with relatively little power but with reasonably high levels of approval. Jennings also suggests that the magnitude of the affected population and the distribution of victims will also be significant. While the magnitude of OHS disasters will vary, in most cases the distribution will be concentrated within a narrow, relatively powerless segment of the population.

Because of these characteristics of the victim population in OHS disasters, it is especially important to inquire into the ways in which a disaster might alter the power and political influence that a group normally exercises. Jennings (1999, pp. 9-10) suggests a number of reasons why activism may be enhanced when it is harm-related: the stakes are all too apparent and immediate for those whose own bodies have been damaged or who are close to someone who has been injured or killed; the propensity for people who have pain and loss experiences to join with others in support groups helps overcome collective action problems; the events are highly emotionally charged and attract media attention; and death and injury provide activists with an accessible stock of vivid representations that resonate with widely held social beliefs about compassion, justice, safety, and health.

As these considerations suggest, OHS disasters may not only enhance the voice of victims, but may also help produce a more receptive environment in which their messages are received. Arthur McEvoy (1995) addressed this phenomenon in his discussion of the aftermath of the Triangle Shirtwaist fire in 1911 that killed 146 workers. One of its most important outcomes was that it "work[ed] a change in the patterns of causal attribution that underlay public thinking about industrial safety" (p. 624). But of course disasters do not naturally produce shifts in common sense views, as this too is a political process, partially influenced by the ability of the victim group to have "[its] account of reality become the reality perceived by others" (Gephart 1984, p. 213). McEvoy (1995, pp. 627-631) identified a number of reasons why the Triangle Shirtwaist fire had such a powerful social effect including: workplace accidents were already a high-profile issue at the time of the fire, in part because of debates about the introduction of workers' compensation legislation; the highly public way in which the victims died; and the fire could not be coded as an accident because of the obvious role of the employer in creating the hazard and obstructing the exits, thereby making visible how employers were extracting wealth from the bodies of workers (also see Bender 2004; Von Drehle 2003).

While the kinds of contingent factors mentioned by McEvoy are no doubt important, other researchers have tried to locate more systemic influences on the politics of causation. Kasperson (1992) and Renn (1992) have developed the concept of the social amplification of risk to explain perceptions of risk and risk behavior. The focus of this analytic framework is on the social processing of information about risks, paying particular attention to the role of groups and non-state institutions in either heightening or attenuating concern. The roles of social movements and the media, for example, have received considerable attention from these analysts.

Of particular interest given the focus of this book are the characteristics of the state institutions in which the politics of response are played out. Wells (1995) examines the legal responses to disaster, paying particular attention to the role of inquiries and inquests, compensation systems, and criminal prosecution. While most of her book discusses specific legal issues, Wells also addresses particular features of the institutions in which legal redress is sought, and their impact on outcomes. In her discussion of corporate manslaughter prosecutions, for example, Wells notes the problem of institutional resistance, which she traces to a number of factors, some internal and others external to the criminal law. Thus, on the one hand, Wells notes, "[a] real tension exists between the paradigm of criminal culpability based on individual responsibility and the increasing recognition of the potential for harm inherent in large scale corporate activity" (p. 173). On the other hand, Wells also recognizes that the criminal justice system is not static and isolated from society, but rather that the social construction of events will shape their legal construction. As Wells (1996) noted in a later article, "[t]he desirability or likelihood of a prosecution for corporate manslaughter, following transport or other disasters caused by management disregard of safety policies or precautions, are not matters that can be assessed from a purely legal standpoint" (p. 57).

Thus, in some ways we have come full circle. State institutions potentially shape the outcome of the politics of disaster but are simultaneously shaped by those politics as they play themselves out in non-state settings. But this should not be surprising given the complexity and interactive nature of legal, social, and political systems. Differences in approach to the politics of response, then, may lie more in the way researchers view social and political systems generally than in their view of the elements that constitute the political terrain. Thus, those who emphasize the salience of unequal power relations in shaping outcomes tend to take a more pessimistic view of the likely aftermath of a disaster. Reich (1991) for example concluded his study of toxic politics by observing that "[d]isaster may provide the opportunity and the impetus for institutional change, allowing for a redistribution of power and a transformation of policy. But the existing distribution of power creates formidable blockages to social change that might benefit the relatively powerless" (p. 281). Gephart (1984) takes a similarly bleak view, noting that, "[t]he primary social change which occurs as the result of [organizationally based environmental disasters] is the normalization of the problems of pollution and environmental degradation" (p. 222). This outcome is explained on the basis that capital, which benefits from certain forms of resource exploitation, is better able to have its view of reality accepted than that of those who bear and are concerned about the cost of that exploitation. Those who are more optimistic operate from a more pluralistic perspective, which sees greater opportunities for those who are relatively less powerful to influence public policy, in part because of openings that disasters may create (e.g., McEnvoy 1995; Renn 1992).

The chapters in this book adopt a case study approach that contributes to these larger debates by providing rich accounts of state response to working disasters across a wide range of times and places. In some of these studies the politics of recognition and response are deeply interrelated. For example, Quinlan and colleagues' study of long-haul road transport in Australia demonstrates that the widespread and incremental nature of fatalities in that industry not only impedes recognition of its disastrous outcomes, but that it also undercuts the ability of regulators to connect these outcomes to their underlying causes related to economic conditions, work organization, and regulatory changes. Indeed, they find that truck fatalities and injuries are not even recognized as an OHS problem, but rather are dealt with through road transport regulation, which character-istically focuses on individual behavior.

Rennie's study traces the slow response of the Newfoundland government to the high levels of industrial disease developing among fluorspar miners in the mid-twentieth century. He identifies a persistent pattern of minimalism: at each stage of the miners' struggle for protection and compensation, the government dragged its feet, doing as little as was politically acceptable at the time. As a result, not only were many disabled workers denied compensation, but also excessively high dust levels persisted in the mines. To explain this phenomenon, Rennie adopts a political-economy-of-knowledge approach that focuses on the processes by which information and opinions about industrial disasters are dis-seminated or suppressed by the parties involved. Medical recognition of the problem was not sufficient to generate an appropriate response and so workers struggled to publicize their plight, but lacked the power to trigger state action. Rather, incremental improvements were made almost exclusively in the aftermath of favorable conjunctures, including findings of public inquiries, heightened levels of industrial conflict, and media attention.

Thörnquist's chapter looks at a similar phenomenon involving Swedish workers suffering from silicosis. She also works from a political economy perspective that focuses on unequal power relations between workers and their employers. These inequalities, however, were mediated in various ways. Ideologically, they manifested themselves in an approach that focused on regu-lating the worker rather than the workplace. Instead of regulating exposure, a matter under the control of employers, regulatory action emphasized medical surveillance of workers. The regulatory response was also shaped by the broader labor market and industrial relations policies of the Swedish social democrats that relied on centralized collective bargaining by a heavily unionized workforce. It was only in the context of growing public awareness of environmental hazards and mounting labor militancy during the 1960s and 70s that stricter controls on the exposure of workers to industrial dusts were introduced.

Separating recognition and response issues is less of a problem when a large number of workers are killed in a single incident: these events are immediately coded as disasters, typically triggering some kind of public inquiry, and often accompanied by prosecutions and civil actions. However, this was not always the case. Patricia Reeves' study (Chapter 6) of the aftermath of the 1860 Pemberton Mill disaster in Lawrence, Massachusetts that killed over one hundred workers— the majority women and girls—examines both the immediate response and the role of the disaster in reshaping popular ideas about work relations that ultimately led to protective legislation. There was neither a formal public inquiry nor legal action taken against the employers. There was, however, an effort to enact protective legislation, but for reasons not transparent from the historical record, this effort failed. Reeve speculates that in the absence of an organized movement of mill workers and supporters, state industrialists opposed to regulation were able to prevent the bill from becoming law. Yet Reeve also finds that in the longer run post-disaster interpretations of the events at Pemberton contributed to the construction of labor narratives of employer avarice and negligence, and of employee susceptibility to bodily harm. While on the one hand this was useful in the fight for protective labor laws, it simultaneously raised doubts about the fitness of industrial workers to participate equally in social and political life, precisely because of their vulnerabilities and lack of independence.

Whyte's study of the aftermath of the Piper Alpha disaster of the British North Sea in 1988, which killed 167 people, also emphasizes the need to take a longer view of the response to disasters (Chapter 7). Here, however, the pattern found by Reeve was reversed. The immediate aftermath of the disaster disrupted the self-regulatory approach to OHS that dominated at the time. Closer monitoring of the scheme of self-regulation was imposed, and some costly safety controls were prescribed. The disruption, however, proved to be temporary. As political and economic conditions changed, the oil industry mounted a cost reduction strategy that led to a loosening of external controls as well as to work inten- sification. OHS regulators accepted these changes notwithstanding consequent increases in injury rates because they accepted the oil industry's argument that it needed to become more "efficient" to survive. As well, their underlying assumption that workers and employers fundamentally have a common interest in safety led them to accept a return to self-regulation without strong worker participation rights. Whyte concludes that because of the ongoing and growing structural advantage enjoyed by capital, the disruption caused by the Piper Alpha disaster to its regulatory agenda was only temporary.

Tucker also takes a traditional disaster, the explosion of the Westray mine in Nova Scotia that killed 26 miners in 1993, and follows the politics of response as they played out in a variety of institutional settings. He begins by constructing a model of the determinants of a working disaster that incorporates interactions between the pre-disaster OHS regime, political-economic context, disaster characteristics, and features of the institutions of redress. Like Whyte, he finds that in the immediate aftermath of the Westray disaster, the legitimacy of the province's OHS regime was struck a severe blow. Public inquiries, administrative and legislative reviews, criminal prosecutions, and civil litigation—all extraordinary responses in the OHS context—were called into play. Yet more than 12 years later, no individual or organization has been held legally accountable despite the obvious reckless disregard for workers lives by the mine operators or for the complete failure of OHS regulators to stop the ongoing and serious violations of the province's health and safety laws. A public inquiry condemned the employer for its neglect of safety and the government for its failure to regulate the mine, but it also endorsed the underlying health and safety model, with its emphasis on internal responsibility, rather than seeing it as a cause of the disaster. That finding, in conjunction with the relative weakness of organized labor in the province, allowed for the re-legitimation of the OHS regime through tinkering.

However, the continuing public perception of Westray as an egregious example of corporate criminality gone unpunished, and more recent corporate scandals such as Enron, put the federal government under pressure to address perceived technical barriers to the successful prosecution of corporate offenders. As a result, in 2003, more than ten years after the disaster, the so-called Westray bill was passed, amending the *Criminal Code.* Overall, the Westray story demonstrates that there may be a multiplicity of responses to a working disaster, some of which legitimate and reinforce pre-existing ideologies and practices, while others hold more promise for effecting meaningful reform and change to popular perceptions.

It is much too early to assess the instrumental impact of the Westray bill, but experience elsewhere suggests caution. Johnstone takes up this issue in Chapter 8 on criminal prosecutions in Victoria, Australia. Although his study does not focus on disasters conventionally understood, the reality is that employers are almost only prosecuted when a worker is killed or seriously injured. Johnstone argues that each one of these events could be characterized as a disaster with the potential to disrupt the "membrane of normalcy" but that, paradoxically, prosecutions have the opposite effect of normalizing the traumatic events that motivate prosecutions in the first place. He explains this outcome as an effect of "pulverization" techniques routinely used by defense lawyers in the criminal process to isolate each event from its broader context, making it appear as something quite unique and unexpected, rather than the outcome of a systemic problem. As well, Johnstone points to the form of the criminal law itself that facilitates decontextualization and individualization through its focus on the immediate event giving rise to the prosecution and its concern with individual wrongdoing, isolated from the underlying social relations in which that action is embedded. As a result, prosecutions are infrequent, and when convictions are secured, sentences tend to be light. According to Johnstone, the current practice of criminal prosecution may unwittingly serve to legitimate inadequate health and safety management and regulation by creating the impression that there are only a few bad apples in an otherwise healthy barrel.

Finally, Dodd (Chapter 9) examines the history of public inquiries into coal mining disasters in Nova Scotia using the techniques of discourse analysis. She shares the view that disasters are potentially disruptive—that multiple deaths challenge people's unreflective acceptance of social and productive relations. The role of inquiries is to resolve these cultural coding problems by constructing a story or explanation of the event that convincingly explains the disaster in ways that reassure the reader that nothing is fundamentally wrong. But in order to succeed, disaster reports must draw on prior plausibility structures and follow literary conventions in order to establish their own legitimacy and definitiveness, establish chains of causation that lead elsewhere than an indictment of exploitive class relations, and make recommendations that if followed provide reassurance that future disasters can be avoided. Prior plausibility structures, however, are historically contingent and change over time. Dodd's investigation of the specific historical practice of writing inquiry reports in Nova Scotia delineates three periods, each dominated by a distinct narrative that, in its own way, ultimately reasserted the underlying harmony within the mining "community."

Overall, these case studies are not meant to be the last word on the study of working disasters, but hopefully they demonstrate the richness of the field and will stimulate further research using a variety of methodologies and disciplinary approaches.

ENDNOTES

1. This definition and the management focus of most disaster research may explain why Merton and Nisbet (1966) chose not to include a chapter on disasters in the second edition of their book, *Contemporary Social Problems.* Fritz's essay appeared in the first edition (1961).
2. For example, his article is not cited by any of the contributors to Quarantelli (1998).

REFERENCES

Barstow, D., and Moss, M. (2003, February 9) Worries over Shuttle's Safety Haunted NASA for Years. *The News Tribune.* Retrieved January 8, 2004, from Tribnet.com, http://www.tribnet.com/news/projects/columbia/story/2594902p-2641716c.html.
Bender, D. E. (2004) *Sweated Work, Weak Bodies.* New Brunswick, NJ: Rutgers University Press.

Broder, J. M. with Oppel Jr., R. A. (2003, February 7) NASA Cedes Authority in Columbia Shuttle Inquiry. *New York Times on the Web*. Retrieved February 21, 2003, from http://query.nytimes.com/gst/abstract.html?res=F00C16FC3E5F0C748CDDAB0894 DB404482

Cherniak, M. (1986) *The Hawk's Nest Incident*. New Haven, CT: Yale University Press.

Clark, C. (1997) *Radium Girls: Women and Industrial Health Reform, 1910-1935*. Chapel Hill, NC: University of North Carolina Press.

Columbia Accident Investigation Board. (2003) *Report*, Volume I, Online at http://anon.nasa-global.speedera.net/anon.nasa-global/CAIB/CAIB_lowres_full.pdf.

Derickson, A. (1998) *Black Lung: Anatomy of a Public Health Disaster*. Ithaca, NY: Cornell University Press.

Fischer III, H. W. (1998) *Response to Disaster* (2nd ed.), Lanham, MD: University Press of America.

Freeman, J. B. (2002) Class and Catastrophe: September 11 and Other Working-Class Disasters. *International Labor and Working-Class History, 62*: 1-6.

Fritz, C. (1961) Disaster. In R. Merton and R. Nisbet (eds.), *Contemporary Social Problems* (pp. 651-694). New York: Harcourt Brace.

Gephart Jr., R. P. (1984) Making Sense of Organizationally Based Environmental Disasters. *Journal of Management, 10*: 205-225.

Gilbert, C. (1998) Studying Disaster: Changes in the Main Conceptual Tools. In E. L. Quarantelli (ed.), *What is a Disaster?* (pp. 11-18). London: Routledge.

Jennings, M. K. (1999) Political Responses to Pain and Loss Events. *American Political Science Review, 93*: 1-13.

Kasperson, R. E. (1992) The Social Amplification of Risk: Progress in Developing an Integrative Framework. In S. Krimsky and D. Golding (eds.), *Social Theories of Risk* (pp. 153-178). Westport, CT: Praeger.

Kreps, G. A. (1998) Disaster as Systemic Event and Social Catalyst. In E. L. Quarantelli (ed.), *What is a Disaster?* (pp. 31-55). London: Routledge.

Kuttner, T. (2003) The Shuttle Spectacle. *Boston Globe* (5 February). Retrieved February 14, 2003, from http://quicksitebuilder.cnet.com/supfacts/id115.html.

Levenstein, C., and Delaurier, G. F. with Dunn, M. L. (2002) *The Cotton Dust Papers*. New York: Baywood.

Lupton, D. (1999) *Risk*. London: Routledge.

Markowitz, G. E., and Rosner, D. (2002) *Deceit and Denial: The Deadly Politics of Industrial Pollution*. Berkeley: University of California Press.

McEvoy, A. F. (1995) The Triangle Shirtwaist Factory Fire of 1911: Social Change, Industrial Accidents, and the Evolution of Common-Sense Causality. *Law & Social Inquiry, 20*: 621-651.

Merton, R. K., and Nisbet, R. A. (1961) *Contemporary Social Problems*. New York: Harcourt, Brace & World.

Merton, R. K., and Nisbet, R. A. (1966) *Contemporary Social Problems* (2nd ed.). New York: Harcourt, Brace & World.

NASA. (1999, January 19) Mission First—Safety Always, Administrator's Message to Employees. Retrieved February 24, 2003 from http://www.hq.nasa.gov/hq/standalone/mshouse/page_183.html.

Oliver-Smith, A. (2002) Theorizing Disasters: Nature, Power, and Culture. In S. M. Hoffman and A. Oliver-Smith (eds.), *Catastrophe & Culture* (pp. 23-47). Oxford: James Curry.

Perrow, C. (1984) *Normal Accidents: Living with High Risk Technologies.* New York: Basic Books.

Prince, S. H. (1920) *Catastrophe and Social Change.* New York: Columbia University Press.

Quarantelli, E. L. (1985) What is a Disaster? The Need for Clarification in Definition and Conceptualization in Research. In B. J. Sowder (ed.), *Disasters and Mental Health: Selected Contemporary Perspectives.* Washington, DC: US Government Printing Office.

Quarantelli, E. L. (ed.) (1998) *What is a Disaster.* London: Routledge.

Reich, M. R. (1991) *Toxic Politics.* Ithaca: Cornell University Press.

Remembering the Columbia Crew. (2003, February 5) *New York Times on the Web.* Retrieved February 21, 2003, http://query.nytimes.com/gst/abstract.html?res=FB0D15F6355C0C768CDDAB0894 DB404482.

Renn, O. (1992) The Social Arena Concept of Risk Debates. In S. Krimsky and D. Golding (eds.), *Social Theories of Risk* (pp. 179-196). Westport, CT: Praeger.

Rosner, D., and Markowitz, G. E. (1991) *Deadly Dust: Silicosis and the Politics of Occupational Disease in Twentieth-Century America.* Princeton: Princeton University Press.

Shuttle Victims Had No Special Insurance. (2003, February 9) *The New York Times on the Web.* Retrieved February 10, 2003, http://www.nytimes.com/apoline/science/AP-Astronauts-Insurance. . . .

Stone, D. A. (1989) Causal Stories and the Formation of Policy Agendas. *Political Science Quarterly, 104*: 281-300.

Turner, B. A. (1978) *Man-made Disasters.* London: Wykeham.

Vaughn, D. (1996) *The Challenger Launch Decision.* Princeton: Princeton University Press.

Von Drehle, D. (2003) *Triangle.* New York: Atlantic Monthly Press.

Wells, C. (1995) *Negotiating Tragedy: Law and Disasters.* London: Sweet and Maxwell.

Wells, C. (1996) Criminal Law, Blame and Risk: Corporate Manslaughter. In C. Hood and D. K. C. Jones (eds.), *Accident and Design* (pp. 50-60). London: UCL Press.

CHAPTER 2

Trucking Tragedies: The Hidden Disaster of Mass Death in the Long-Haul Road Transport Industry

Michael Quinlan, Claire Mayhew, and Richard Johnstone

In the early hours of October 20th, 1989, a semi-trailer carrying canned fruit on Australia's main east-coast highway between Brisbane and Sydney veered onto the wrong side of the road and collided with a interstate commuter bus at Cowper, 800km north of Sydney. Twenty people were killed. The truck driver (among those killed) was a subcontractor for a large transport company. Viewed by colleagues as a reliable operator, he had been booked for over 29 traffic offenses (mainly speeding) over the previous three years and was found to have a blood ephedrine level many times that of a chronic user. This incident and a bus collision on the same highway less than two weeks later lead to a swathe of new regulatory controls (including new speed limits and speed governors). However, the regulatory response in no way addressed the economic pressures on truck drivers, exacerbated by the subcontracting system, to drive excessive hours, to speed, or to use drug stimulants. Within a short period there was evidence of drivers evading the new controls by, for example, tampering with governors.

Further, while a public outcry drove the regulatory response, apart from a coronial inquiry there was little in the way of an official investigation into the incident or safety issues in the long-haul road transport industry more generally. In coal mining, such an incident of mass death would have occasioned a royal commission or judicial inquiry (but see Hopkins 1999). In road transport it did not. This may seem surprising for a number of reasons.

First, as the Cowper incident highlights, safety problems in the road transport industry have considerable potential to extend to persons using the road system who are not commercial drivers. That is, death and serious injury involving long-haul road transport is not confined to drivers but also has a public safety dimension. Although incidents as serious as Cowper are unusual, the death of other road users in collisions with trucks is not. Indeed, around two-thirds of those killed in crashes involving articulated trucks are not truck drivers but other road users (mainly the occupants of cars but with smaller numbers of truck passengers and pedestrians). There is some evidence that risks have grown in tandem with the increasing size of rigs. In air transport it is arguable that the public safety rather than occupational safety considerations have been a major force for regulatory intervention. Why has the combination of public and occupational safety concerns been less powerful in road transport?

Second, leaving public safety issues entirely to one side, it can still be noted that the toll of dead and maimed drivers is of a scale that might be expected to warrant more significant investigation and regulatory intervention. In Australia, the United States, and probably some other industrialized countries, road transport is one of the most dangerous industries and truck driving among the most dangerous occupations in terms of the incidence of death and serious injury. As will be argued in this chapter, the death toll in trucking is substantial and can readily be conceived of as a creeping occupational health and safety disaster— one marked by numerous violent deaths rather than clustering into a few highly · visible incidents. The question remains as to why this toll fails to arouse a more concerted response.

Part of the reason lies in the fact that widespread death in the trucking industry is viewed as normal rather than disastrous and demanding concerted action. The labeling of a phenomenon as a disaster, or more specifically as an occupational disaster, is not determined on the basis of objective criteria but rather is shaped by community perceptions and, in particular, the media. For the community at large, the media is the primary source of public information on disaster and therefore exerts an influence on how these incidents are defined and interpreted (Fischer 1994, p. 23).

Occupational disasters are generally viewed, like natural disasters, as being the results of specific incidents, events or at least closely related series of incidents. However, researchers have readily acknowledged that some incidents will have long-term, direct impacts on health, with the Seveso and Bhopal incidents (see Jasanoff 1994) being prime examples—in the latter the long-term toll far exceeds those killed in the immediate aftermath of the toxic chemical release (Shrivastava 1987; 1994; Jasanoff 1994). Further, researchers have used the term "occupational" or "public health disaster" where there has been no significant single incident but rather a large number of individual exposures to a hazardous substance. For example the term has been used in relation to the thousands of deaths (and with the notable exception of the Gauley Bridge disaster, usually over a number of years if not decades) associated with exposure to coal dust, silica, and asbestos (Corn 1992, pp. 118-120; Derickson 1998; Rosner and Markowitz 1994).

Finally, when we examine research into the underlying causes of both specific incident-based disasters and those attributed to a longer-term phenomenon it can be noted that many of the researchers just mentioned (see for example

Derickson 1998; Jasanoff 1994; Shrivastava 1987; Turner 1976) have identified an essentially similar array of long-running political, regulatory and organizational failures often fueled by financial pressures or incentives—or what Carson (1989) has labeled the political economy of OHS. With regard to the single incident-based disaster there is more of an inclination for some to portray it as technological failure but careful research by Shrivastava (1987), Jasanoff (1994) and others has argued technological failures were the outcome of organizational or social shortcomings that accumulated over time. As Jasanoff (1994, pp. 5-6) has observed, research into Bhopal confirmed Perrow's (1984) argument about the mixing of technologies and social properties (including "tight coupling" and complex interactions) that made them unforgiving of error and whereby the combination of engineering defects like faulty valves with human elements such as poorly trained staff, communication problems, and inadequate expert support could produce catastrophic incidents. Leaving this observation aside, the other point to be made is that single-incident based phenomena cannot be meaningfully differentiated from those occurring in the course of years by reference to distinctive patterns of causation.

Perceptions and representations of risk also shape the determination of disasters. Drawing on the work of Beck (1992), Adam and van Loon (2000, pp. 3-4) note that the concept of risk is socially constructed and that perceptions of risk are linked to understandings about what constitutes a hazard and to whom. They go on to argue that risk definition entails political processes and that risks have, in turn, become a significant force for political mobilization. An essential connotation of disaster is that it affects groups and communities (i.e., it impacts collectively) and is not a risk that workers can both cause and manage as individuals. Applying these observations to the trucking industry, two points can be made.

First, as will be emphasized later in this chapter, by and large the regulatory regime employed in trucking—as in road transport more generally—focuses on individual driver behavior thereby diminishing the notion of shared causes and impacts. Public perceptions of individual control and responsibility are reinforced by both the advertisements of road safety authorities and most media coverage of particular incidents (though broader causal patterns are identified on occasion—see below). On the other hand, OHS regulation, where commercial structures and differences of power receive explicit recognition and an individualized discourse on causation is not promoted (even if there is evidence that the growth of contingent work arrangements may be weakening this message [Quinlan 2003]), plays a minimal role. The death of truck drivers in highway incidents is rarely investigated by OHS authorities let alone forming the subject of a prosecution. As a result, the relationship of the incident to work—including arrangements placing a broad group of drivers at risk—is accorded little regulatory or social significance. In some respects, what has been achieved by this regulatory bifurcation is analogous to Carson's (1979) conventionalization thesis in relation to earlier factory crime. Treating trucking incidents via transport legislation rather than OHS legislation diminishes the chances that operators (or load owners) will be prosecuted for even the most serious offenses (see Perrone 2000) and also effectively results in a lower level of penalties.

Second, at a broader societal level the growing influence of neo-liberal ideology within industrialized societies promotes the notion of individual agency, responsibility, and risk management and correspondingly corrodes notions of collective welfare and state protection (see O'Malley 1996). This ideology—which is increasingly infiltrating public policies at all levels—emphasizes the need for individuals to take personal preventative actions whether in terms of their employment, retirement, or safety at work. In long-haul trucking, the increasing influence of market relationships on work arrangements (through the use of elaborate subcontracting chains, owner/drivers and trip-based payment) has created a climate where individualism flourishes and more collective notions of the origins and management of risk are difficult to foster (note too the problem of reconciling conflicting identities [Beck 1992, p. 7]). Trucking can be seen as an exemplar of the neo-liberal ideal of a competitive industry where contingent work arrangements are pervasive.

The remainder of this chapter will try to explain why the death toll in road transport has attracted so little attention. While recognizing the interaction between public safety and occupational health concerns, its primary focus is on the latter. In so doing, the chapter looks critically at the regulatory response, examining recent experience in North America, Europe, and New Zealand as well as Australia. It will be argued that changes to work organization and competition in the trucking industry have contributed to a high rate of fatality among drivers in the United States and Australia if not elsewhere. In particular, outsourcing, reward systems, and the growth of contingent forms of employment have contributed to dangerous levels of work intensity and disorganization. There is growing international recognition that the expansion of contingent work is undermining OHS standards. Unlike some other industries, contingent work arrangements are not new to the road transport industry but the extent of precarious employment has nonetheless expanded in recent decades. In this sense the road transport industry may be a barometer of the implications of this shift.

What is of critical importance is that thus far the response of regulators in Europe, the United States, and Australia has failed to address the underlying causes just identified. At best, regulators have focused on driver fatigue, evasion of road rules, failure to maintain vehicles, and drug use. We would argue that these regulatory responses are doomed to fail because they are essentially dealing with symptoms, not the underlying cause of these practices, namely the economic pressures on drivers to compete and survive, and the disorganization that arises from widespread outsourcing. A primary factor here appears to be the unwillingness of road transport agencies to accept lessons learned in other areas of occupational safety and an unwillingness to confront either vested interests or the externalities and other consequences of neo-liberal policies. For their part, OHS agencies have demonstrated a similar reluctance to enter the terrain. Much of the commissioned research on the industry remains disarticulated, picking up a limited array of issues and failing to make any connection between the economic organization of the industry and OHS. In coal mining, periodic disasters provide an often-limited opportunity to make connections between economic structures, work organization, regulatory activity, and OHS. In road transport the dispersed and incremental nature of fatalities is even less conducive to making such connections.

The chapter is divided into three parts. Part 1 briefly summarizes evidence on poor safety in the long haul road transport industry in Australia, with some comparisons to the United States and Europe. Part 2 critically examines the regulation of safety in long-haul road transport. It identifies the regulatory framework pertaining to long-haul road transport and public concerns over safety. Two subsections then try to explain why existing regulatory interventions have failed. In the first it is argued that the dominant road transport model of regulation has been hamstrung by vested interests and fails to address the underlying reasons for non-compliance: namely the combination of industry structure and commercial practices with market-based regulatory reforms. Though the focus of the chapter is on Australia, evidence is presented indicating parallel problems and trends in the road transport industry in the United States, European Union, and New Zealand. Despite important institutional/regulatory and other differences between Europe, the United States, and Australia it is concluded that policies to remove restrictions on the movement of goods and promote competition have contributed to an expansion of precarious employment and a parallel deterioration in safety. The final subsection in Part 2 examines the circumscribed input of OHS legislation into long-haul road transport. It is argued that this approach has been crucial in obfuscating the occupational connections in truck-related fatalities because, unlike OHS legislation, commercial pressures are only partly/incidentally recognized and enforcement is focused on drivers rather than their employers, freight forwarders, shippers, and other parties to road freight.

1. PAYING THE TOLL: DEATH, INJURY, AND ILLNESS IN LONG-HAUL TRUCKING—A "SLOW BURN" DISASTER?

Measured in terms of the overall number of injuries and fatalities, as well as the incidence per 1000 employees, road transport ranks as a very dangerous occupation. In Australasia, North America, and the European Union the road transport industry accounts for the highest number of work-related fatalities in any given year and the occupation of truck driver usually ranks in the top six most dangerous occupations. For example, annual censuses of fatal occupational trauma in the United States consistently show truck drivers constitute the largest number of deaths (well over 10% of the total) and rank in the 6 to 8 most dangerous occupations, accounting for employment share (Knestaut 1997; Toscana and Windau 1998; Windau and Jack 1996). Almost 70% of truck drivers who die as result of work are killed in highway crashes and around half the drivers killed are in control of semi-trailers and thereby overwhelmingly involved in long-haul freight tasks (NIOSH 2000; Toscano 1997; Toscano and Windau 1998, p. 37). The National Institute of Occupational Safety and Health (NIOSH 2000, p. 41) recently identified an upward trend in the number of truck driver fatalities and the fatality rate per 100,000 workers (truck driving also accounted for the highest number of non-fatal injuries in 1995—a by no means atypical year). In short, long-haul truck driver is the most dangerous occupation in road transport industry, as well as being one of the most dangerous occupations per se.

There is no annual census of fatal occupational traumas in Australia but the National Occupational Health and Safety Commission (NOHSC) has produced periodic fatality censuses. The most recent of these (1989-1992) indicated that transport and storage accounted for 22% of all fatal injuries. Transport and storage had the third highest death rate of any industry (23 deaths per 100,000 employed) and of the 370 transport and storage workers killed between 1989 and 1992, 308 were truck drivers (NOHSC 1999, p. 3). Truck driver ranked as the sixth most dangerous occupation (41 deaths per 100,000 employed, behind fishermen, forestry workers, drilling plant operators, mining laborers, and ship pilots/ deckhands)—seven times the all-industry average (5.5 per 100,000 employed). More recent data (1993/94-1996/97) for one state (Victoria) confirms this pattern.

Using virtually any measure trucking is a major source of traumatic death and serious injury in the Australian community. While the long-haul sector (defined as a single-delivery trip of more than 100 kilometers) represents a small part of the total road transport task (about 20% in Australia) highway incidents involving heavy vehicles account for a disproportionate number of deaths and serious injuries. Official statistics rarely distinguish between crashes involving short-haul and long-haul trucks, but crashes involving articulated vehicles can be taken as a partial proxy as the great majority of articulated trucks are used in long-haul tasks. Table 1 indicates deterioration in truck-related fatalities during the 1980s followed by a sharp improvement in the early 1990s. In absolute terms there has been no trend improvement in either the number of fatalities (truck driver or other road user) or the number of fatal crashes involving articulated trucks after 1991. By way of contrast, since 1991 there has been an improvement in the total number fatal all-vehicle crashes and fatalities (see Table 1). Crashes involving articulated trucks constitute almost 9% of crashes and account for almost 10% of all vehicle fatalities.

Of course, such figures do not take account of the substantial increase in the total road freight being hauled since 1988. This can be done by analyzing the number of fatal crashes and fatalities per 100 million kilometers traveled. This data indicates there was a substantial improvement in both the rate of crash-related fatalities and fatal crashes per 100 million kilometers traveled for articulated

Table 1. Fatal Crashes and Fatalities, All Crashes and Articulated
Vehicles, Australia 1981 to 2003

	Crashes			Fatalities		
Year	All crashes	Articulated vehicles	Articulated vehicle crashes as percentage of all crashes	All fatalities	Articulated vehicles	Articulated vehicle deaths as percentage of all fatalities
1981	2914	236	8.1	3321	N/A	—
1982	2872	251	8.7	3252	N/A	—
1983	2485	216	8.7	2755	N/A	—
1984	2508	232	9.25	2822	N/A	—
1985	2627	218	8.3	2941	N/A	—
1986	2577	194	7.5	2888	232	8.0
1987	2487	199	8.0	2772	243	8.8
1988	2572	260	10.1	2887	320	11.1
1989	2406	250	10.4	2801	335	12.0
1990	2050	205	10	2331	263	11.3
1991	1874	156	8.3	2113	183	8.7
1992	1736	154	8.9	1974	181	9.2
1993	1737	171	9.8	1953	204	10.4
1994	1702	151	8.9	1928	179	9.3
1995	1822	165	9.1	2017	199	9.9
1996	1768	161	6.2	1971	194	9.8
1997	1603	146	9.1	1768	171	9.7
1998	1580	151	9.5	1763	179	10.2
1999	N/A	163	N/A	N/A	191	N/A
2000	N/A	165	N/A	N/A	208	N/A
2001	N/A	146	N/A	N/A	178	N/A
2002	N/A	171	N/A	N/A	200	N/A
2003	N/A	144	N/A	N/A	173	N/A
Average			8.8			9.9

Source: *Road Fatalities Australia: 1998 Statistical Summary,* Federal Office of Road Safety, Canberra 1999; ATSB *Articulated Truck Crashes,* Monograph No. 8, Australian Transport Safety Board, Canberra, 2001; and ATSB *Fatal road crashes involving articulated trucks,* Road Safety Working Paper No. 2, Australian Transport Safety Board, Canberra, 2004.

trucks between 1988 and 1999, and the improvement was greater (though coming from a much higher base) than for all other vehicles. However, after 1995 the improvement in crash-related fatalities (for both vehicle categories) Australia-wide is marginal and the improvement in the rate of fatal crashes is arguably greater for other vehicles than articulated trucks (Quinlan 2001). If anything, the NSW specific data after 1995 paints a slightly worse picture for articulated trucks. Most important, perhaps, while both the gap between articulated trucks and other vehicles in terms of the crash fatality and fatal crash rate per 100 million kilometers traveled has narrowed, it still remains substantial (at around three times that of all other vehicles), and since 1995 this trend has slowed if not stalled (Quinlan 2001).

Long-haul trucking is an important public safety as well as occupational safety issue. The risks associated with long-haul trucking extend well beyond truck drivers to other road users. Table 2 provides a breakdown of fatalities involving articulated trucks for both Australia and New South Wales—the latter constituting the most populous state and a hub for the trucking industry (especially the eastern mainland corridor which accounts for over 90% of all long-haul trucking). In 1999, 189 Australians died in crashes involving articulated trucks (or about one-tenth of all road fatalities that year), 51 of whom were truck drivers.

Table 2. Fatalities Involving Articulated Trucks in NSW and Australia, 1990 to 1999

Year	Arctic drivers killed		Other road users killed[a]		Total killed	
	NSW	Aust[b]	NSW	Aust[b]	NSW	Aust[b]
1990	18	46	76	216	94	263
1991	13	30	65	153	78	183
1992	18	40	66	141	84	181
1993	21	42	48	143	69	204
1994	9	27	58	140	67	179
1995	10	31	53	168	63	199
1996	13	33	43	160	56	194
1997	15	36	56	135	71	171
1998	23	N/A	48	N/A	71	179
1999	13	N/A	51	N/A	64	189

[a]In crashes involving at least one articulated truck.
[b]Source for Australian data: Australian Transport Safety Bureau, Transport Safety Statistics Unit. Supplied by RTA.

Consistent with Table 1 after 1991, there is no clear trend of improvement in relation to either the number of truck drivers or other road users killed in crashes involving articulated trucks for both NSW and Australia. Overall, truck drivers constitute about one-third of all those dying in such crashes.

It is difficult to compare safety performance in the industry across countries due to differences in truck configuration and categorization (in terms of official statistics) as well as reporting and other differences. Nonetheless, with these caveats in mind, it appears the safety performance of the Australian long-haul road sector is below that of countries in Europe and North America for which we have data. Comparisons in the 1980s indicated the rate of fatal accidents per 100 million kilometers traveled by trucks in Australia was 1.75 times the Finnish rate and 1.85 times the U.S. rate (Cairney 1991, p. 10). Using data for the year 1998, the fatal crash rate involving articulated trucks in Australia was 3.07 per 100 million vehicle/kilometers traveled while the road fatality rate involving articulated trucks was 3.63 per 100 million vehicle/kilometers. U.S. National Highway Traffic Safety Administration data for the year 1996 (the most recent available) indicates there were 1.63 fatal crashes involving large trucks (i.e., over 4.5 tons GVM) per 100 million kilometers traveled and 1.75 fatalities in crashes involving heavy trucks per 100 million kilometers traveled. The most comparable U.K. data for 1998 indicates there were 1.2 fatal crashes involving heavy gross vehicles (i.e., over 3.5 tons GVM) per 100 million kilometers traveled and 1.79 fatalities in crashes involving heavy gross vehicles per 100 million kilometers traveled (Quinlan 2001). Overall, it appears that the fatality/fatal crash rate involving heavy vehicles is almost twice that of the United States and several European countries and there has been no discernible improvement over the past decade.

Notwithstanding these apparent differences, there are serious shared concerns about safety in the long haul trucking industry in Europe, Australia, and North America. Fatigue and, to a lesser extent, speeding and drug use have been identified as major safety issues in all. The U.S. Department of Transportation (US DOT 2000) recently reported that truck driver fatigue was the main contributing factor in 15% of all commercial vehicle accidents, accounting for 755 deaths and 19,000 injuries each year. In the largest Australian state (New South Wales) the Roads and Traffic Authority (RTA) estimated that in the years 1993 to 1998 fatigued heavy truck drivers accounted for 80.8 casualty crashes (or 7.6% of total casualty crashes) and fatigued articulated truck drivers accounted for 58.7 (or 5.6%) casualty crashes. The RTA identified an upward trend in both the numbers of crashes and casualties over time (Quinlan 2001). Figures for 1999 indicate that of 1595 persons killed or injured on NSW roads in heavy truck crashes, truck driver speeding contributed to 170 casualties, driver fatigue to 98 casualties, and insecure loads to 25 casualties. Of the 830 persons killed or injured in crashes involving articulated trucks, truck driver speeding contributed to 130 casualties, driver fatigue to 70, and insecure loads to 15 deaths or injuries. Ignoring single-vehicle incidents, truck drivers were deemed at fault in roughly one quarter of crashes, Australia-wide, for the years 1990-1996. Truck driver fault exceeded 90% in single-vehicle incidents (a significant number were fatigue-related).

Crashes resulting in death and serious injury represent the tip of the iceberg. A survey of 300 long-distance truck drivers (Mayhew and Quinlan 2001) found about 14% had experienced a crash in the past 12 months, with the figure being highest for small fleet employee drivers (17.3%) and owner/drivers (13.1%). Small fleet drivers and owner/drivers were around twice as likely as large fleet drivers to report serious crashes. Almost a quarter of drivers reported a crash in the last five years, with small fleet drivers again reporting most (26%). In explaining these differences it is perhaps more than coincidental that small fleet and owner/drivers worked longer hours and faced increased competitive pressures in comparison to large fleet drivers. It is hard to get comparable international data. A survey of 1006 French heavy vehicle drivers (Hamelin 2000, p. 23) asked them whether they had *ever* been involved a traffic accident causing injury. Just over 14% indicated they had been involved in an injury-causing crash. Given differences in the questions posed it is difficult to compare the survey results. A notable finding from the French survey was that reported crashes were significantly higher for for-hire carriers (17% overall and 22.7% for drivers under 40 years of age) than drivers working for companies transporting their own goods (9.2% with no significant age variation). An earlier Australian study (James [Mayhew] 1993) found that long-haul drivers over age 45, and more particularly 50, were at an exponentially increased risk of having a fatal crash.

As this survey evidence suggests, official statistics on death or serious injury in collisions is only a partial indicator of the incidence of health and safety problems in long-haul trucking. Since many drivers are self-employed—a group for which coverage under workers' compensation is problematic in many countries—injury/illness statistics based on compensation claims data need to be treated with extreme caution. The just-mentioned survey of 300 drivers (Mayhew and Quinlan 2001) found over 15% of owner/drivers lacked/were uncertain about their workers' compensation or private insurance coverage. Similarly, 15.4% of small fleet employee drivers were uncertain about their coverage. The survey found over a quarter of drivers reported an acute injury or illness, with owner/drivers being far more likely to report minor injury ("usual little things") than small or large fleet drivers. Well over half the drivers reported a chronic injury, a response that should be of grave concern to those concerned with the long-term health and well-being of drivers. Over a third of owner/drivers and small fleet operators reported a chronic back injury (the figure for large fleet drivers was 23.5%). On the other hand, more large fleet drivers reported hearing loss (29.4%) than small fleet (19.2%) and owner/drivers (16.2%), though this difference could reflect more testing of the former. The incidence of acute and chronic injury is well above the norm in Australia but, again, international comparisons are difficult. A French study of 1006 heavy vehicle drivers (Hamelin

2000, p. 23) asked them whether they had experienced a work-related accident without specifying a time limit. Just over one third of drivers (33.6%) stated they had experienced an accident. There was no significant difference in the response of drivers with for-hire carriers and those working for not-for-hire carriers, but over half of the drivers under 40 years of age reported an accident (with a slightly higher figure for for-hire carrier drivers).

Beyond injuries there are also disease, psychological stress, and occupational violence. We are unaware of accurate data pertaining to disease or hazardous substance exposures among truck drivers. The driver survey (Mayhew and Quinlan 2001) provided information on the latter two issues. Driver psychological well-being was assessed using the General Health Questionnaire (GHQ). Results revealed an overall mean score of 10.3, which is in the high range (a score of 8.59 is relatively normal), with owner/drivers having the highest mean score (11.5), especially those working on the Hume Highway (mean of 13.1). Nearly 16% of drivers had scores of 14 or more (almost half were owner/drivers), which is deemed to constitute an extreme health risk. In short, long-distance truck drivers operate under considerable stress. The survey also indicated low-level occupational violence was a serious problem for truck drivers. About half the drivers surveyed reported experiencing occupational violence, most commonly verbal abuse or threats, although around 1% of owner/drivers and large fleet drivers had been physically assaulted. Owner/drivers experienced more occupational violence (54.5%) than small fleet (45.2%) and large fleet drivers (42.3%). About 20% of all drivers had experienced "road rage," mostly at the hands of other road users and several had been shot at (Mayhew and Quinlan 2001a).

2. PUBLIC CONCERN, INCOMPATIBLE POLICIES, AND MUTED REGULATORY RESPONSES

The safety of long-haul road transport is a source of serious and growing public concern in Europe, North America, and Australia. Such concern is evidenced in prominent media coverage of serious truck crashes, incidents of drug use by drivers, coronial reports, and truck safety inquiries and special investigative features. For example, the inquiry into trucking safety conducted in 2000 for the Motor Accidents Authority of New South Wales got hundreds of media *hits* both in Australia and overseas, and in the United States in recent years there have been a number of special multi-part features in newspapers detailing the long hours and dangers encountered by truck drivers (see for example *Kansas City Star* 15, 16, 17 December 2001). Another indication of these concerns has been the formation of community bodies lobbying for improvements in trucking safety in Australia (Concerned Families of Australian Truckies or CFAT), Canada (Canadians for Responsible and Safe Highways or CRASH), the United States (Citizens for Reliable and Safe Highways or CRASH), and elsewhere. These bodies have publicized the industry's shortcoming and have lobbied for more stringent regulation on issues like truck size and fatigue as well as calling for more vigorous/better resourced enforcement. In recent years transport unions have conducted high-profile national and international campaigns on trucking safety (on issues like fatigue as well as commercial pressures and low pay). Some community bodies (like CFAT, whose activists are mainly the wives of drivers) have emerged with union support or have forged links with unions. At the same time, reflecting broader concerns about public safety on highways, other community bodies have been established without union input or have pursued policies including ones that would be problematic for unions representing road transport workers (such as moving more freight by rail). At the very least, these bodies have provided an additional input into policy deliberations and sharpened awareness of the human impact of truck crashes (both in terms of the families of injured truck drivers and other road users).

The level of public interest in trucking safety is readily understandable. The sheer scale of death and serious injury in truck-related crashes (making personal knowledge of incidents more likely), graphic media reporting of serious incidents (media reports both reflect and accentuate community concerns), and the capacity to identify based on their own experience of sharing a road with the intimidating presence of a much larger vehicle, all result in a heightened level of risk perception. What is significant, however, is how seldom these concerns have translated into effective regulatory intervention. A number of factors may help explain this.

First and most obviously, while far more people die as a result of truck crashes than any other type of work-related incident, in most cases the actual number killed or maimed in a single incident is small in comparison to, for instance, a mine explosion. Where large numbers of deaths have occurred in a single incident (such as the Cowper and Clybucca crashes in 1989 which together killed 35 persons) significant regulatory responses have occurred, but such incidents are rare. Further, to a great extent deaths in trucking incidents are subsumed into the general road toll and while in one sense this seems logical and appropriate, this approach ignores that trucking is a commercial undertaking subject to pressures that arguably make it largely immune from the sorts of deterrent prompts used to modify the behavior of other drivers (in relation to drinking, speeding, etc.). These presumptions mean fatal truck incidents are seldom seen as requiring the investigation and explanation that accompanies multiple workplace deaths in other industries. At best, as in the Cowper NSW (1989 where 20 died) and Blanchetown South Australia (1996 where six motorists died) a coronial inquiry is held. By way of contrast, Royal Commissions or other large (in terms of budget, scope, and time taken) formal investigations were recently undertaken to investigate and make recommendations on the drowning of four miners in 1996 due to an inundation at the Gretley Colliery in the Hunter Valley north of Sydney and the 1998 death of two workers following an explosion at Esso's Longford gas facility in Victoria (in this case the fact the explosion shut down the gas supply in Victoria for several weeks played a part).

In short, truck-related deaths usually occur as a slow but regular *burn* of mortality and even in those rarer instances where large numbers die the incident is still not viewed as an occupational disaster in the same way as a mine explosion, factory fire, or bridge collapse. Indeed, regulators seldom view truck-related deaths as occupational fatalities. The deaths may be recorded for OHS statistics as occupational fatalities—and even here there will be a large number will be missed unless census or a coronial database is used in preference to workers' compensation claims (which will miss many self-employed drivers)—but from a regulatory perspective OHS is very much a bit player. It is worth exploring this point in some detail.

In Australia and most other industrialized countries the long-haul trucking industry is subject to a complex web of overlapping regulation composed of road transport legislation (including both general provisions as well as some specifically applying to the road freight industry), dangerous goods/environmental protection legislation, OHS legislation, industrial relations laws, and, of more importance lately, competition/trade practices laws. As will be demonstrated below, each of these bodies of regulation can affect safety. While most countries have moved to establish coordinating agencies in the last decade if not before, each body of legislation is often administered by a separate agency. In formal terms road transport legislation holds the pre-eminent position and, notwithstanding attempts at co-ordination, other agencies and in particular OHS agencies have deferred to it and its enforcement arms (traffic inspectors and the police) as the lead agency where they have not largely abdicated the field. The idea of recognizing a lead agency in areas of overlapping responsibility and agency claims is a long-established practice within government that has obvious bureaucratic and policy consistency benefits. However, when it comes to the long-haul trucking industry the reluctance of OHS agencies to take on a stronger role has been nothing short of disastrous.

2.1 Problems with Existing Road Freight Safety Regulatory Regimes

At present in Australia, as in most other countries, maintenance of safety in the trucking industry is overwhelmingly reliant on road transport legislation and the agencies responsible for enforcing this (namely the police/highway patrol and Department of Transport officers—including specialist units—or their equivalent like the RTA in New South Wales). The long-haul road freight industry is thereby subject to the rules governing all vehicles on public roads but with a number of additional requirements. The latter include specific licensing of drivers to operate heavy vehicles, provision for drug testing, the keeping of logbooks, and the maximum allowable work hours for 24 hour/7 day periods as well as regulations governing vehicle inspection/registration, size/specifications, load/load restraint, and safety control devices (such as compulsory tachographs or speed governors). Most countries impose some regulatory controls directly on operators (i.e., trucking firms or owner/drivers) in terms of revocable privileges (to operate on highways within a jurisdiction) or mandatory licensing (based on financial and OHS performance). Finally, in recent years there have been moves to place legal responsibilities on operators and other parties (like clients) via chain of responsibility provisions in road transport legislation.

Without gainsaying the need for on-road enforcement, in Australia and it would seem elsewhere, the devotion of considerable (if arguably still inadequate) resources to compliance has failed to prevent widespread, persistent and systemic breaches of both special regulations and basic road-rules applying to speed etc.

For example, under current regulations truck drivers in Australia are permitted to work up to 12 hours (in some cases 14 hours) in a day and 72 hours a week (a similar limit applies in Canada) while slightly more stringent limits apply in the United States (where the maximum is 60 hours per week) and the European Union. In Australia and the United States (see Belman, Monaco, and Brooks no date) surveys spanning well over a decade indicate that the bulk of the truck driving workforce work close to these limits, with a sizable portion exceeding it on a regular basis. A survey of 573 U.S. long-haul truck drivers undertaken by Belman et al. (no date) in 1997 found the majority of drivers were working at or above the 60 hour maximum specified by hours of service regulation. In Australia, a survey of 820 drivers Hensher et al. (1991, p. 61) found 41% had received logbook fines in the past year, the incidence being highest among small fleet drivers (53.5%) and lowest among large fleet drivers (31.1%). An inquiry into safety in the long haul trucking industry (Quinlan 2001) received submissions from the NSW Police, the NSW Roads and Traffic Authority, and other agencies attesting to widespread breaches of driving hour limits. Long hours behind the wheel do not capture the full workload of long-distance drivers. In addition to driving, drivers often spend considerable time loading/unloading, waiting in queues at depots/client warehouses, and undertaking vehicle maintenance. Williamson, Feyer, Friswell, and Sadari (2000) surveyed fatigue among 1000 long-distance drivers and benchmarked their findings against an earlier (1991) survey. There had been increase in the work required of long-distance drivers, entailing longer trips and a reported earlier onset of fatigue. Most drivers did some midnight-to-dawn driving (when there are far higher risks of crashing), over 20% had exceeded the 72 hour working hour limit in the last week, and around a quarter admitted breaking driving hours regulations on every trip. In short, many drivers worked excessive and dangerous hours and despite the use of devices including video cameras to record truck movements (Safe-T-Cam), the situation was, if anything, getting worse.

A direct consequence of the long hours worked by drivers is resort to stimulant drugs to combat fatigue and stay awake at the wheel. The precise level of drug use in long-distance trucking is unknown but available evidence indicates it is widespread (most surveys and vehicle testing suggest at least 20 to 30% of drivers regularly use illegal stimulants (see Hartley 1999; Quinlan 2001). Aside from long-term health effects, the consequences of drug use by drivers have been graphically illustrated by incidents such as a truck/bus smash at Cowper NSW in 1989 already referred to and a truck/multiple car smash at Blanchetown (South Australia) in 1996 where six motorists died (see below). Drug-use is a long-term feature of the industry and is structured into the work process in a way found in no other occupation aside from prostitution. Efforts to combat this practice in Australia and elsewhere, including compulsory drug testing in the United States, seem to have yielded limited results at best. In the United States compulsory drug testing appears to be unable stop drivers moving to another firm and has also been seen as contributing to a rapid turnover of drivers (with consequent effects on safety; see Belzer et al. 2000).

Speeding is another serious enforcement issue. Heavy vehicles are significantly over-represented in crashes. Despite the use of speed limiting devices and other compliance tools (like a "three strikes and you're out" rule in NSW), speeding by long-distance trucks remains widespread. Hidden Culway detection sites used by the NSW Roads and Traffic Authority indicated that the proportion of trucks exceeding the speed limit ranges from 30 to 50%, depending on the route/highway (Quinlan 2001). Blitzes have a limited effect and stringent enforcement within particular areas has often led to a relocation of speeding (aided by experience and rapid radio/phone communication among drivers).

Hours/logbooks, the use of drugs, and speeding are not the only areas where enforcement has proved problematic (overloading and "cuts" in routine maintenance are other problems) but they do illustrate limitations with the current regime. The obvious questions are: why is regulatory evasion so widespread, and why has the present approach failed to have more effect? The answer to these questions is that the current regulatory regime is too driver-focused, penalties are not commensurate with the incentive to commit offenses, and regulatory intervention fails to address the pressures underpinning safety breaches. In Australia the overwhelming majority of enforcement activity targets truck drivers, with relatively few prosecutions of operators and virtually no compliance activity in relation to clients or other parties whose behavior may affect safety.

While on-road enforcement of safe driving behavior is a critical component of any strategy to achieve safety in the long haul trucking industry, by itself such activity is unlikely to change behavior if incentives/pressures to breach legislation are not addressed. During the long-haul trucking safety inquiry even some industry associations pointed to inadequacies in this regard:

> Penalties are manifestly inadequate and do not properly target the prime offenders. The possibility of being detected versus the additional revenue dollars achieved by cheating the system outweighs any real concerns about

current penalties applied. Too often the driver is the easy target to bear the burden of penalty. (written submission, Victorian Road Transport Association cited in Quinlan 2001)

There is a strong body of evidence that systemic safety breaches by drivers are a direct outcome of pressures from shippers/clients, freight-forwarders, intense competition for work among operators, and exploitative subcontracting arrangements. In Australasia, North America, and Western Europe road freight is the dominant mode of internal transport and has been steadily increasing its share of the total freight task relative to other modes, most notably rail. Given expansion in the overall task this has not meant an absolute decline in rail freight but the shift is important. This shift is a direct consequence of the increasing competitiveness of road freight, assisted by changes in regulatory arrangements as well as technology. By and large, rail freight has not been similarly advantaged. It is worth noting that influencing the balance of competitiveness between industries can have serious health and safety consequences that are seldom if ever considered by the neo-liberal reform agencies. In 1998 the ARRB estimated road freight averaged 3.8 fatalities per billion gross ton kilometers while the comparable figure for rail was 0.55 fatalities (ARRB 1998).

While regulators in Australia and other countries have focused their attention on fatigue, speeding, drug use, overloading and the like, there are grounds for arguing these are symptoms of more deep-seated problems affecting the industry. There is growing evidence that industry structure, commercial practices, and regulatory policies shaping this have had profound effects on safety in long-haul trucking. These features include the large number of operators (many small and only marginally viable); relatively easy entry into the industry; intense competition for work; and increased pressure (in terms of timing, service quality, etc.) from customers, loading agents, and freight forwarders. Intense competition has kept freight rates at marginal levels in recent years, encouraging cost-cutting devices (via subcontracting work/leased labor, speeding, long hours etc.) that compromise safety.

Evidence of the role of commercial factors in safety is not new. In Australia problems with subcontracting and an oversupply of marginal operators were recognized by the early 1980s. In 1984 the May Inquiry into the federal road freight industry recommended compulsory operator licensing (as is the case in the European Union) but while the requisite legislation was passed it was never implemented. In the 1990s Hensher and colleagues undertook a series of surveys that tested the role of commercial factors in encouraging unsafe driving practices. In their first major survey Hensher et al. (1991, p. 101) found drivers spent considerable time (an average of 3.5 hours) on off-road activities (loading/ unloading, maintenance, etc.) before commencing a trip. Sampling particular trips, Hensher et al. found 35% of drivers were traveling to a set schedule but another 60% reported having set a self-imposed arrival time due to concerns about queuing and getting the next load. Of those drivers on a set schedule, few were offered incentives (2.7%) but a quarter indicated they would be penalized for late arrival (Hensher et al. 1991, p. 48). Around half the drivers felt freight companies demanded unreasonably tight schedules (Hensher et al. 1991, p. 51). Average trip speed was highest among small fleet (82.01 kph) and younger drivers aged 17-24 years (84.72 kph) compared to an overall average of 81.06 kph.

Econometric analysis revealed that economic rewards were a major influence on the propensity to speed among owner/drivers and employers of drivers:

> There is very strong evidence to support the primary hypothesis that the trip rate received by the owner driver (i.e., gross earnings) and the freight rate obtained by the company using an employee driver have a significant influence on the propensity to speed. The negative relationship is stronger for owner drivers as might be expected...The main impetus of this study has been confirmed: on-road performance is strongly linked to economic reward. (Hensher et al. 1991, p. 96)

They drew a particular bead at the safety consequences of trip-based payment:

> Any deviation from a fixed salary tends to encourage practices designed to increase economic reward which are not synergetic with reducing exposure to risk. (Hensher et al. 1991, p. 102)

It is worth noting that Hensher et al. were by no means the first to point to the hazards of trip-based payments. Further, the use of subcontracting and trip-based payment can be seen as an attempt by operators to both intensify work and spread their economic risks in a context of intense competition. Again, the connections had been repeatedly identified but never acted on. In its 1989 report, *Concerning Alert Drivers and Safe Speeds for Heavy Vehicles*, the NSW Parliamentary Committee on Road Safety STAYSAFE pointed to the frequent use of bonus/ penalty systems (including threats of losing further work) in relation to delivery schedules which necessitated speeding and inadequate rest. The Committee urged that the Roads and Traffic Authority take action to render such inducements both illegal and subject to substantial penalties (*STAYSAFE* 1989). Within a year the Coronial Inquest into the 1989 Cowper tragedy raised an essentially identical raft of issues including unreasonable trip schedules, arrival time penalties/ bonuses, requiring drivers to load, and using refusal to renew contracts to pressure owner/drivers to engage in unfair dangerous practices. The Coroner observed that the truck driver causing the incident was

> paid a fee per trip plus a fee per kilometre travelled. The more trips he fitted in, and the further he drove each day, the more he was paid. Such a method of remuneration is decidedly unhealthy. (Coroners Court of NSW 1990, p. 27)

The Coroner also drew attention to the commercial pressures on safety arising from the subcontracting system and the vulnerability of subcontractors (including owner/drivers):

It is those drivers most dependent on loading contractors for their livelihood who are susceptible to unreasonable demands.

In this regard it has been submitted that these loading contractors should themselves be licensed, so that the opportunity by them of breaches of safety laws could result in they themselves being punished, and having their own licenses suspended.

Both Mr McPhee and Mr Robertson of the Road Transport Association were critical of loading agencies, which act as middle men, getting jobs done as cheaply as possible and taking his margin. It often follows that the owner-driver who is so dependent on them is forced to his own loading in addition to his own driving, so adding to the risk of fatigue.

The evidence at the inquest showed that the arrangements between the deceased truck driver and the owners of the prime mover and semi trailer were very loose, and not conducive to safe, careful driving. Tragedy resulted.

A case has been made out for the licensing of loading agents to ensure that they carry out their work in a responsible way, with a concentration on driver welfare as well as profit margins.

It has been reported (SMH 29-2-1990) that at a road safety summit organised by the major trucking companies the setting of unrealistic delivery schedules was criticised, and it was decided that freight consignors should be made accountable for checking that drivers can make their journeys with speed and time limits.

In view of other recommendations made, I do not recommend that action in this regard commence immediately, but rather that the RTA give the matter earnest consideration with a view to implementing such a scheme in the future. (Coroners Court of NSW 1990, pp. 28-29)

Again, while an array of regulatory interventions were introduced following the Cowper tragedy these represented the traditional array of tougher laws on speeding plus the mandatory fitting of speed governors and vehicle monitoring devices (VMDs). None addressed payment systems, subcontracting arrangements, or other commercial practices that were seen to impinge on safety.

Six years later little had changed. If anything subcontracting had grown and trip-based payment systems remained pervasive. The Coroner into the Blanchetown crash (see below) echoed the comments of his Cowper disaster counterpart:

The extent to which the current system, whereby drivers are paid by the trip, or by the kilometre represents an incentive to break the law (the evidence from this inquest certainly proves that it does), and whether it is possible to design a different system which provides drivers with more incentive to comply with the law, and with safe work practices. (cited in House of Representatives Standing Committee on Communications, Transport and the Arts, 2000, p. 96)

Returning to Hensher et al. (1991, pp. 28-29), their study also considered the insecurity of owner/drivers without contracts or regular load arrangements and the problem of backloading (involving heavily discounted freight rates) where two-way freight movement imbalances made return loads scarce. The combination of competition, low freight rates, and uncertainty of loads and consequent uncertainty of earnings had other safety-related effects. Most notably, it encouraged self-imposed schedules and the use of drug stimulants to extend work time. Hensher et al. advocated a more regulated system of bidding for contracts in preference to complete economic deregulation "... *primarily because of the inability of deregulation to manifest an acceptable program of internalising the negative externalities of unfettered competition*" (Hensher et al. 1991, p. 102).

A later survey of 402 drivers by Golob and Hensher (1994) reaffirmed these findings. Golob and Hensher (1994, p. 29) rejected a simple dichotomy between owner/drivers and employee drivers as small company drivers had some of the worst practices in terms of speeding, drug-use, and traffic fines. They argued the nature of contracts, work practices, and the ability to secure loads provided a more useful explanatory classification. Thus, drivers on regular contracts were less likely to use drugs or exceed the speed limit. Over a third (37%) of drivers had a schedule imposed by an employer or freight forwarder and these drivers were more likely to be fined for speeding. For the remainder, propensity to self-impose a schedule, and speed/attract fines, was associated with the time spent securing a load and final delivery (carrying perishable goods also influenced scheduling and other behavior). Self-imposed schedules were the most important influence on the propensity to take stimulant drugs. Golob and Hensher (1994, p. 25) found the greatest influence on average trip speed was earning rates of owner/drivers and employee drivers. Drivers with higher earnings exhibited lower speeds, particularly in the case of owner/drivers:

> There appears to be a case for much more stringent safety regulations centred on the health of the driver as distinct from the "health of the rig." There is a great temptation for commentators to argue if someone wants to enter this industry, get burdened with high debts and work excessive hours to "make a quid" then they should be allowed to. This may be acceptable wisdom if safety of human resources at large were not at risk. It is precisely because of the negative externalities aligned to safety that changes are required in the competitive practices in the industry. (Golob and Hensher 1994, pp. 28-29)

More recent research has reached similar conclusions to those of Hensher et al. A survey of 300 (Mayhew and Quinlan 2001) long-haul drivers found they rated freight rates/low pay and delayed payment as the single most serious safety issue. Another survey of more than 1000 drivers by Williamson et al. (2000) found that, in addition to scheduling pressure from freight forwarder and customers, the trip-based payment system was a significant influence on drivers' work schedules. Comparing results to a survey undertaken a decade earlier, Williamson et al. (2000) argued:

> Both surveys reveal that payment by results was the predominant method of remuneration for all drivers, even company employees, and this form of payment increased markedly across the period of the two surveys. . . . Analysis of the relationship between payment type and experience of fatigue demonstrated that drivers who were paid in a payment-by-results mode were more likely to report fatigue as a substantial or major personal problem and to experience fatigue more often than drivers paid under other payment regimes. In addition, a significant percentage of drivers volunteered the strategy of standardising or regulating minimum payment rates as a way of managing fatigue.
>
> The pressures exerted by the payment by results system can also be seen in the influences on drivers to break the working hours regulations. The factors that distinguish drivers who frequently break the working hours regulations from those who do not are related to organisation of work such as the need to do enough trips to earn a living and to get in early to get the next load rather than personal reasons. This is further evidence that the way drivers are remunerated clearly has an adverse effect on the ability to manage fatigue well. This is another factor that should be examined further if fatigue management is to be truly achieved in this industry. (p. 111)

Williamson et al. (2000, p. 113) note that tying earnings to driving hours meant drivers were liable to resist attempts to limit/enforce maximum hours of work. On the other hand, a significant number of drivers believed a regulated minimum payment system would be a more effective means of managing fatigue by obviating the need to work long hours. There is evidence from other countries that improving payment may be the most effective way to improve safety (Belzer et al. 2000).

These observations need to be placed in context. Unlike the United States, there was never any formal regulatory restriction on the interstate movement of trucks or particular types of goods in Australia. However, over the past 20 years competition in the interstate trucking industry has arguably intensified for a number of reasons, all linked to dominant neo-liberal philosophy.

First, prior to the 1980s regulation of trucking was entirely a matter for each state jurisdiction. However, since this time there have been increasing efforts to coordinate long-haul trucking throughout Australia, beginning with a federal interstate registration scheme (FIRS) and more especially following the creation of the National Road Transport Commission (NRTC) in 1991. The NRTC was a product of a neo-liberal economic reform agenda, having as its key objectives enhancing efficiency and reducing industry costs as well as improving environmental and occupational health and safety. The NRTC sponsored the introduction of uniform national regulations governing heavy vehicles and a substantial increase in vehicle mass (to well over 40 tons GVM in the case of the 22-wheel semi-trailer—the workhorse of the industry—and over 60 tons in the case of the double-articulated B-Double). The NRTC has not ignored safety but it would be fair to say this aspect did not receive the same level of attention until recently. Indeed, it has been argued that commercial considerations dominated the reform process. The recent inquiry into safety in the long haul trucking industry (Quinlan 2001) heard evidence that insufficient attention had been given to the safety effect of larger trucks (including fatigue, vibration, and steering problems; for relevant U.S. research, see Apparies, Riniolo, and Porges 1998). Other criticisms of the NRTC's approach to safety included its flirtation with even longer driving hours in the mid-1990s, its support for voluntary rather mandatory operator accreditation, and its failure to encourage use of OHS legislation. While the NRTC has encouraged fatigue management and developed "chain of responsibility" legislation that could address commercial practices (including customer pressure) the latter is still demonstrably inferior to the regulatory option of OHS legislation. In a sense this continued a trend set in the previous decade where safety-related aspects of federal reform, especially proposals for operator licensing and the compulsory fitting of tachographs, were not adopted. Judged in hindsight, industry interests and especially the Australian Trucking Association (aided by the dominance of neo-liberal ideology), have successfully resisted mandatory operator licensing for over a decade. This has been achieved even though the major industry association in at least one jurisdiction (Victoria) has taken a contrary view and—more importantly, perhaps—the alternative option of voluntary accreditation has consistently failed to attract the level of membership necessary to alter safety practices across the industry. The fact that the NRTC has itself consistently promoted voluntary accreditation as the preferred model has undoubtedly assisted in achieving this outcome.

Second, the combination of easy entry of small and often marginal operators, pressure from customers, and intense competition among operators has "squeezed" freight rates. Virtually all efficiency gains have been passed on and there are indications of long-term economic viability problems (as seen in large numbers of bankruptcies among small operators and instability even among large transport companies). Subcontracting has become an integral part of the tendering process with large freight-forwarding and transport companies using low labor cost owner/drivers and small fleets to undertake work rather than using directly employed drivers. This pressure explains why performance payment systems have become more pervasive in the industry. With some minor exceptions no legal minimum payment pertains to owner/drivers, a contrast with employee drivers whose wages and other conditions are subject to state or federal awards and agreements. Competition between employed drivers and often "underpaid" owner/drivers has encouraged widespread evasion of the legal entitlements of employee drivers, especially those working for small fleets.

Third, underpayment of owner/drivers is a longstanding problem (hardly surprising given their weak bargaining position, often exacerbated by indebtedness to finance truck purchase etc.), with periodic cycles of bankruptcy. There have been attempts to set up Australia-wide agreements on minimum rates, most notably the Interstate Owner-Driver agreement reached in the aftermath of the 1979 Razorback truck blockades. Based on a minimum 22 ton load and updated every six months by a costing committee of both employer and union representatives, the agreement ultimately failed to have a serious effect. Crucial limitations were its status as a "recommendation" rather than having legislative backing and the consequent lack of enforcement/compliance (the rates were only adhered to in "union" yards), problems in costing (escalation provisions), determining market rates, and the failure to cover specialist trucks such as refrigerated trucks and tankers. Moreover, the agreement was seen to clash with the deregulation/free market philosophy of the 1980s and received little if any endorsement from government. It was further undermined by the targeting of anticompetitive (co-operation on pricing) arrangements among the major freight forwarding companies by the Trades Practices Commission in the early 1990s. The Transport Workers' Union lost a considerable number of owner/driver members in the long haul sector as a result of the decision.

In sum, there is compelling evidence that a combination of structural characteristics of the long-haul trucking industry, intense competition, and commercial practices have exerted a significant influence on safety over a number of years. Put simply, there were powerful pressures on operators to breach regulations and the accompanying penalty regime often made calculated evasion an economically rational response. The introduction of competition policies has exacerbated the situation by intensifying economic pressures on operators. The regulatory response to this has been muted to say the least. The NRTC, a body with the unenviable task of simultaneously promoting efficiency and safety, accumulated evidence on the impact of commercial practices but refused to endorse mandatory operator licensing. More recently, it has promoted the notion of *chain of responsibility* in road transport legislation that would see a greater focus on operators and other parties. Similar in concept to the general duty provisions in OHS and environmental protection legislation, *chain of responsibility* is currently at a much less developed state, applying to only some types of offenses (like those pertaining to loading and driving hours), carrying penalties that are still much lower than those found under OHS or environmental protection laws, and with very few prosecutions (and at the time of writing virtually none above operator level).

Notwithstanding some important regulatory differences (including differences in the extent and starting point of competition policies) there is evidence of similar problems with regard to long-haul road freight in Europe, the United States, and New Zealand. While it is beyond the confines of this chapter to provide a detailed set of international comparisons some brief observations based on recent studies/inquiries are warranted.

For example, in 1995 the Transport Committee of the New Zealand House of Representatives undertook an inquiry into truck crashes (Storey 1996) following the death of 118 people in 105 crashes involving trucks in the previous year. The Committee identified a number of disturbing practices including signing of contracts by owner/drivers that effectively required them to breach traffic laws, requiring drivers to work excessive hours, and setting work schedules that encouraged excessive speeds (Storey 1996, p. 9). The Report found breaches of law were widespread and a direct consequence of the commercial advantage pertaining to such behavior:

> Until truck drivers and management start respecting and obeying the law, no attempts to reduce truck crashes will succeed. At present, lawbreakers are being given an economic advantage which will not disappear until a commitment to safety has a greater economic benefit. This severely handicaps the majority of responsible operators. (Storey 1996, p. 9)

The Report argued trucking safety was the responsibility of all involved in the road freight task, including fleet managers, owner/drivers, tradespersons operating their own truck, freight forwarders, and all those "who set delivery times, rates and other terms and conditions" (Storey 1996, p. 19). In explaining an increasing level of risk taking the report emphasized commercial pressures and policies that had intensified competition over freight rates and work. Three quotes illustrate this. An experienced trucking operator observed:

> The real fact of the matter is that those who keep the rates down are doing so by not paying their fair dues and cheating the system. The competition is not being done on a fair playing field. Uneconomic units on the road go a long way to contributing to the accident problem simply because drivers have to work long hours, they get tired or they don't have the cash flow to effect repairs to their vehicles. (Storey 1996, p. 21)

The Insurance Council of New Zealand expressed concern at the safety implications of intensified competition, arguing:

> . . . [it]has resulted in drivers extending driving hours in order to maintain their income. The problem is especially acute for owner drivers who have been forced to reduce their charge out rate to maintain business. The Council understands many fleet operators add to the problem by pressing drivers to drive beyond legal hours or ignore the issue when their drivers do. (Storey 1996, p. 21)

An experienced transport manager offered the following views on deregulation:

> Road transport operations in New Zealand have undergone significant change over the last ten years. Deregulation and the competitive NZ business environment have allowed transport operators to extend their operations over large geographical areas . . .

The effect of these changes has caused many operators to stretch their operations to within fine limits in order to gain a competitive edge. This includes tight control on operating costs and the expectation of drivers to work to the limits of regulation.

In some circumstances, those (i.e., freight forwarders, dispatchers) who cause the use of heavy motor vehicles are unaware of the regulations and transport management factors controlling the use of heavy motor vehicles. Under these circumstances the level of risk is extremely high.

In many situations drivers are compelled to work under conditions that fail to have adequate control measures applied to those who are responsible for transport operations. Operators with strong internal policies, controlled procedures and reasonable expectations of their drivers are better equipped to operate within the current environment. (Storey 1996, pp. 21-22)

The report recommended measures be taken to enforce a level playing field so that "an economic advantage is not given to those who break the law and those who play by the rules can compete fairly" (Story 1996, p. 32). In the aftermath of the 1996 parliamentary report there was crackdown of sorts on truck operators with 21 having their licenses canceled over the next three years for offenses such as faulty brakes, damaged steering, and overweight loads (Pickmere 2000). However, the enforcement of operator licensing has been arguably insufficient to affect change. An investigation undertaken by the New Zealand Office of the Controller and Auditor General (1996) found that with the exception of one region (Hamilton) little action had been taken to review the "fit and proper" status of operators. The report also identified an emerging problem of unlicensed operators openly flouting the system.

Similarly, in the United States in 1977 a restructuring of the trucking industry initiated by the Interstate Commerce Commission removed regulations limiting market entry, collective rate-making, and allowing carriers to favor larger clients. Increased competition reduced rates, especially for larger manufacturers and shippers, but thousands of carriers went bankrupt and the wages of non-supervisory trucking employees fell by 26.8% between 1978 and 1990 (Belzer 1994, p. 1). Non-union drivers suffered the largest loss in wages plus a significant increase in unpaid hours (for waiting, etc.). This widening gap encouraged an increase in the non-union workforce and more pervasive patterns of low payments and evasion of work rules (relating to driving hours, drug use, etc.). Like other neo-liberal reforms, economic gains mostly derived far less from efficiency improvements than a combination of crude work intensification and a massive transfer of wealth from workers and small business to large owners of capital. Further, while environment and safety laws were retained (and indeed strengthened in areas like transporting hazardous substances and drug testing of drivers), economic deregulation exacerbated risks to drivers and public road users in general. Belzer (1994) argued it made compliance with rules more costly for carriers, also observing that:

> Since economic deregulation, hundreds of thousands of owner-operators and drivers working for small, unregulated carriers have become harder to locate, supervise, train and monitor. . . . In addition, the highly competitive market fostered by regulatory restructuring provides a daily incentive to violate rules designed to encourage safe operations. (p. 20)

Updating his analysis, Belzer (2000a, p. 150) argued the collapse of wage rates in trucking at an absolute level and in relation to other industries (like manufacturing) helped to explain high labor turnover (sometimes exceeding 200% per annum) and perceived driver shortages. As in Australia, Belzer (2000, p. 139) found U.S. truck drivers were overwhelmingly paid on a performance-related basis, most commonly on a mileage basis (equivalent to the per kilometer rate in Australia) which rewards driving but not other work activities. According to Belzer (2000a, p. 142), these pay systems are popular because they enable trucking companies to shift some of the risks they encounter from market pressures and customer scheduling demands, loading delays etc. onto the driver. The tight margins applying after deregulation meant that any miscalculation by a trucking firm could prove disastrous, helping to explain an increasing number of bankruptcies (Belzer 2000a, pp. 100-102). His analysis of the return on equity and bankruptcies has striking parallels with Australian research by Croke (1998) showing a downward trend throughout the 1990s (with a sharp fall in 1995 following intrastate deregulation). Belzer (2000a) argued the combination of customer pressure and intense competition has offset benefits that might otherwise have followed industry concentration (through mergers etc.):

> Even though the industry is more concentrated, competition remains very high because customers are cost driven and competitors can engage in "destructive" competitive practices. . . . The carrier making the back haul sets the rate, in this case, and nobody makes a profit. In other words, variant capacity utilization may systematically justify very different rates, and since at equilibrium every carrier is hauling freight at the lowest possible rate, profits remain chronically low. Controlling for information asymmetry, each customer will purchase its preferred bundle of lowest rate and highest service, keeping competition intense. (p. 87)

Belzer's analysis has been supported by other researchers such as Engel (1998, p. 40) who argued intense competition following deregulation had resulted in strong benefits to consumers but had dubious effects on the industry itself as firms strove to reduce average variable costs.

Further research by Belzer and colleagues confirmed a strong relationship between reward levels and safety. In 1995 JB Hunt, the second biggest trucking company in the United States, announced a substantial wage increase for its drivers that placed it well above the norm for the industry. Belzer (2000b) assessed the impact of this, finding that it had a significant effect in reducing both the incidence of crashes and labor turnover. Higher pay enabled the company to select more desirable driver characteristics and crash likelihood also progressively decreased with additional tenure. In another study Belzer (2000b) examined the hours of service issue, especially the impact of unpaid working time (e.g., time spent waiting for a load). Like Hensher et al. (see above), they found that the more wasted (i.e., unpaid) time drivers had the more likely they were to squeeze too many hours into a day, forcing schedule irregularity and excessive hours. Indeed, they found the number of unpaid hours was the best predictor of work in excess of 60 hours per week. In terms of a policy response, Belzer (2000b) argued charging shippers and consignors for delay time and paying drivers for this time could reduce the consequent safety risks.

As in Australia, little use has been made of OHS legislation to address safety in long-distance trucking although, with all its faults, this law is more suited to addressing the commercial practices that are at the heart of safety problems. Writing on the United States (Belzer 2000a, p. 70) observed ". . . truckdriver safety seems to have fallen between the cracks as critics charge that neither DOT nor OSHA has taken clear responsibility for truckdriver safety and health" (see also Jeffress 1999). In Australia, there have been recent moves to rectify this by using the general duty provisions in OHS legislation but even so, few serious on-road incidents are investigated to identify criminality on the part of transport operators, clients and the like (Perrone 2000; Quinlan 2001).

The promotion of competition by the European Commission is having a similar effect on road transport in the European Union. According to Hamelin (2000, p. 5), subcontracting, business start-ups, and failures spread at the height of the deregulation "fever" from the mid 1980s. Competition between freight forwarders held freight rates down, with many transport firms, some barely viable, taking contracts at "rock-bottom" prices just to stay in business and the turnover of firms enabling the embedded costs of the haulage system (including those associated with economic swings) to be farmed out. Hamelin (2000, p. 5) argues fierce competition between haulers has been instrumental in making anti-social working hours the norm for drivers. This can be seen as one aspect of a broader question as to whether the social costs of road transport, including public safety, should be borne by the industry and passed on in haulage rates, or regarded as a cost to the community.

By the mid 1990s, if not before, regulators (and others) were expressing serious concern at the safety implications of the growth in the volume of road freight at the same time as freight rates and profit margins were being squeezed. Derek Gibbons from the British Department of Transport (Bousfield 1996) observed:

> As profit margins get smaller, we are worried about the "cowboy" companies that aren't properly licensed and don't train their drivers correctly. (p. 66)

As in Australia (Quinlan 2001), there have been recurring complaints from drivers and operators that the pressure from customers and the just-in-time (JIT) system is undermining safety (Bousfield 1996, p. 66). This is consistent with Stoop and Thissen's (1997) finding that highly articulated transport systems with narrow windows for service/delivery are not conducive to safety. This aspect of JIT is seldom considered.

From 1998 onward the level of competitive pressure was intensified as a direct result of the European Commission's economic reform process. The first (anti) cabotage regulation on road transport introduced in July 1998 effectively removed license requirements to drive in particular countries, enabling drivers to not only take loads into countries where they were not licensed but also to do domestic trips within these countries on an "occasional" basis. Precisely what "occasional" means is yet to be decided with individual countries reluctant to make a move that might jeopardize their own transport operators. Given significant disparities in licensing requirements and safety legislation, wage rates, working conditions, and union density between countries (especially between southern and northern Europe) the cabotage regulation has intensified competition between transport operators in different regions in Europe. According to Hamelin (2000, p. 25) this competition has led to a further cut in already low freight rates. This has occurred in a context where the only common legal provisions governing labor management among European hauliers is EEC Safety Regulation 3820/85 (passed in 1985) and there are serious disparities and omissions in the legal framework governing driving hours. In other words, there is a mismatch between direct competitive pressures and a patchwork quilt of regulatory protection to prevent anti-social outcomes.

Even the largest operators in the Netherlands have sought ways to cut operating costs by changing their employment practices and manipulating legal categories. Analogous to the maritime industry, it has also led to emergence of companies using drivers from Eastern Europe at low *flag of convenience* wages. This practice has already caused concern among representatives of British haulage industry. A recent inquiry into the industry by the House of Commons Environment, Transport and Regional Affairs Committee (2000, p. xxvii) heard evidence that drivers from Hungary, Romania, and Slovakia were receiving between 16 and 23% of the pay of a driver from the United Kingdom. These low wages enabled companies to *double man* their lorries and so operate for much longer hours and more cheaply.

Like its Australian counterpart the British industry includes a large number of small companies and self-employed drivers (90% of fleets have fewer than five trucks and 50% have one truck) and a very small number of large operators. Like Australia, the standard workhorse of the industry is a 38-42.5 ton articulated lorry and these vehicles make a disproportionate contribution to the overall road toll (although the toll is low by Australian standards), accounting for 7% vehicle kilometers traveled but 15% of all road fatalities. As in Australia, there has been debate about the sustainability of freight rates and serious concern that ease of entry into the industry and a consequent over-supply of operators has compromised safety. As the National Road Freight Industry Inquiry (May, Mills, and Scully 1984) argued for Australia, operator licensing was introduced in an effort to address these issues.

The British report found that the profitability and viability of the road haulage industry had been undermined by a longstanding problem of very low haulage or freight rates (Committee of Environment, Transport and Regional Affairs 2000, p. xxii). The report enumerated three factors that had kept rates so low: namely, entry into the industry was too easy, creating an oversupply of operators; there was competition from other European competitors following the 1998 EU cabotage regulation; and some companies routinely ignored regulation to secure a commercial advantage. The Committee (2000, pp. xvi-xvii) accepted evidence from industry and other witnesses that deregulation had made the industry too easy to join, creating an oversupply of operators that depressed haulage rates and compromised safety. It found that the profitability and viability of road haulage companies had been undermined by the longstanding problem of very low haulage rates. The Committee believed it was essential for hauliers to be able to pass on their true costs to customers, and ultimately to the consumer. A key recommendation was to substantially raise the financial requirements for entry into the industry under the operator-licensing scheme.

The Committee found that, despite the efforts of the Vehicle Inspectorate and police, a significant minority of operators flouted regulations relating to driving hours, vehicle maintenance/defects, and other safety-related issues. The Committee (2000, p. xxxi) strongly supported the application of the European Union Working Time Directive but believed the exemption of self-employed drivers was unjustified, creating a loophole that induced movement of drivers into this category. European unions have long pressed for an extension of the 1993 European Working Time Directive to cover self-employed workers including those in road transport (another European Regulation 3820/85 sets maximum driving hours for self-employed and employee drivers but did not include activities like loading). The Union of Industrial and Employer's Confederations (UNICE) has strongly resisted this measure, arguing that all member states already had some form of working-time regulation and advocating a voluntary/ non-binding, sector-specific approach. Yet, as a 1997 European Commission White Paper had noted, there was no consistency in member-state regulations (with these differences being exacerbated by variations in compliance activity) and the competitive advantages derived from perpetuating such differences warranted a Community-wide approach. Yet the regulatory gap remains.

The aforementioned issues have also caused concern in Sweden (with around 35,000 long- and short-haul truck drivers). In Sweden with its highly unionized transport workforce (paid under a single collective agreement despite pressure for separate enterprise agreements from the Swedish Competition Authority) and (unlike other parts of Europe) relatively few self-employed drivers, the effects are liable to be most profound. Already, a number of Swedish transport firms have sought to relocate their operations. As elsewhere, researchers (see Frick 2000) have pointed to the fragmented nature of the industry, a poor understanding of OHS, the inability of operators to resist customer demands, the impact of deregulation (especially the right of cabotage and leasing of Eastern European drivers), and lack of enforcement of minimum standards. Cost savings achieved through inferior working conditions and compromises on safety have emerged as major means of competition. There is growing evidence of undercutting of working conditions by smaller operations and drivers accepting below-agreement rates or individual (i.e., kilometer rate) contracts in an effort to safeguard their jobs, as well as an increase in hazardous work practices (Segerdahl 2000). The Swedish Transport Workers Union has countered the threat by pursuing a Scandinavia-wide collective agreement and more effective EU Directives to govern the industry.

As in the United States, there is growing concern in Europe about retaining a solid core of trained and experienced truck drivers at the same time as intensified competition is leading to a more volatile, younger and inexperienced workforce. As in the United States, there is evidence that inexperienced entrants have significantly higher rates of crashes and work-related injuries than their more experienced counterparts (Hamelin 2000, p. 22). In short, the shift to a more volatile workforce means a more hazardous workforce.

2.2 The Failure to Treat Truck-Related Deaths as Work-Related

One consequence of the current regulatory approach is that truck-related deaths, let alone other serious incidents, are by and large not investigated for breaches of OHS law or related corporate criminality. Obviously, without some level of investigation, serious breaches of OHS and other legislation are likely to go undetected. When there is evidence that the (surviving) driver of a heavy vehicle may have caused the death or serious injury to road users or other parties it is almost certain that charges will be laid by road traffic regulatory agencies (in cases of death a charge of manslaughter is common). While charging the driver may be appropriate, this response is unbalanced on three grounds. First, the focus on culpability on drivers and failure to explore let alone pursue the legal responsibility of employers and other parties sends very poor signals to the industry and its clients about appropriate modes of behavior on their part. Second, if regulatory strategies are to be successful in preventing injuries and fatalities from long-haul trucking activities, regulatory measures must focus on the sources of hazards, which as we have shown are usually the demands placed on drivers by consigners, freight forwarders and other clients, and employer trucking companies. Third, at least equally important, when a truck driver dies in an highway/on-road incident there is very seldom an investigation of possible corporate responsibility, let alone the launching of a prosecution.

The failure to investigate work-related deaths with a view to identifying corporate criminality or to follow up on such investigations is by no means confined to road transport. However, there is clear evidence that, with the possible exception of farming, road transport stands in a league of its own in this regard. Criminologist, Dr. Santina Perrone carried out a thorough investigation of the circumstances surrounding regulatory response to all work-related fatalities that occurred in a four-year period (1987-1990) in the state of Victoria. Perrone (2000) carefully sifted WorkCover, coronial inquests, court proceedings, and other records of investigation. She found that of 258 deaths occurring in a corporate context, in 55 cases there was insufficient information to determine the negligent contribution of the employer, and transport fatalities comprised almost three quarters of these (74.5%). Perrone's (2000) examination of the reasons for this and its implications are particularly pertinent. She noted the following about the relevant OHS agency (then known as the HSO):

> [HSO did] not investigate traffic fatalities as a matter of course, particularly those involving trucking collisions occurring en route during the course of transporting livestock and other freight. This is despite the fact that as previously stated, transport fatalities constituted the largest single category of overall fatalities in the sample.

> This lack of attention to trucking fatalities is particularly concerning in the light of findings relating to the involvement of alcohol and other drugs in such incidents. Whilst in total, only nine cases were identified whereby it was ascertained through the course of toxicological examination that prescription stimulants and/or illicit drugs (amphetamines, cannabanoids, morphine etc) were present in the body of the deceased worker at the time of the fatality, six of those cases (66.7%) involved the trucking industry. Similarly, of the twenty-two cases where alcohol consumption was an issue, nine of those (41%) were situated in the trucking industry. (p. 45)

Perrone argued these problems were mirrored in terms of police and coronial investigations:

> Compounding such regulatory disregard is the observation that police investigations conducted into such fatalities almost invariably fail to delve into the deceased's routines and responsibilities, working conditions and employer demands. Although witnesses at the scene of a collision are routinely questioned, police investigations are invariably concerned predominantly with peripheral issues such as road measurements and configurations, the visibility of road safety/speed sign, weather conditions, the mechanical soundness of the vehicle and the like. This technical focus on immediate cause basically serves to decontextualise the incident, so that it simply becomes another road "accident" rather than a work-related harm; a purely unplanned and unintentional occurrence. Only on rare occasions were

depositions sought from employers, and when interviews did transpire, the line of questioning adopted proved inadequate, with relevant organisational issues not ordinarily canvassed. (For similar arguments regarding the short-sightedness of investigations in the United States, see for example Knestaut, 1997)

. . . The dissimilarities in investigative rigor further extend in the coronial arena. Unlike the mandatory requirements to conduct an inquest into the circumstances surrounding a suspected homicide . . . coroners have a considerable degree of discretionary latitude where work death is concerned and that discretion is regularly exercised. During the period under review, coroners chose to dispense with a formal inquiry in 32% of work-related fatalities ($N = 112$ cases).

Of those cases which underwent a review short of formal inquest, the transport industry once again featured prominently, surpassed only by the farming industry. Unfortunately, those transport cases that were the subject of coronial review often failed to yield vital information that would have shed light on systemic shortcomings. Pertinent organisational questions often remained unexplored: for example, were unscrupulous employers subjecting workers to unrealistic work schedules that discouraged sufficient rest periods and perhaps encouraged substance abuse? Were regulations mandating the possession and maintenance of logbooks enforced? Were logbooks doctored and/or speed-limiting devices circumvented? Were correct loading procedures observed? Was the employee provided with a roadworthy vehicle, adequate training, instruction and supervision? (Perrone 2000, pp. 46-47)

Perrone examined her sample of work-related fatalities to identify instances where the available evidence indicated prosecutable corporate negligence and categorized this according to whether the negligence was of a minor, intermediate, or extreme nature. With regard to the transport industry cases where evidence was sufficient to make an assessment Perrone determined that 23 of the 24 fatalities involved intermediate company negligence. In construction and manufacturing, by way of contrast, 50% and 40% of cases respectively were determined to involve extreme negligence (Perrone 2000, pp. 69-70). However, Perrone added an important rider to this that is consistent with observations above about the number of transport cases where evidence was too poor to make any determination whatsoever as to negligence (2000):

It is imperative here that we recapitulate the poor state of investigative scrutiny extended to the transport industry and stress the urgent need for ameliorative measures. The failure to thoroughly consider the circumstances surrounding trucking has meant that in most cases not even a minimum degree of corporate responsibility could be ascribed, despite the fact that information suggested differently. For example, in a number of instances, long-distance truck drivers appear to have suffered fatigue and consequently fallen asleep at the wheel. The circumstances are suggestive of objectionable time schedules blindly followed in the impetus to undercut competitors, but investigations

> almost invariably failed to explicitly address this issue. Had such issues been
> considered, then perhaps more of these fatalities would have been categorised
> as extreme negligence cases. (p. 70)

Examining the number of cases where a prosecution actually occurred, Perrone found that the transport sector constituted a problem area. Perrone (2000, p. 193) identified 89 fatalities containing a degree of negligence warranting prosecution, 24 of which were in transport. Only 14 or around 60% of these transport cases were known to the OHS agency (comparable to services but far below the 90-100% figure for all other industries) and prosecution occurred in only six cases. The latter represented only 42% of known transport cases or 25% of all relevant transport cases and, again, both figures were well below the comparable figure for all other industries aside from services. In sum, while transport and service sectors contributed a greater volume to Perrone's sample of work-related fatalities than manufacturing or construction the latter two—both a traditional jurisdictional focus OHS agency activities—attracted far more investigation and prosecutorial activity. In other words, Perrone found a substantial inadequacy in OHS agency responses to work-related fatalities in the transport industry. A study of road transport fatalities in New South Wales by Hopkins (1992) reached essentially similar conclusions. He argued that while excessive hours/inadequate rest breaks due to pressure from freight forwarders, etc. could constitute a breach of general duty provisions to provide a safe system of work under the NSW *Occupational Health and Safety Act*, none of the incidents had been investigated by the OHS agency (WorkCover).

Perrone's analysis also found support in submissions made to an Inquiry into safety in the long haul road transport industry commissioned by the Motor Accidents Authority of New South Wales (Quinlan 2001). Aside from insurers, the union and CFAT, one state industry association, and a number of operational police could not understand why WorkCover did not investigate serious on-road incidents involving heavy vehicles with a view to laying charges.

> . . . in my mind all heavy vehicle accidents, I am talking about all heavy
> vehicle accidents—they are industrial accidents. (oral submission, police
> traffic coordinator based in southern NSW cited in Quinlan 2001)

The officer stressed that he was not advocating more enforcement per se, as the pattern of offenses seemed to have changed little over time, but rather more carefully targeted enforcement that would deal with those elements, such as freight forwarders, who were at the heart of the problem. The same highway patrol commander expressed surprise that the families of drivers who were killed did not take civil action against companies, arguing there would be enough evidence in the majority of cases to suggest the work practices imposed on them were responsible for the incident:

I'm really surprised that family members of drivers who are killed on the road, haven't under civil law, sued the pants off companies. I believe that families of drivers would have so much evidence to offer . . . to say that work practices by their husbands [were to blame]. (oral submission cited in Quinlan 2001)

On the rare occasions when the option of using OHS legislation to proceed against employers and other responsible parties has been canvassed by coroners or judges in criminal trials of truck drivers these comments were ignored. The coronial inquest into the Blanchetown incident is one such case. On August 3rd, 1996 a semi-trailer (the prime mover being federally registered) belonging to WRB Transport Pty Ltd. that had been traveling erratically for some time collided with two cars near Blanchetown, South Australia resulting in the deaths of six people. The semi-driver, who survived the smash, was later found to have drug residues (Phentermine—a derivative of amphetamine, Ephedrine, and Tetrahydro-cannabinol, found in Cannabis). Subsequently the coroner found that a number of company personnel (named in the inquest) had knowingly supplied drugs to the driver and this was a common practice in response to the "ludicrous hours many of the drivers spent at the wheel" (Coroners Court of South Australia 1999, p. 32). During the Inquest Coroner Chivell undertook the time-consuming and unusual step of interviewing many of the drivers for WRB, enabling him to corroborate the existence of the practice (and despite an unsuccessful appeal by the company to have the Supreme Court rule the evidence inadmissible). Interviews with drivers by the coroner also identified the reasons for this drug use, namely, a situation where drivers employed by the company were regularly making trips that should take two and half days (if logbooks were properly abided by) in a day and a half. Drivers were encouraged to undertake trips in this time by a mixture of reward pressures (receiving $440 for Adelaide/Sydney return trip) and scheduling pressure imposed by the company (in relation to the Blanchetown crash an early arrival was specified on both the written manifest and on an envelope). Blanchetown provided further evidence that evasions of awards (minimum wage rates) compromised safety and were essentially an outcome of competitive pressures on transport operators (low freight rates and lower labor costs charged by owner/drivers) and employee driver fears that demanding award entitlements would place their job at risk. The coroner formed the view that, despite management claims to the contrary, unrealistic schedules that breached both road transport and OHS legislation were the norm.

In his findings the coroner addressed the culpability of two managers under the *Occupational Health, Safety and Welfare Act, 1986*. Specifically, the coroner believed both men had abrogated their responsibility as employers and then referred to duties under Section 19(1)(a) to provide a safe working environment and a safe system of work, and to provide adequate information, training and supervision (Section 19(1)(c)). The coroner also referred to Section 19(3) that requires employers to monitor employee health and wellbeing, keep injury records and provide information at the workplace (Coroner's Court of South Australia 1999, p. 23). It should be noted that very similar general duty provisions are found within the principal OHS Act of every jurisdiction in Australia. The coroner noted that the Act also provided for detailed regulation identifying how these objectives could be achieved in particular industries. In concluding his observations on this point the coroner observed:

> The time has long passed when employers can take the "hands off" approach described by Mr. Bunker and Mr. Cushnie. I do not seek to suggest that WRB or its managers are in breach of the Act—to do so may contravene Section 26(3) of the Coroners Act. I merely observe that the attitudes displayed by both these witnesses are not consistent with modern concepts of the duty of employers to their employees.
>
> In this regard, it seems to me that the Office of Workplace Services, part of the Department of Administrative and Information Services, has a substantial role to play in ensuring, by training, information and policing, that this legislation is complied with. I do not know what action has been taken by that department in relation to the heavy vehicle industry to date, but it seems to me that there is plenty of scope for them to play a more active role in relation to this industry, assuming they have the resources to do so. (Coroners Court of South Australia 1999, p. 24)

In many respects the coroner's findings in relation to the Blanchetown incident mirrored earlier comments of District Court Judge Lowrie when sentencing the truck driver (Brian Douglas Snewin) charged with causing death by dangerous driving. It is worth reproducing some of these comments, as they highlight the interconnection between low pay/trip based payment and scheduling pressures/long hours with safety, and the judge's view that these problems were by no means atypical:

> It is not the first time I have heard how wage rates relate kilometres driven and the physical demand at times put on drivers by irresponsible employers to comply with schedules. I am not surprised with those submissions. It was said that you worked for one major trucking company, an interstate company, and found you could not financially survive because of the long hours and the small amount of remuneration and, of course, not assisted by vehicle breakdowns.
>
> I am told you resigned from a number of positions because of the nature of these driving schedules and turn around times and delays. You clearly could not cope financially. Again I have heard of these difficulties with these so-called log books. It was mentioned that in one State, for instance, there is no requirement for log books and subsequently there is the impossibility of monitoring driving situations.
>
> These matters really must be addressed by not only legislation but the industry. . . . The details of your driving in the prior week from Adelaide to Sydney are simply unbelievable but no doubt you accepted the tasks as

directed by management of this firm. And, indeed, looking at those hours and schedules it always spelt disaster.

I am told it was a common practice with this company to supply you with stimulants. When I look at these schedules. . . [it] is no wonder you had no concentration on that day or the next day. . .The conduct of those companies and the schedule is extremely culpable conduct. (*R* v *Brian Douglas Snewin* 1997, sentencing decision, pp. 1-2)

A similar set of circumstances can be found in relation to a Victoria case where the 22-year-old driver was killed in February 1996 when his small cattle truck was rear-ended by a semi-trailer. It was later revealed that at the time of the incident the semi-driver had been working up to 14 hours a day for 18 consecutive days. In sentencing the driver to three years jail (with a minimum two-year non-parole period) the County Court Judge observed:

Caught up in a very competitive, aggressive industry whose habits all too frequently spill over onto roadway behaviour, Mr. Braun (the driver's employer) was, in my belief, negligent in his supervision, clearly had little interest in the log book and left too much to driver discretion. (Age 1998, cited in Perrone 2000, p. 160)

Despite these comments, no charges were laid against the employer.

For its part the Transport Workers Union has pushed for OHS agencies to become more involved. In 1997 WorkCover NSW investigated Scott's Refrigerated Freightways. In his 1997 inspection WorkCover inspector Ron Keelty examined evidence from Safe-T-Cam, interviews with drivers, logbooks and manifests. After examining all these records (especially Safe-T-Cam) was he was able to determine that the logbooks had not been filled in correctly. Keelty concluded that "[t]he company did not have any systems in place for ensuring employees and contractors who [drove] the company vehicles took the required rest breaks" (WorkCover Investigation, Scotts Refrigerated Freightways, summary).

Keelty concluded that there was evidence of drivers working excessive hours contrary to RTA requirements. From the evidence compiled for the report he concluded that it appeared the company was not complying with the employer's duty to employees in section 15 of the *Occupational Health and Safety Act 1983* (NSW) by failing to provide adequate supervision to ensure workers got adequate rest breaks. In his view, the evidence also suggested that the company was not complying with s.16, putting the contractors it employed at risk by requiring them to work excessive hours (for a detailed discussion of these general duty provisions, see what are now Sections 8 and 9 of the amended *Act*, 2000).

Although the NSW Branch of the TWU pressed for a prosecution in relation to Scott's Refrigerated Freightways, there was no follow-up. In November 1999 branch officials met with WorkCover General Manager John Grayson to discuss their concerns over driving hours and in January and February 2000 wrote to him asking WorkCover to investigate specific fatal/serious on-road incidents and to inform it of current investigations. In February the General Manager responded stating that the agency investigated work-related accidents in any industry, had always investigate traffic accidents on a road works site or where there were indications inadequate systems of work contributed to the accident. He then added:

> WorkCover recognises that for some workers in the road transport industry a truck or motor vehicle is a place of work. I have therefore issued a media release reminding employers in the transport industry of their obligations to report workplace incidents, which in their case may include road traffic accidents.
>
> WorkCover acknowledges however that the NSW Police Service, which provides the emergency response is the lead agency in regard to the investigation of road traffic accidents. WorkCover also acknowledges the role and responsibility of the Roads and Traffic Authority (RTA) in this regard.
>
> The RTA has primary responsibility for the regulation of the long-distance trucking industry, including making provision for or with respect to the management and prevention of driver fatigue in connection with the driving of heavy trucks and coaches. WorkCover is advised that it is the practice of an RTA Officer to attend the majority (85%) of road traffic accidents involving heavy vehicles.
>
> Arrangements like these are accepted practice among government agencies where there is potential for more than one agency to be involved because of overlapping legislation and/or responsibilities. (Correspondence, John Grayson, General Manager of WorkCover, to Tony Sheldon, Secretary of NSW Branch TWU, February 24th, 2000)

It might have been expected that the WorkCover NSW approach would be endorsed by the other enforcement agencies most directly involved, namely the police and the RTA. However, this was not the case. What is perhaps most telling is that the RTA itself did not share WorkCover's views. In its submission (executive summary) to the trucking inquiry the RTA stated that "[t]here would be advantages in WorkCover taking a stronger role in insuring safe working practices in the industry given that trucks are clearly workplaces of their drivers."

Consistent with this position, the RTA recently adapted its *Heavy Vehicle Drivers Handbook* to include a section, approved by WorkCover, making the relevance of this legislation explicit.

The position adopted by WorkCover NSW was not unique, with OHS regulatory agencies in other countries adopting a similar position. However, OHS agencies elsewhere in Australia had begun to adopt a more proactive role. In its written submission to the NSW trucking inquiry (given the interstate nature of the industry the inquiry took evidence from all jurisdictions) WorkCover Victoria stated that issues of driving hours, drug use, and speeding were interrelated and it was currently undertaking research to develop a frame-work for prevention. The submission noted that in 1997 the Transport Industry Safety Group (TSIG) had produced a guide explaining the OHS duty of care (with a video version) in order to address a lack of knowledge within the transport industry. The TSIG has also produced a video guide on fatigue management entitled *How the hell can you take a break?* More recently WorkCover funded the development of TransCare—a transport-specific performance-based management system designed to achieve a more comprehensive and due-diligence approach to OHS—by the Victorian Road Transport Association. The Victoria agency made it clear it believed it had a strong enforcement role to play in road transport, one made especially important by advantageous features of OHS legislation and corresponding problems with the existing road transport regulatory framework. It noted that road transport was an extremely competitive low-margin industry with many small operators and subcontractors, but the OHS legislation had regulatory requirements, especially those within the general duty provisions, to deal with this. The agency referred to section 21(3) of the Victoria *Occupational Health and Safety Act 1985* that extends employer duties to independent con-tractors and their employees and section 22 that imposes a duty on employers and self-employed persons to ensure that the conduct of their undertaking does not to expose other persons (such as road users and truck drivers themselves) to risks to their health or safety. Further, it noted that OHS responsibilities extended along the full vertical chain of responsibility from consignor/supplier through transporter to client (see further, Quinlan 2001, appendix 2). There is evidence of a growing interest in prosecuting on-road transport incidents in Victoria although the trend is still insufficient to invalidate Perrone's overall assessment.

For example, in 1999 a long-distance trucking company, Don Watson Transport, was successfully prosecuted in the Victorian County Court for a contravention of the employer's duty to its employees in section 21 of the Victorian *Occupational Health and Safety Act 1985*. Thanks to the perseverance and skill of the investigating inspector, the prosecution was able to prove that the company did not have a system of work in place that monitored the hours drivers worked, to ensure against driver fatigue. The court found that the system was conducive to log book or drug offenses by drivers, and fined the company $12,000 (Victorian WorkCover Authority 1999, p. 34).

Agencies in other states have also made initiatives at least consistent with building the role of OHS regulation in long haul road transport. In the same year the trial connected to the Blanchetown case the WorkCover Corporation of South Australia produced a detailed 25-page guide to meeting the OHS duty of care in the road freight transport industry (WorkCover South Australia 1998 and since updated 2001). Western Australia, which unlike other jurisdictions had not pre-scribed truck driver hours under road transport legislation, introduced a voluntary (and later, mandatory) fatigue management code based on the general duty provisions of OHS legislation (and which had the added advantage of "roping in" subcontractors employed by transport firms). In Queensland, the Division of Workplace Health and Safety (1994) issued a guide on health and safety in the road freight industry in 1994 that has recently been updated. Even the 1994 version identified the relevant general duty provisions covering employers, employees, self-employed persons and others (sections 9, 10, 13, and 14) under the Queensland *Workplace Health and Safety Act, 1989*. The guide contained a fairly detailed and (for the time) advanced section on fatigue, which among a number of others, was clearly directed at the long-haul sector.

The need to bring OHS legislation into play in the trucking industry has also begun to be recognized in other countries. For example, a New Zealand inquiry into truck crashes recommended that:

> The *Health and Safety in Employment Act 1992* should be applied imme-
> diately to truck operations by the Occupational Safety and Health Service,
> in conjunction with the Police, especially for serious offending where the
> full force of the *Act* is justifiable. (Storey 1996, p. 12)

The New Zealand report noted that OHS legislation provided that employers, including company directors, who breached the *Act* could be fined up to $NZ 100,000 or jailed for up to one year. In other words, the penalties available were fare more significant than those normally applied under road transport legislation and could also consider systemic offenses. The New Zealand report also made recommendations in relation to the appointment of inspectors (both in the short and long term) to facilitate enforcement under the *Health and Safety in Employment Act, 1992* (Storey 1996, pp. 84-85). A more recent inquiry into health and safety problems in Tranz Rail (New Zealand 2000) reinforced this point, arguing that rail employees should be afforded the protection of general duties in the principal OHS Act:

> There is, in our view, no justification for rail employees having a lower level
> of occupational health and safety protection than the work force generally. We
> therefore recommend that the provisions of Part II of the HSE Act that set out
> the duties of employers relating to health and safety in employment should
> apply without restriction to all rail employees. (p. 46)

The New South Wales Trucking Inquiry (Quinlan 2001) saw no reason why an analogous argument should not apply to road freight. Indeed the Tranz Rail Inquiry made specific reference to road transport, and the recommendations of the 1996 inquiry into truck crashes, to support its argument with regard to rail freight.

The reluctance of OHS agencies to get involved in road transport could be explained in terms of the large logistical demands this would make on already constrained resources or (and this point was made to the New South Wales Trucking Inquiry) evidentiary problems. As noted in passing, logbook records made by drivers are unreliable documents, and pressure to exceed driving hours can be informal (relying on "understandings" of what is required among drivers, the tone and demeanor of managers, etc.) and difficult for an outside agency to establish. It also clear that, especially with small to medium operators, "last minute jobs" may leave little in the way of a "paper trail" and the increasing use of electronic tendering exacerbates this. However, as indicated above (see the *Scott Refrigeration* case) such evidence can be collected and OHS legislation provides a far more effective vehicle for pursuing "system" offenses. There are also ways to create paper trails and replace logbooks (see Quinlan 2001). While evidentiary and resourcing issues are legitimate concerns they are not insurmountable, nor are they the main reason that more use has not been made of OHS legislation to investigate truck-related fatalities. On any objective assessment the toll of dead and maimed in the long-haul trucking industry warrants an allocation of even scarce resources.

We argue that OHS, road traffic, and industrial relations regulators need to work together to ensure that a more systematic approach is taken to the regulation of long-haul trucking, since the source of the enormous risks in this industry are directly attributable to the *modus operandi* of consignors, forward freighters, other clients, and trucking companies themselves. A regulatory approach that merely focuses on individual crashes and the responsibility of drivers for those crashes will routinely ignore the systemic causes of road injuries and death, and will persist in the isolation of each incident from its underlying causes and the tendency to underestimate the disastrous nature of the road toll attributable to long-haul trucking. OHS regulators are best suited to investigate the systemic nature of long-haul trucking-related road hazards, and should play a central part in their prevention.

Over the past three years there is evidence of further attempts to bridge this gap, with OHS regulatory agencies, including WorkCover NSW, launching "big ticket" prosecutions and compliance campaigns against trucking operators. For example, in October 2004 an employer, Jim Hitchcock, was convicted under the *Occupational Health and Safety Act* of failing to provide safe conditions, resulting in the death of long haul driver, Darri Haynes, in a two-semi collision on the Pacific Highway (and close to where the Cowper smash occurred in 1989). Further echoing the Cowper incident, the case revealed that Haynes had not slept in two days, was "fuelled" by methamphetamine and was struggling to adhere to a timetable, fearing he would lose his job if he complained. Justice Walton found Hitchcock's company failed to manage fatigue (apart from the use of often falsified logbooks) and provided pay incentives to increase driving hours. The test case decision also confirmed that a driver's truck is their workplace (and therefore falls clearly within the domain of OHS legislation). Further, in her inquest into the death of three truck drivers in separate incidents (two in single vehicle crashes and one due to drug induced cardiac arrhythmia) Deputy NSW Coroner Dorelle Pinche took the unusual step of issuing a supplement highlighting the common features, namely fatigue, drug-use, falsified log books, pressures for deliveries, and an the absence of medical testing. More particularly, Pinche drew on guidance material and the findings of two government inquiries to stress the need to deal with the underlying problem (Coroners Court of New South Wales 2003):

> As long as driver payments are based on a (low) rate per kilometer there will always be an incentive for drivers to maximize the hours they drive, not because they are greedy but simply to earn a decent wage. I anticipate that this incentive will remain an overriding concern for drivers irrespective of legal and safety considerations. This is obviously a structural matter for the road transport industry that has already been placed on the agenda . . . However, structural changes do not feature prominently in current initiatives as far as I can ascertain . . . I intend to forward my findings . . . to the (sic) WorkCover NSW, the Road Transport Authority and any other relevant body to be taken into consideration in future policy development. (pp. 4-5)

In 2004 WorkCover released a draft fatigue management regulation for long-haul trucking that included imposing obligations on clients and suppliers using road freight but (as of October 2004) this had yet to be implemented following vigorous criticism from business groups (WorkCover NSW 2004 and ABL 2004). In sum, while there is a clear trend toward OHS regulators taking a greater interest in truck driver health and safety the shift is slow and being fiercely contested by parties who benefit from the existing approach.

CONCLUSION

The notion of occupational disasters normally conjures up images of mine explosions or inundations, factory fires, or, less often, the large-scale exposure to hazardous substances such as in Bhopal, Seveso, or asbestos mines and towns. Yet in terms of its absolute and relative toll on both workers and the community, long-haul road transport represents an ongoing tragedy of magnitude equal to the worst of these types of catastrophe. Despite evidence of public concern, truck-related injury and death is not viewed as an OHS problem, principally because regulators have chosen not to treat it as an OHS problem. Even the most serious incidents of mass death have for the most part not resulted in OHS regulatory interventions but rather modification of road transport legislation. The latter, while having some regard to commercial pressures that evidence shows are at the root cause of dangerous practices, do not by themselves provide a framework to effectively combat the causes of drug use, long hours, speeding, and so on. Indeed, the promotion of deregulation and competition policies has arguably increased the mismatch between the power of particular interest groups and economic imperatives that drive industry work practices on the one hand and the array of legislative controls that seek to combat the adverse effects of these on the other.

In most industrialized countries road transport was highly competitive even prior to these changes, but now the level of competition has intensified to the point where there are strong inducements to employ exploitive work arrangements and evade or avoid minimum regulatory standards. These include subcontracting work to low cost owner/drivers and paying employee drivers minimal wages based on driving time (and using immigrants in the case of Europe and the United States). The implications of this for safety are becoming increasingly clear even though the effects are hidden or understated by the shift to the self-employed and small operators. In road transport, competition between different categories of workers (employee driver, self-employed driver, large fleet driver, and small fleet driver) is direct and intense, and so the adverse OHS effects have spread across the entire industry. The situation is also obfuscated by the conspicuous failure of the regulatory apparatus to investigate deaths and other serious incidents in terms of corporate criminality. While some OHS agencies are taking more interest in the industry it is unlikely this situation will change in the near future.

Shrivastava (1994) argues there is logic to industrialism that legitimates the externalization of dysfunctional effects of production onto the public. He goes on to say:

> This contradiction creates a vicious circle in the context of competition. The more competitive an industry becomes, the more pressure its firms face to cut costs to maintain rates of profit. This goal is often achieved by reducing manpower and cutting back non-production services, such as worker training, maintenance, safety and environmental protection. Competition thus creates and externalizes still more hazards. (p. 258)

In other words, adverse OHS outcomes can be seen as just one of an array of production externalities that have long been legitimated within industrial societies but in industries where competition is intense or is made more so by government competition policies, changes in the labor process and then the pressures to make yet further sacrifices in terms of OHS will mount. Long-haul trucking arguably provides an illustration of this phenomenon.

REFERENCES

ABL. (2004) *Submission in Response to a Proposed Amendment to the Occupational Health and Safety Regulation 2001.* Australian Business Limited.

Adam, B., and van Loon, J. (2000) Introduction: Repositioning Risk; the Challenge for Social Theory. In B. Adam, U. Beck, and J. van Loon (eds.), *The Risk Society and Beyond* (pp. 1-31). London: Sage Publications.

Apparies, R., Riniolo, T., and Porges, S. (1998) A Psychological Investigation of the Effects of Driving Longer Combination Vehicles. *Ergonomics, 41*(5): 581-592.

ARRB. (1998) *Towards a Methodology for Comparative Resource Consumption: Modal Implications for the Freight Task.* Australian Road Research Board Transport Research Report, 1998, ARR318.

ATSB. (2001) *Articulated Truck Crashes.* Monograph No. 8. Australian Transport Safety Board.

ATSB. (2004) *Fatal Road Crashes Involving Articulated Trucks.* Road Safety Working Paper No. 2, Australian Transport Safety Board.

Beck, U. (1992) *Risk Society: Towards a New Modernity.* London: Sage Publications.

Belman, D., Monaco, K., and Brooks, T. (no date, 1998) *Let It Be Palletized: A Portrait of Truck Drivers' Work and Lives From the 1997 Survey of Truck Drivers.* Trucking Industry Program, University of Michigan.

Belzer, M. (1994) *Paying the Toll: Economic Deregulation of the Trucking Industry.* Washington, DC: Economic Policy Institute.

Belzer, M. (2000a) *Sweatshops on Wheels: Winners and Losers in Trucking Deregulation.* Oxford: Oxford University Press.

Belzer, M. (2000b) *The Relationship Between Pay and Safety: The Case of Truck Drivers.* Unpublished paper presented to Wayne State MAIR Faculty, 2 February. Trucking Industry Program, University of Michigan.

Belzer, M., Burks, S., Monaco, K., Fulton, G., Grimes, D., Lass, D., Ballou, D., and Sedo, S. (2000) *Hours of Service Impact Analysis: Benefit-Cost Analysis of Proposed HOS Changes.* Unpublished paper. Trucking Industry Program, University of Michigan.

Bousfield, G. (1996) EU Road Transport Safety Suffers as Companies Compete. *Safety and Health, 153*(1): 66-69.

Cairney, P. (1991) *Improving Truck Safety in Australia.* Special Report No. 46. Australian Road Research Board.

Carson, W. (1979) The Conventionalisation of Early Factory Crime. *International Journal of the Sociology of Law, 7*: 37-60.

Carson, W. (1989) Occupational Health and Safety: A Political Economy Perspective. *Labour and Industry, 2*(2): 301-316.

Corn, J. (1992) *Response to Occupational Health Hazards: A Historical Perspective.* New York: Van Nostrand Reinhold.

Coroners Court of New South Wales. (1990) *The adjourned hearing into the Inquest touching the deaths of David Keith Hutchins and nineteen others which occurred as the result of a collision between a semi-trailer and motor coach at Cowper, near Grafton, on 20 October 1989,* Coroners Court, Glebe, 20 April.

Coroners Court of New South Wales. (2003) *Supplement to the Findings into the Deaths of Barry Supple, Timothy Walsh and Anthony Forsyth,* Dorelle Pinch, Deputy State Coroner, 30 January.

Coroners Court of South Australia. (1999) *Finding of Inquest concerning the deaths of Susan Margeret Duffy, Walter Edward Duffy, Vida May Claxton, Christopher Verdun Claxton, Nita Claire Hastwell and Ivy Nell Hastwell on 3rd day of August 1996,* Coroners Court, Adelaide, 17 March.

Correspondence, John Grayson, General Manager of WorkCover to Tony Sheldon, Secretary of NSW Branch TWU, 24 February 2000 (copy included in NSW Branch, TWU submission to Long Haul Trucking Inquiry).

Croke, D. (1998) *1998 Road Transport Viability Report.* Monash Consultancy Services Ltd.

Derickson, A. (1998) *Black Lung: Anatomy of a Public Health Disaster.* Ithaca: Cornell University Press.

Engel, C. (1998, April) Competition Drives the Trucking Industry. *Monthly Labor Review,* 34-41.

Fischer, H. (1994) *Response to Disaster: Fact versus Fiction and Its Perpetuation— The Sociology of Disaster.* Lanham: University Press of America.

Frick, K. (2000) *Regional Safety Reps and the New Economy in Road Transport.* Paper presented to Working without Limits? Re-organising Work and Reconsidering Workers' Health TUTB-SALTSA Conference. Brussels, 25-27 September.

Golob, T., and Hensher, D. (1994) Driving Behaviour of Long Distance Truck Drivers: The Effects of Schedule Compliance on Drug Use and Speeding Citations. *Institute of Transportation Studies Working Paper.* ITS-WP-94-12.

Hamelin, P. (1987) Lorry Driver's Time Habits in Work and Their Involvement in Traffic Accidents. *Ergonomics, 30*(9): 1323-1333.

Hamelin, P. (2000) *The Working Time of Professional Drivers as a Factor of Flexibility and Competitiveness in Road Haulage and Passenger Transport.* Paper presented to Working Without Limits? Re-organising Work and Reconsidering Workers' Health TUTB-SALTSA Conference. Brussels, 25-27 September.

Hartley, L. (1999) *Patterns of Drug Use in the WA Road Transport Industry.* Murdoch University Western Australia.

Hensher, D., Fildes, B., Cameron, M., Parish, R., Taylor, D., and Digges, K. (1991) *Long Distance Truck Drivers on Road Performance and Economic Reward.* Federal Office of Road Safety, Canberra.

Hopkins, A. (1992) Trucking Deaths: A Suggestion. *Journal of Occupational Health and Safety—Australia and New Zealand, 8*(3): 243-249.

Hopkins, A. (1999) *Managing Major Hazards: The Lessons of the Moura Mine Disaster.* Sydney: Allen and Unwin.

House of Commons. Environment, Transport and Regional Affairs Committee (2000) *The Road Haulage Industry: Report together with Proceedings of the Committee and Minutes of Evidence Appendices taken before the Transport Sub-committee.*

House of Representatives Standing Committee on Communications, Transport and Arts. (2000) *Beyond the Midnight Oil: Managing Fatigue in Transport.* Commonwealth of Australia, Canberra.

James, C. (Mayhew). (1993) Self-Employed and Employee Transport Workers: Labour Process Determinants of Occupational Injury. *Labour and Industry, 5*(3): 75-89.

Jasanoff, S. (ed.). (1994) *Learning from Disaster: Risk Management After Bhopal.* Philadelphia: University of Pennsylvania Press.

Jeffress, C. (1999) *Building a Bridge between Trucking Industry Safety Practices and OSHA Safety and Health Program.* Speech to American Trucking Association, Executive Committee Winter Meeting, San Francisco, 16 February.

Kansas City Star, December 15-17, 2001.

Knestaut, A. (1997) Brief: Fatalities and Injuries Among Truck and Taxicab Drivers. *Compensation and Working Conditions, 2*(3).

May, T., Mills, G., and Scully, J. (1984) *National Road Freight Industry Inquiry.* Report of Inquiry to the Minister for Transport, Commonwealth of Australia, Canberra.

Mayhew, C., and Quinlan, M. (2001) Occupational Health and Safety Amongst 300 Long Distance Truck Drivers: Results of an Interview-Based Survey. Report prepared for Quinlan, M. (2001) *Report of Inquiry into Safety in the Long Haul Trucking Industry,* Motor Accidents Authority of New South Wales, Sydney.

Mayhew, C., and Quinlan, M. (2001a) Occupational Violence in the Long Distance Transport Industry: A Case Study of 300 Truck Drivers. *Current Issues in Criminal Justice, 13*(1): 36-46.

New Zealand Office of the Controller and Auditor General. (1996) *Transport Services Licensing Act 1989—The "Fit and Proper Person" Test*. Office of the Controller and Auditor General, Wellington.

New Zealand. (2000) *Ministerial Inquiry into Tranz Rail Occupational Safety and Health: Report to the Ministers of Labour and Transport*. Wellington, August.

NIOSH. (2000) *NIOSH Work Health Chartbook, 2000*. Washington, DC: U.S. Department of Health and Human Services.

NOHSC. (1992) *Strategies to Combat Fatigue in the Long Distance Road Transport Industry*. Federal Office of Road Safety, Canberra.

NOHSC. (1999) Submission to House of Representatives Standing Committee on Communications, Transport and the Arts Inquiry into Managing Fatigue in Transport.

O'Malley, P. (1996) Risk and Responsibility. In A. Barry, T. Osborne, and N. Rose (eds.), *Foucault and Political Reason: Liberalism, Neo-Liberalism and Rationalities of Government* (pp. 189-207). London: UCL Press.

Perrone, S. (2000) *When Life is Cheap: Governmental Responses to Work-Related Fatalities in Victoria 1987-1990*. Unpublished Ph.D. thesis. Department of Criminology, University of Melbourne.

Perrow, C. (1984) *Normal Accidents*. New York: Basic Books.

Pickmere, A. (2000) Heavy Metal, Big Damage. *New Zealand Herald*. 20 September, p. A13.

Quinlan, M. (2001) *Report of Inquiry into Safety in the Long Haul Trucking Industry*. Motor Accidents Authority of New South Wales, Sydney.

Quinlan, M. (2003) *Developing Strategies to Address OHS and Workers' Compensation Responsibilities Arising from Changing Employment Relationships*. Research Report Commissioned by WorkCover Authority of New South Wales, Sydney.

R v Brian Douglas Snewin, No. 1293/96 District Court of South Australia, Criminal Jurisdiction, Adelaide, Sentencing by Judge Lowrie, 31 January 1997.

Rosner, D., and Markowitz, G. (1994) *Deadly Dust: Silicosis and the Politics of Occupational Disease in Twentieth Century America*. Princeton: Princeton University Press.

Segerdahl, M. (2000) *Swedish Transport Union*. Personal Interview 10 January 2000.

Shrivastava, P. (1987) *Bhopal: Anatomy of a Crisis*. Cambridge: Ballinger Publishing.

Shrivastava, P. (1994) Societal Contradictions and Industrial Crises. In S. Jasanoff (ed.), *Learning from Disaster: Risk Management After Bhopal* (pp. 248-267). Philadelphia: University of Pennsylvania Press.

Stoop, J., and Thissen, W. (1997) Transport Safety: Trends and Challenges from a Systems Perspective. *Safety Science, 26*(½): 107-120.

Storey, W. Chair. (1996) *Report of the Transport Committee on the Inquiry into Truck Crashes*. New Zealand House of Representatives, Wellington.

Toscano, G. (1997) Brief: Dangerous Jobs. *Compensation and Working Conditions, 2*(2).

Toscano, G., and Windau, J. (1998) Profile of Fatal Work Injuries in 1996. *Compensation and Working Conditions*, 37-45.

Turner, B. (1976) The Organizational and Interorganizational Development of Disaster. *Administrative Science Quarterly, 21*: 378-397.

U.S. Department of Transportation. (2000) *US DOT Press Release*, 9 August 2000.

Victorian WorkCover Authority. (1999) *Recent Prosecutions*, VWA, Melbourne.

Williamson, A., Feyer, A., Friswell, R., and Saduri, S. (2000) *Driver Fatigue: A Survey of Professional Heavy Drivers in Australia.* Draft of Report Prepared for the National Road Transport Commission.

Windau, J., and Jack, T. (1996) Highway Fatalities Among the Leading Causes of Workplace Deaths. *Compensation and Working Conditions,* 57-61.

WorkCover NSW. (2004) *Draft amendment to the OHS Regulation 2001: Fatigue Management in the Long Distance Road Freight Industry* —Consultation Paper.

CHAPTER 3

The Australian Epidemic of Repetition Strain Injury: A Sociological Perspective

Andrew Hopkins

In the early 1980s Australia saw a rapid rise in reports of work-related upper limb disorders, largely among workers whose jobs involved repetitive hand movements. Although assembly line workers are most at risk in this respect, the greatest publicity was given to keyboard workers, among whom the problem seemed to occur in epidemic proportions. "Repetition strain injury" (RSI), as it was called, became a focus of media attention and professional concern, and the term "RSI" became a household expression. The epidemic reached its peak in 1985 and then slowly waned. By the end of the decade, although new cases continued to be reported, RSI was no longer a major issue in the public consciousness. One very concrete indicator of this rise and fall in public concern was the number of articles about RSI appearing in *The Canberra Times*, the daily newspaper in the national capital: 1 in 1982, 5 in 1983, 31 in 1984, 47 in 1985, 54 in 1986, 30 in 1987, 20 in 1988, and 11 in 1989 (Bammer 1990).

The causes of this extraordinary phenomenon have been hotly debated. The central point of contention in the debate concerned the nature of the condition: was it an injury, diagnosable and possibly treatable by conventional medicine, or was it a neurosis with no physical cause, susceptible only to psychiatric treatment?

RSI AS INJURY

The standard view was that RSI was an injury (Bammer and Martin 1992). This view was given authoritative expression in the much-cited article by Browne and co-workers in the *Medical Journal of Australia* in 1984:

> RSIs are . . . musculotendinous injuries of the upper limbs, shoulder girdles,
> and neck caused by overload of particular muscle groups from repeated use,
> or by the maintenance of constrained postures, which result in pain, fatigue
> and a decline in work performance. (p. 330)

Browne and colleagues acknowledged that there might be a psychological component: one of the factors they cited as possibly contributing to RSI was "increased muscle tension associated with mental stress." This psychological component may sometimes be relevant to an understanding of variations in individual susceptibility to the problem. Moreover, some work environments are systematically more stressful than others, leading to higher rates of injury (Hopkins 1990a). But it needs to be emphasized that acknowledging a psychological component is in no way inconsistent with the notion of RSI as a real injury.

The two major government reports on the matter, one by the Public Service Task Force on RSI and the other by the National Occupational Health and Safety Commission, both accepted the standard view of the problem. Indeed, the fact that the complaint was generally known in Australia as repetition strain *injury* and not, for example, as occupational neurosis, or as regional pain syndrome, as advocated by some medical authorities, is indicative of the dominance of the standard view.

The standard view naturally gave rise to an explanation of the epidemic in terms of changes in work practices. The rise of the problem coincided with the progressive introduction of word processing equipment in office environments and the deterioration of working conditions with which this was associated. Managers purchasing the new equipment assumed that it would lead to greater work output and consequently increased their expectations of keyboard operators and pushed them to work faster. At the same time, particularly in the public service, staff cutbacks were resulting in increased workloads for remaining staff. According to the injury theory the rise in RSI was directly attributable to these changes.

In response to the epidemic, the government promulgated guidelines placing limits on the speed of work and requiring regular rest breaks. Moreover, in many workplaces jobs were redesigned so that staff members were no longer classified as keyboard operators but as administrative assistants, with correspondingly broader duties. Finally, a great deal of attention was paid to ensuring that keyboard workers were provided with "ergonomically" designed furniture to facilitate correct posture. The decline in the epidemic corresponded with the implementation of these changes (Ellis 1988, p. 13). Indeed, this is the standard explanation of the decline in the problem of RSI in Australia (Emmett 1992, p. 303).

On the assumption that RSI is an injury, this explanation in terms of changing office technology and changing work practices fits the facts reasonably well. It does however leave certain questions unanswered, most importantly: why did similar epidemics not occur in other countries when the new word processing technology was introduced? Another unanswered question is, why is it that RSI among blue collar workers in Australia did not receive the same attention in the 1980s even though processes of technological change and employee cutbacks were increasing the pace of work in much the same way as was occurring in white collar work, in particular, public service white collar work?

RSI AS NEUROSIS

The most prominent competing explanation of the epidemic is based on the assumption that RSI is a form of neurosis. This view was energetically advocated by various psychiatrists and, surprisingly, by a number of orthopedic surgeons, who were of the view that if the symptoms of which patients complained were not detectable using conventional medical equipment then the pain could have no physical basis and must be psychological in origin.

According to one psychiatrist, RSI complainants suffered from unresolved psychological conflicts that might be work-related but might also originate in domestic or other areas of life. These conflicts were for some reason too painful to consciously acknowledge and were "converted" to acceptable symptoms with absolutely no physical basis. The choice of symptoms was determined by considerations of psychic or even financial reward (provided by the system of workers compensation which exists in Australia—see below):

> As long as compensation is paid for functional (i.e. non-physical) symptoms as if they were the result of a hypothetical 'injury', symptoms are rewarded and reinforced, and the epidemic will continue to spread . . . Control of this epidemic will require a complete withdrawal of the injury theory and its mythology and terminology. (Lucire 1986, p. 32)

This is close to a theory of straight out malingering, the major difference being that the latter assumes conscious motivation whereas the conversion neurosis theory presupposes unconscious processes. Certain orthopedic surgeons came even closer to accusing suffers of bad faith by diagnosing "compensation neurosis."

The theory of RSI as a conversion disorder provides an easy explanation for the epidemic nature of the problem, for the choice of symptoms is influenced by what people see going on around them. In a sense, RSI spread because it became fashionable. The theory accounts also for the fact that the epidemic appeared to be a purely Australian phenomenon: workers in other countries would not have been aware of what was happening in Australia and so could not have imitated their Australian counterparts.

Lucire goes further to suggest that RSI spread by a process of "hysterical contagion" (1986, p. 325) and that the epidemic of RSI was an epidemic of hysteria. Mullaly and Grigg (1988, p. 21) have shown, however, that RSI does not conform to other historical instances of epidemic hysteria, which are normally sudden in onset, building to a climax within a few weeks and abating just as quickly.

A further argument against the neurosis theory is that it has now been established that people who complain of RSI have physically detectable damage to their nerve pain pathways. This is evidence, in other words, that their pain is not "all in the mind" but has some real physiological basis (Helme, LeVasseur, and Gibson 1992).

The fact that, despite its many inadequacies, the neurosis theory achieved such prominence in Australia in itself deserves explanation. Legislation in every Australian state and territory requires employers to compensate their employees for work-related injuries and illness, particularly when these involve time off work. Furthermore, the law requires employers to take out insurance to cover this liability. The RSI epidemic thus cost employers and their insurers dearly, and in the mid 1980s, they began to contest compensation claims in courts and to argue that RSI was not work-related and, therefore, not compensable. They found it expedient to require long-term claimants to undergo examination by psychiatrists and other medical specialists who were known to be inclined to the view that RSI was a conversion neurosis. These specialists could then be called upon to expound their views in court. There is no doubt that this process resulted in these views gaining far more prominence than they would otherwise have had.

A SOCIOLOGICAL PERSPECTIVE

The neurosis theory is flawed in too many ways to be regarded as a satisfactory explanation. But in suggesting a connection with the compensation system and in raising the possibility that RSI might involve some element of fashion or contagion, it did point to the possibility that social factors might have influenced the epidemic in ways not encompassed by the injury theory. A sociological approach allows for the possibility both that the injuries of which sufferers complained were real and work-related, and that there were social processes at work, quite apart from the injury-producing processes, which contributed to the epidemic. Perhaps the most important insight to be derived from sociology in this matter is that regardless of the incidence of the underlying problem it is only socially recognized as an epidemic if it is observed and reported. The processes of observation and reporting are thus crucial in understanding the progress of an epidemic. As Willis observes, citing Figlio,

> [recognition of an epidemic depends on] the appearance of observers of the disease or injury who set in operation various medical, legal and administrative apparatuses to "cope" with the disease or injury. (Willis 1986, p. 212)

THE IMPORTANCE OF NAMING

Interestingly, one of the factors that facilitated the recognition of the problem of RSI was the name itself—"RSI." Tendonitis, tenosynovitis, bursitis, etc. had long been known in Australian compensation statistics. However, in the late 1970s, newly established workers' health centers began to use the term "tenosynovitis," or "teno" for short, to describe all the repetition injuries they were finding among their predominantly blue-collar clientele.

Subsequently, as reports of problems among keyboard workers began to appear, the term "repetition injury" emerged—for example, the Australian Public Service Association published a pamphlet with this title in 1980. Then, in 1982 the National Health and Medical Research Council put out guidelines on how to deal with "repetition strain injuries." The new term was legitimated by its use in article titles in the *Medical Journal of Australia* in 1983 and early 1984, and the term "RSI" quickly passed into widespread use, replacing all other terms. Newspaper headlines invariably spoke of RSI and such was the acceptance of the term that many doctors simply diagnosed RSI in cases of work-related upper limb disorders, rather than seeking a more precise medical diagnosis. Despite complaints in some quarters that RSI was a term unknown to medicine, it became a very concrete malady in the public mind. In short, the existence of a simple and universally used term in Australia facilitated the social recognition of the problem.

The significance of naming becomes more apparent if we contrast the situation in Australia with that in the United States, a country in which I did comparative research on the problem of RSI in the late 1980s and where at the time RSI appeared to be almost unheard of. The specialist literature in the United States had tended to employ the term *cumulative trauma disorder,* the meaning of which is far less clear to the general public than *repetition strain injury.* For this reason, newspaper articles that appeared in the United States sometimes confused the issue by using the term *repetitive motion injuries* in their headlines and then writing about *cumulative trauma disorders* in the text. The influential Bureau of National Affairs wrote about the problem under its Australian name of *repetition strain injury,* while the National Council on Compensation Insurance referred to *musculo-skeletal problems.*

But the matter was even more confused than this. In individual cases, the specific medical diagnosis was often *carpal tunnel syndrome* (nerve damage in the area of the wrist known as the carpal tunnel). As a result, a number of unions issued pamphlets describing carpal tunnel syndrome and sometimes the related problems of tendonitis and tenosynovitis.

Clearly, none of these more precise medical terms had the easy appeal of RSI. But more importantly, the absence of any consistently applied terminology in the United States hindered the widespread public recognition of the problem of injuries caused by repetitive motion.

WORKERS' COMPENSATION

The naming issue is really only a preliminary matter. The real power of the sociological approach is revealed when we turn to the question of recording and reporting. Let us consider what actual evidence there is that an RSI epidemic occurred. There are in fact no statistics on the incidence of occupational disease or injury in Australia. The only quantitative data we have on RSI is of incidence of compensation claims. These data show a dramatic increase in the early 1980s. For instance, in the five years from 1979 to 1984 the number of new cases of *musculo-skeletal* disease recorded in the NSW workers compensation statistics jumped from 980 to 4,550 per year, a nearly five-fold increase. This trend was apparent at the level of particular enterprises with many employers recording sharp increases in the number of RSI claims and—more importantly—sharp rises in their workers' compensation premiums. It was the premium increases more than anything that drew the attention of employers to the problem. Clearly, at least for some workers, it was relatively easy to get compensation for RSI during the early 1980s. Furthermore, the rising number of workers' compensation claims for RSI provided *objective* evidence of the epidemic. In turn, this evidence generated public concern and stimulated governments to take action, initially by conducting inquiries and then by promoting the changes in work practices discussed earlier.

It is useful to look in more detail at the situation of one particular group of workers, federal government employees, to understand the role of compensation in the social recognition of RSI. The Australian federal public service seemed in the mid 1980s to be the employer hardest hit by the problem of RSI. Indeed Canberra was sometimes labeled the RSI capital of Australia. The government— a Labor government—was very sensitive to the interests of its employees, and had issued the following instruction to claims officers dealing with federal employees:

> Claims for compensation because of RSI should generally be granted where a claim is supported by medical evidence from the treating doctor that the employee is unfit to work because of RSI and the [claims officer] considers that the condition is work-caused or work-related. *In most cases, where the employee has been engaged in work of a manual, repetitive nature and the treating doctor certifies the condition to be consistent with the stated cause, [a claims officer] can accept that the condition is work-caused or work-related.* (Emphasis added)[1]

The result of this policy was that compensation claims were accepted on the basis of certificates provided by the claimant's own doctor, which often simply stated that the claimant was suffering from RSI and needed a specified period off work. The system thus offered little resistance to those making claims.

Of course, making a claim was not without risk. Sufferers often had few if any signs of the problem they could show to others, which meant that they were vulnerable to accusations by workmates and bosses that they were fabricating symptoms. But they could see that many who had made claims had not on the whole been discriminated against and this encouraged them to come forward and claim compensation themselves, rather than continuing to suffer in silence. Here then was the element of contagion hypothesized by the neurosis theory.

The federal government went even further in generating evidence of the extent of the problem. It began a quarterly census of all staff "involved in any RSI-related action." This phrase was largely interpreted by those responsible for providing the information as meaning "being in receipt of compensation for RSI." Although medical certificates did not always specify the complaint as RSI, government departments seemed to be in no doubt about which were RSI cases and had little difficulty in providing the information required. The figures were published four times a year, providing much publicized evidence of the epidemic. According to this census, the numbers of new cases of RSI peaked in late 1985 and then began to decline steadily.

In order to emphasize the role of the compensation system in bringing the problem to light, it is useful to refer again to comparative research in the United States (Hopkins 1990b). As previously noted, RSI among keyboard operators was unrecognized in the United States when the Australian epidemic was occurring. This is in large part due to the fact that although workers' compensation systems operate in the United States, it was difficult if not impossible to get compensation for repetition strain injuries. In some states, such ailments were simply excluded by legislation from workers' compensation coverage on the grounds that they are "ordinary diseases of life" suffered by much of the population. Furthermore, in some states patients were required to go to doctors selected by the compensation authorities. Should they choose to go to their own doctor that doctor's report would not be recognized and the bill would not be paid. Doctors selected by the authorities were naturally cautious about concluding that the problem was work-related. Finally, where an employer contested a claim, as would often happen with RSI cases, the matter was decided in a formal hearing before a board or court, and claimants felt compelled to hire legal counsel. Even if the decision was in favor of the claimant the employer was free to appeal and was strongly motivated to do so, to avoid what could be a costly precedent. In all these circumstances it was clear that regardless of the number of people suffering from RSI, the number receiving workers' compensation would be negligible.

Let us focus specifically on the way in which federal employees were treated in the United States in order to draw comparisons with their Australian counterparts. Claims adjudicators for federal employees were instructed to deal with claims for "occupational stress or strain"—and this would have covered many RSI cases—as follows:

The claimants are prone to generalise in stating the basis of their claim, whereas there is a great need for specific allegations. In all cases, the claims examiner must be particularly careful to require detailed allegations of the claimant which are sufficiently specific.

The disabilities are not peculiarly of industrial origin. They may, *and in many cases do* (emphasis added), have their origin in the employee's structural makeup or personal life activities. In all cases, the claims examiner must be particularly careful to develop the facts about the prior medical and industrial history and possible causes in the employee's personal life and activities.[2]

The contrast between the extreme caution of the above statement and the liberal position of the Australian authorities could hardly be more striking. It is obvious that no matter how widespread the problem of RSI might have been among federal employees in the United States at the time of my research, it would have been largely invisible in the compensation statistics.

This comparison with the United States illuminates the particular role played by the compensation system in generating claims and hence statistics on RSI in Australia and in this way contributing to the social recognition of the problem.

A further comparison is germane to this discussion. The Australian epidemic was most apparent among white-collar workers, particularly in the public sector. This reflects the fact that the compensation system was far less encouraging of claims from manual workers. Manual workers in Australia are disproportionately from non-English-speaking backgrounds. Consequently, they are less able to lodge compensation claims. Moreover, the early 1980s was a period of high unemployment among manual workers and many feared, rightly or wrongly, that making a compensation claim might jeopardize their job. The result was that while RSI was known to be a problem among assembly line workers—many attended union-run workers' health centers for treatment—it did not generate corresponding numbers of compensation claims. In short, the fact that RSI seemed to be a problem afflicting keyboard operators in particular was at least in part an artefact of this differential tendency to make claims. Since compensation claims were really the only hard indicator of the problem, RSI among blue-collar workers remained relatively invisible.

Just as the compensation system in Australia contributed to the recognition of the problem of RSI among keyboard operators, it also contributed to its apparent decline. From about the mid 1980s onwards, employers and insurers alike began scrutinizing claims more carefully. No longer was RSI a sufficient diagnosis. Doctors were asked to be more specific. They were asked to indicate why they thought the problem was work-related and not simply the result of repetitive activity at home. And they were asked to say just what it was that employees could and could not do, so that an employer might have the option of providing alternative work to an injured employee. In cases where this was possible an employee might not need any time off work at all. Faced with this increasing scrutiny patients' own doctors were less inclined than formerly simply to accept the patient's word. Furthermore, compensation agencies were given responsibility for rehabilitation and became far more interested in the fate of employees who were off on compensation. Given this rather more interventionist approach, the numbers of workers suffering from RSI actually needing time away from work declined, and those who did need time off work found themselves returning to work sooner. Thus the decline in the number and duration of claims was in part attributable to changes in the way compensation policy was being administered. Put another way, even if the underlying incidence of the problem had remained unchanged, the compensation system would have recorded a drop in the incidence and cost of claims, thus contributing to the apparent decline of the problem.

The changes were particularly dramatic in the case of federal government employees. In 1988 an entirely new federal compensation and rehabilitation authority was established with a brief to intervene far more actively in the ways described above. Moreover in 1987, without explanation, the government ceased conducting its census of RSI among its own employees, thus eliminating the publicity about the problem generated by these figures. This significantly reduced the visibility of the problem in the public sector.

CONCLUSION

repetitive strain injury (RSI)

The sociological perspective that I have provided on the RSI epidemic is superior to both the straight injury account and the neurosis explanation provided earlier. It acknowledges both that RSI is an injury, as most authorities would agree, and that there are social processes, even an element of contagion, involved in the reporting of the phenomenon. This is yet another demonstration of the well-known sociological insight that statistics often tell us more about collection procedures than they do about the phenomena they are supposed to reflect. To give a rather different example, an increase in arrests for a particular offense may be the outcome of an administrative decision to focus police resources on the behavior in question, rather than an indication of any real increase in the incidence of the offense in question.

The rise and demise of the RSI problem in Australia had a great deal to do with the fact that the statistics on RSI are in fact statistics of compensation claims and that the number of claims is very sensitive to the way in which the compensation system operates. This is not to deny that there was a real increase in the underlying incidence of the problem in the first half of the 1980s and a real decline in the second half of the decade. There is a great deal of anecdotal evidence to suggest that such changes in fact occurred. Moreover, sociology can tell us much about the processes that produced these injuries—technological change, the organization of work, and so on. But the reporting of the phenomenon is itself a variable process, subject to social influences, with the result that it cannot always be assumed that changes in reported rates necessarily bear any relationship to the phenomenon of interest. In particular, the fact that the numbers of claims for RSI are now low in Australia should not be taken as indicating that the problem has been resolved. Anecdotal evidence suggests that RSI remains a problem, particularly among certain groups of blue-collar workers who are frightened to make claims for fear of losing their jobs (Hopkins 1995). In such situations the absence of claims reflects not the absence of the problem but its suppression. Moreover, RSI sufferers' groups continue to function and large organizations continue to report new cases. What this analysis suggests is that while the true incidence work-related upper limb disorders may rise and fall over time there are also social processes at work which render the problem visible or invisible at various times. Those who wish to understand an apparent change in the extent of such disorders must understand that the appearance of change may reflect both change in the real incidence of the problem and, independently, change in the way it is reported and socially recognized.

ENDNOTES

1. Unpublished document provided to author.
2. Unpublished document provided to author.

REFERENCES

Bammer, G. (1990) *Occupational Disease and Social Struggle: The Case of Work-Related Neck and Upper Limb Disorders.* (Working paper #20). Australian National University: National Centre for Epidemiology and Population Health.

Bammer, G., and Martin, B. (1992) Repetition Strain Injury in Australia: Medical Knowledge, Social Movement, and Defacto Partisanship. *Social Problems, 39*(3): 219-237.

Browne, C., Nolan, B., and Faithful, D. (1984) Occupational Repetition Strain Injuries. *Medical Journal of Australia, 140*: 329-332.

Ellis, N. (1988, June) Occupational Overuse Syndrome. *Patient Management, 133.*

Emmett, E. A. (1992) New Directions for Occupational Health and Safety in Australia. *Journal of Occupational Health and Safety—Australia and New Zealand, 8*(4): 293-308.

Helme, R., LeVasseur, S., and Gibson, S. (1992) RSI Revisited: Evidence for Psychological and Physiological Differences from an Age, Sex and Occupation Matched Control Group. *ANZ Journal of Medicine, 22*: 23-29.

Hopkins, A. (1989) The Social Construction of Repetition Strain Injury. *Australian and New Zealand Journal of Sociology, 25*(2): 239-259.

Hopkins, A. (1990a) Stress, the Quality of Life and Repetition Strain Injury in Australia. *Work and Stress, 4*(2): 129-138.

Hopkins, A. (1990b) The Social Recognition of Repetition Strain Injuries: An Australian/American Comparison. *Social Science and Medicine, 30*(3): 365-372.

Hopkins, A. (1995) *Making Safety Work: Getting Management Commitment to Occupational Health and Safety*. Sydney: Allen and Unwin.

Lucire, Y. (1986) Neurosis in the Workplace. *Medical Journal of Australia, 145*: 323-327.

Mullaly, J., and Grigg, L. (1988) RSI: Integrating the Major Theories. *Australian Journal of Psychology, 40*: 19-33.

Willis, E. (1986) Commentary: RSI as a Social Process. *Community Health Studies, 10*: 210-219.

CHAPTER 4

"All Part of the Game":
The Recognition of and Response to
an Industrial Disaster at the
Fluorspar Mines, St. Lawrence,
Newfoundland, 1933-1978

Richard Rennie

In 1933, a New York entrepreneur offered the people of St. Lawrence, a remote community on the south coast of the island of Newfoundland, an opportunity to escape the economic hardship that accompanied the Great Depression and the recent collapse of the cod fishery by establishing an industry to mine the veins of fluorspar buried in the barren hills around the town. Over the ensuing years, many men from St. Lawrence and neighboring communities were lured to work in the mines by the promise of a steady paycheck. Fifty years after the first mine was opened, nearly 200 of them were dead from industrial diseases such as lung cancer and silicosis.

While in the sheer number of victims indicates that what transpired at St. Lawrence was undeniably an industrial disaster, the process by which it was recognized as such was in fact long and convoluted, spanning several decades of controversy and struggle. In fact, for more than two decades, until official confirmation of the cause and extent of the tragedy began to emerge during a pivotal period in the late 1950s and early 1960s, this disaster garnered little notice from either authorities or the general public despite the efforts of the miners' union and others to draw attention to the mounting toll of disease and death. Furthermore, even as the toll steadily mounted and further understanding of the cause and extent of the tragedy emerged throughout the 1960s, it tended to attract attention only as a result of lobbying efforts on the part of the union or community activists, or in the context of such events as industrial accidents and the 1967 appointment of a Royal Commission to study the situation.

The response to that Royal Commission, which tabled its final report in 1969, became the catalyst that drew provincial and national attention to the

St. Lawrence disaster, bringing into sharp relief what Bayer describes as the polarization of the "minimalist" and the "maximalist" positions, so often a feature of disasters involving industrial disease, and a constant source of controversy in the case of St. Lawrence. The minimalist position (usually adopted by government and industry) attempts to limit as much as possible the recognition of diseases as industry related, while the maximalist position (usually adopted by unions and activists) attempts to extend that recognition as much as possible (Bayer 1988, p. 7). In the case of St. Lawrence, this dispute was central to the question of who would qualify for workers' compensation benefits, and became particularly intense in the wake of the Royal Commission, fueling political squabbling, labor unrest, and public protests throughout the 1970s, and thus generating widespread recognition of the St. Lawrence tragedy.

Fluorspar is used in the production of steel, aluminum, and glass, and while the deposits around St. Lawrence were known about as far back as the 1870s, they did not attract commercial attention until the 1920s, when world demand for the mineral sharply increased (Fellman 1926; Murray and Howley 1881, p. 235). The first mines were established by the St. Lawrence Corporation of Newfoundland, incorporated and owned by New York entrepreneur Walter Seibert (Farrell 1983, pp. 70-71; Howse and Fischer 1939; Martin 1985, pp. 66-67). In 1939, a second company entered the St. Lawrence mining industry when the Aluminum Company of Canada (Alcan) established a subsidiary, Newfoundland Fluorspar Limited (Newfluor), to supply fluorspar to its aluminum smelter at Arvida, Quebec. By the early 1940s, there were over 500 men from St. Lawrence and neighboring communities employed at several mines around the town (Newfoundland 1942, p. 2).

While the mines generated much-needed employment and brought a certain degree of prosperity to the community, especially during the industry expansion associated with the Second World War, they also brought a host of health hazards. The air in the shafts, some of which were nearly 1,000 feet deep by the 1940s, was thick with dust and smoke. There was no ventilation of any kind and workers had nothing in the way of basic facilities such as protective clothing and clean drinking water (Slaney 1975, pp. 14-15).

The legislative regime provided no protection from such hazards. The Commission of Government, an unelected body of bureaucrats and colonial administrators that had taken over the affairs of Newfoundland in 1934 in response to the economic and political crisis that had gripped the colony (Neary 1988, pp. 44-52; Overton 1990), was loath to do anything that might jeopardize industry and threaten jobs. It refused to update the obsolete mines regulations and inspection regime that had been introduced in 1908, despite being urged to do so on several occasions by mines inspectors brought in from Ontario.[1]

Less than a decade after the start of mining, workers were convinced that conditions at the mines were beginning to damage their health. Shortly after forming the St. Lawrence Workers' Protective Union (SLWPU) in 1941, for instance, workers complained to a government tribunal appointed to investigate a labor dispute that dust in the mines was beginning to affect their lungs, and asked to be x-rayed. The town had no medical facilities to carry out such tests and the nearest hospital was about 20 kilometers away, a trip that could only be made on foot, by boat, or by horse and sled. The tribunal did not recommend any action be taken on the workers' request, but wanted to "place the Union's wishes on record, as they were expressed very strongly" (Newfoundland 1942, pp. 49-51).

Throughout the 1940s, indifference on the part of the government and the employers, geographic isolation, and the absence of medical facilities in the community continued to play a role in the lack of understanding about the health impacts of conditions at the mines, though it was increasingly obvious that there was a problem. For instance, in the context of an industry slump and associated layoffs in 1948, the local Public Relief Officer made the unexplained but highly suggestive observation that in assessing the eligibility of relief applicants, "it is questionable that some applicants are really able-bodied but there is no way for them to secure medical certificates."[2] One resident recalled that during the late 1940s, "We knew men were dying, but we didn't know what they were dying from" (Ed Ryan, personal interview, February 7, 2000).[3]

The exact connection between working conditions and respiratory ailments began to become clearer in 1950, but was complicated by the co-existence of tuberculosis, which was still rampant in Newfoundland at this time. In 1950, Dr. J. J. Pepper, one of a number of itinerant doctors who had come to the community over the years, and who had set up practice in a recently constructed makeshift clinic, became alarmed after viewing lung x-rays of a St. Lawrence miner taken by a traveling health clinic that visited isolated communities as part of the government's anti-tuberculosis campaign. Pepper believed that while the man had tuberculosis, he also had silicosis (Aylward 1969, p. 34), an incurable respiratory disease caused by the inhalation of fine dust, which can be created by the grinding or drilling of hard rock such as the granite that surrounded the St. Lawrence fluorspar veins (Gibbs and Pintus 1978, pp. 76-78). Pepper sent the x-rays to a colleague in Ottawa, who agreed with his diagnosis. Pepper suspected that several other miners and former miners were also silicotic (Aylward 1969, p. 34).

The co-existence of multiple ailments, sometimes related to each other in complex ways, is a common impediment to readily identifying diseases as work-related (Ison 1978, p. 2). Tuberculosis was a common culprit in this regard, often creating confusion about the connection between lung ailments and working conditions, as it did among miners in the United States and in Great Britain during the early 20th century (Bryder 1985, pp. 108-109; Derickson 1988, p. 39). Tuberculosis and silicosis are not entirely separate conditions, however, as a definite pathological connection between the two was well established by the early 20th century. It had been recognized that silicosis reduces the capacity of the respiratory system to combat the effects of tuberculosis-causing germs, and in fact the term "silico-tuberculosis" had evolved to describe the resulting condition (Raffle 1994, pp. 423-424; Rosen 1943, pp. 125-128; Rosner and Markowitz 1992, pp. 15-38; Schepers 1964).

This explains the issue that perplexed people in St. Lawrence in the early 1950s: St. Lawrence miners seemed to have not only a higher incidence of tuberculosis, but also a lower rate of recovery from the disease compared to others who received similar treatment at a sanitorium 400 kilometers away in St. John's. One St. Lawrence resident recalled that St. Lawrence miners released from the sanitorium "had come home and died, while men from other places treated for TB were recovering" (Ed Ryan, personal interview, February 7, 2000). The situation began to become clearer when the man whose x-rays had initially alarmed Pepper in 1950 died in December 1952, at the age of 46 after spending considerable time at the sanitorium. Pepper sent a lung sample he obtained from the corpse to an expert in the United States, who confirmed that it was silicotic (Harry Spencer, personal interview, October 13, 2000).

The evidence that a serious work-related health problem existed among St. Lawrence miners emerged just as the political and legislative regime was undergoing a major transformation as a result of Newfoundland having joined the Canadian Confederation in 1949. One legislative development that had direct implications for the St. Lawrence situation was the introduction of a new workers' compensation regime. The new *Workmen's*[4] *Compensation Act,* which became law on 31 March 1951, replaced a law passed in 1908 based on the British model in effect at that time, under which employers could pay compensation directly to injured workers (or in the case of death, their dependents) through a private arrangement or a court settlement (Newfoundland 1909). In Newfoundland, the majority of the very few claims ever made under this system were settled "to the detriment of the worker" (Fogwill 1950, pp. 2-3). The 1951 Act was, like those which had been adopted by other Canadian provinces over the first half of the 20th century, a collective, compulsory system under which employers paid premiums which were then used to compensate disabled workers or the dependents of deceased workers. For several reasons, however, the application of the new Act in the St. Lawrence case was far from straightforward. Because the Newfoundland Act, like those in other Canadian jurisdictions, treated illnesses the same way as accidents, it considered the time of disablement to be the time at which the worker ceased employment, rather than the time the illness developed or was diagnosed. Therefore, the Act did not apply to those cases where the worker had ceased employment before the Act came into effect, on 31 March 1951.

In addition to potential complications resulting from the inapplicability of the Act in many cases, and the possibility of each claimant having to pursue legal action outside the Act, there were also problems arising from the co-existence of tuberculosis. A survey conducted in 1954 showed that the incidence of tuberculosis among the general population in St. Lawrence was twice that of nearby fishing communities.[5] How to deal with cases where more than one condition existed simultaneously, but only one was covered by the Act, was a pressing problem for the Workmen's Compensation Board (WCB), since determining the amount of the benefit due to a disabled worker depended on the degree of disability that could be shown to be work-related. Similarly, while compensation would be paid in cases where it could be shown that a worker had died from a compensable illness, the coexistence of two illnesses made such a determination difficult. As the Chairman of the WCB remarked to St. Lawrence Corporation manger Donald Poynter in 1954, "The whole silicosis thing is very complicated from the legal standpoint."[6]

Another factor that complicated the government's decision about how best to approach the problem was the potential impact of industrial disease and any response to it upon the industry and the employment situation. Officials of the WCB, the Department of Mines, and the Department of Health and Welfare were concerned that "the welfare of the residents . . . be weighed against the possible financial liability of the mine owners should silicosis become prevalent to the point where heavy compensation is necessary."[7] Concern over possible job losses at St. Lawrence also influenced the government's decision to not introduce pre-employment screening and annual chest x-rays for applicants and employees in underground mines, as had been suggested by the Ontario Department of Health.[8]

While authorities did little to assist in such matters as detecting industrial disease, the community finally got a hospital, though not through any effort or concern on the part of the government or mine operators. The hospital, opened in 1954, was a gift from the United States government in gratitude for the efforts of people in St. Lawrence and neighboring communities in rescuing men from two naval vessels that had run aground near the community in 1942 (Brown 1979).

Lacking a clear course of action on how best to approach the industrial disease question at St. Lawrence, the government apparently chose to do nothing. The extent of the bureaucratic delay that marked the government's handling of the issue is indicated by the fact that in February 1957, the Chief Inspector of Mines reminded the Deputy Minister of Health and the Chairman of the WCB of a three-phase plan that had been formulated in 1953, and informed them that phase two, a meeting with mine operators to discuss the possibility of establishing a system for screening applicants and employees, had now been completed—four years after the plan was adopted.[9]

At a meeting held to discuss this issue in February 1957, the management of both Newfluor and the St. Lawrence Corporation suggested that annual examinations were unnecessary and that workers found to be suffering from a respiratory disease should simply be taken off the job by a physician. In an obvious attempt to prevent mass disqualifications among St. Lawrence miners and to allow workers with silicosis to remain on the job, the Department of Mines suggested that only tuberculosis be used grounds for disqualification from continued employment.[10] The proposed changes did not get past the dis-cussion stage at this point, and the matter was again dropped.

Shortly after abandoning the most recent proposals for medical screening, the government brought in J. P. Windish, an industrial hygienist from the Occupational Health and Safety Division of the federal Department of National Health and Welfare, to conduct dust surveys at St. Lawrence. Like much else about the St. Lawrence situation, this move grew out of a long and convoluted course of bureaucratic stonewalling. After concluding in 1950 that miners were developing silicosis, Dr. J. J. Pepper had written the Department of National Health and Welfare asking for help in investigating the possibility of industrial disease among St. Lawrence miners. He had been told that the federal department would act on such a request only if put to it by the provincial Department of Health. Six years later, the same request was made by the provincial Department of Mines, and the same answer received. The provincial Department of Mines then asked the provincial Department of Health to request the survey, and the federal Department complied (Aylward 1969, p. 34).

The 1957 study confirmed dust levels up to 700 times the allowable limit throughout Newfluor's "Director" mine, which Windish attributed to substandard equipment and inadequate ventilation (Windish, Sanderson, and Newfoundland Fluorspar Limited 1958). The survey was carried out only at Newfluor's operations, since the St. Lawrence Corporation had—conveniently—shut down most of its operations shortly before Windish's visit, when a supply contract with the U.S. government ended.

In addition to helping further explain the link between the workplace environment and respiratory ailments, the results of the 1957 dust study revealed the complete ineffectiveness of the new legislative regime that had been introduced in 1951 to govern health and safety in mines. The 1951 regulations required, among other things, ventilation sufficient to remove dust and other harmful impurities from underground air and to ensure an adequate flow of oxygen (Newfoundland 1952). These standards were to have been enforced by the Inspection Division of the provincial Department of Mines, but the 1957 dust study revealed that this was far from the case.

The results of the dust study prompted the government to finally introduce legislation regarding medical screening, but of a very attenuated nature. A regulation drafted in September 1959 and due to come into effect on 1 April 1960 required that all applicants for employment in dust-exposure occupations, which included underground mining and any surface work involving the crushing or grinding of rock, undergo an examination by a designated Medical Examiner to ensure that they were free from "active disease of the respiratory organs," had no known history of active tuberculosis, and were otherwise fit for the job. To keep a certificate in good standing, the holder was required to undergo an annual examination. No certificate was required for those already employed underground when the legislation came into effect, or for anyone continuously employed underground in a dust exposure operation after that date (Newfoundland 1959, September 29). In other words, only job applicants who had not been employed in a dust exposure occupation at some point after 1 April 1960 were subject to the regulation, a restriction no doubt designed to prevent many disqualifications among St. Lawrence miners, but which did little to assist in assessing the full extent of the industrial disease problem.

While the 1957 survey provided yet more evidence of the link between dust and respiratory ailments, and brought some limited legislative change, it did not explain another, even more disturbing phenomenon: an abnormally high rate of lung cancer among the mining population. SLWPU president Aloysius Turpin indicated growing local awareness of this problem when he told the chairman of a cancer convention being held in St. John's in January 1958 that "a large number of our miners died with Cancer and Silicosis."[11]

By June 1958, government authorities had also become concerned about a possible cancer problem in the community. The province's Deputy Minister of Health, Leonard Miller, contacted federal health authorities and Alcan's Chief Industrial Medical Officer, Frank Brent, informing them that "an altogether disproportionate number of deaths from carcinoma of the lung have emanated from the town of St. Lawrence" and requesting any information or advice they could offer.[12]

Neither Brent nor federal authorities could offer an explanation, since there seemed to be no obvious connection between cancer and the mining of fluorspar, which was not known to be radioactive. Brent was eager to note, however, that although some of the men so far believed to have died from lung cancer had worked for Newfluor, all of them had also worked for the St. Lawrence Corporation at some point.[13] Already, the corporate interests were moving to limit their liability for the unfolding disaster.

In response to the growing concern about lung cancer and the union's demand for an investigation, in 1959 the provincial Department of Health brought Windish back to St. Lawrence to search for a possible link between cancer and working conditions. While obviously relieved that officials planned to investigate the issue, the union pointed out that since it had begun trying to draw attention to industrial diseases more than 20 years previous, a disaster had been unfolding virtually unnoticed by authorities and the general public.

Assuming that the source of lung cancer was some form of radiation, Windish conducted tests for radiation that revealed concentrations of the radioactive gas radon-222 as well as "radon daughters" created by radioactive decay of R-222 well in excess of the Safe Working Level (SWL) in nearly every area of Director mine (Windish 1960, pp. 1-2). While many areas of the St. Lawrence Corporation's main mines had by now been rendered inaccessible by disuse and flooding, the accessible sections of those mines, as well as some small-scale shafts the company had re-activated, were tested and also found to contain deadly levels of radiation.[14]

Since there was no uranium within the mines, and tests did not indicate any radioactivity in the fluorspar itself, the radon gas was assumed to have originated in a source outside the mines and then been carried into the mines in the groundwater—the same water miners had been forced for years to drink—in which R-222 is highly soluble (Windish 1960, p. 23). The main health hazard arising from the radiation arose from the fact that the solid radon daughters created by the decay of R-222 became attached to dust or to condensation in the air and were deposited on the lungs when inhaled, and often eventually led to lung cancer (Windish 1960, pp. 12-13). Windish concluded that inadequate ventilation was the primary reason for the build-up of radon gas to lethal levels. (Windish 1960, p. 13).

Revelations regarding the presence of radiation and its link to cancer among workers had several immediate repercussions. First, the union pulled all underground workers (84 from Newfluor and 22 from the St. Lawrence Corporation) off the job, agreeing only to allow some men to enter the underground on a rotating basis to install ventilation equipment (Miners back request, 1960, March 11).

Secondly, the media took an unprecedented interest in the St. Lawrence situation. St. John's newspapers, for example, were soon reporting that workers had been unwittingly exposed to radiation up to 200 times the permissible level and that an average of three St. Lawrence miners had died of cancer each year since 1948 (Government officials, 1960, March 2, and Miners get more cancer, 1960, March 2). The national media also picked up the story at this point, with the *Financial Post* running a piece on cancer among St. Lawrence miners, though it shied away from drawing a definitive link to radiation in the mines (McArthur 1960, March 12).

Thirdly, company officials moved to exercise control over the flow of information to the public, to limit corporate liability, and to in effect normalize the situation. For instance, immediately after the revelations concerning radiation were made public, Alcan's Chief Medical Officer, Frank Brent, contacted provincial Health Minister James McGrath seeking confirmation that McGrath had earlier agreed that should he be called upon to make a public statement, he would "advise [the company] in advance of the situation and of [your] proposed statement."[15] Brent also sought agreement from McGrath that there was no "proof positive" of a link between cancer and working conditions at St. Lawrence. The fact that a physician employed by a private corporation and the province's highest-ranking public health official were discussing such arrangements privately is indicative of the kind of actions that had inhibited an adequate investigation of the St. Lawrence situation. Newfluor manager R. Wiseman, meanwhile, attributed much of the fear and negativity associated with the situation to "distortion of the facts by the press" (*St. John's Daily News,* Radiation picture, 1960, March 18).

As for the St. Lawrence Corporation, one of its supervisors, Theo Etchegary, who was also the mayor of the town, stated publicly "the men knew all along this condition existed and considered it an ordinary hazard of mining" (*St. John's Evening Telegram,* Miners wait and see, 1960, March 3). Despite the fact that this statement defied all evidence and reason, St. Lawrence Corporation Mine

Captain Murdock Judson supported it, claiming that the men knew that such hazards were "all part of the game" (*St. John's Evening Telegram,* Miners wait and see, 1960, March 3). Furthermore, representatives of the St. Lawrence Corporation continued to insist that there was no conclusive proof that radiation in the mines was linked to cancer deaths among miners (Miners stay out, 1960, March 24). Amazingly, St. Lawrence Corporation manger Donald Poynter continued to blame illness and death among miners on tuberculosis.[16]

About a month after the revelations regarding radiation, both companies had reportedly installed ventilation equipment (*St. John's Evening Telegram,* Ventilation system, 1960, April 1) and Windish confirmed that the radiation had been reduced to safe levels.[17] Underground workers then began returning to their regular duties.

As it turned out, the controversy that followed disclosure of the results of the radiation survey coincided with the date of the coming into effect of the legislation regarding medical screening of applicants—1 April 1960. Anticipating a problem hiring recruits once the amendment came into effect, on 25 March Wiseman asked the provincial Department of Health to designate a Medical Examiner at St. Lawrence to fulfill the requirements of the legislation.[18] With a swiftness that bore a striking contrast to its dilatory response to requests from the union and others for attention and action over the years, a few days later the Department appointed Dr. Cyril Walsh, resident physician at St. Lawrence, as Medical Examiner as of 31 March.[19] To further accommodate the employers' need to hire and retain men unimpeded by the requirements for medical screening, on 29 March the regulation was amended so that now no certificate was required for anyone *employed* in a dust exposure occupation *before* the regulation came into effect on 1 April, or anyone *not employed* in a dust exposure occupation *since* the Regulation came into effect. The only group for whom the certificate was now required, therefore, was applicants who had worked in a dust exposure occupation at some point after April 1960 (Newfoundland 1960, March 29).

By the time dust and radiation surveys had confirmed the presence of lethal contaminants in the St. Lawrence mines, they had already exacted a heavy toll. A study undertaken in response to the discovery of radiation in 1960 confirmed that lung cancer among St. Lawrence miners was nearly 29 times the provincial average. Between 1933 and 1960, 26 miners had died from lung cancer and 17 from other types of cancer, 22 from silicosis and/or tuberculosis, and over 30 from conditions unknown because of a lack of medical information. The average age of death for lung cancer victims among the mining population up to that point was 46.8 years, the youngest being just 33 years old. In addition, because the average time from first exposure to death was 19.1 years, many others would undoubtedly develop cancer in the future (de Villiers and Windish 1964). In terms of such characteristics as mortality rates and average age at death, the St. Lawrence disaster was worse than even some of the most notorious cases known up to that time, including the lung cancer among uranium miners in

Germany, Czechoslovakia, and South Africa (de Villiers and Windish 1964; Thompkins 1944).

In the wake of confirmation of the toll that working conditions had taken and would continue to take, attention switched to the issue of compensation for victims and their families, and the ensuing controversy fueled the dispute over the true dimensions of the problem. Restrictions on the applicability of the *Workers' Compensation Act* meant that, of the many St. Lawrence miners who had been afflicted by various diseases up until 1960, only six cases had ever been awarded compensation benefits, all for silicosis (Workmen's Compensation Board of Newfoundland 1953-1960). As a direct response to the St. Lawrence situation, the Act was amended in July 1960 to make "carcinoma or malignant disease arising from radiation" a compensable illness (Newfoundland 1961).

While the 1960 amendment extended coverage to some cases that were previously excluded, the WCB continued to deny coverage to many potential claimants because the Act still did not apply to cases where the victim had left employment before the Act had come into effect in 1951. Claims were also denied because of other limitations on how the Act was applied. For instance, though the 1960 amendment made "carcinoma or malignant disease" compensable, the Act was applied so that in the St. Lawrence case this was limited to lung cancer. Claims for other types of cancer were not recognized, nor were claims for respiratory diseases other than silicosis. Claims were also rejected because of an inability to determine conclusively the relationship between working conditions and various ailments.

Throughout the early 1960s, the SLWPU continued to lobby for increased recognition of diseases as work-related and therefore compensable. In 1963, the union moved to strengthen its hand by affiliating with a larger organization, the Quebec-based Confederation of National Trade Unions (CNTU), making it one of the very few unions outside of Quebec to ever do so. The decision to seek such an affiliation was likely based on the fact that on several occasions during the late 1950s and early 1960s, the drawbacks of being a small, independent organization had been made apparent. For instance, the SLWPU had no strike fund to support workers during the wildcat strike of 1960 and several shorter job actions thereafter, and when the union had learned of radiation in the mines in 1960, it had contacted the International Union of Mine, Mill and Smelter Workers seeking information on the hazard. The decision to affiliate with the CNTU in particular was likely motivated by the fact that the CNTU represented workers at many Alcan operations in Quebec, including the Arvida smelter to which the St. Lawrence fluorspar was shipped and where, the SLWPU had learned in 1959, workers were paid considerably more than workers at St. Lawrence.

While the victims and their families coped daily with the impacts of industrial disease and the lack of compensation coverage, the issue only began to draw wider attention in 1965, when it was raised before a committee appointed to review the

Workmen's Compensation Act. The Review Committee received a submission which it described as so "extraordinary and startling" as to require immediate attention (Winter 1966, p. 42). It came from St. Lawrence resident Rennie Slaney, a former miner, supervisor, and clerk with the Corporation for many years, who later worked with Municipal Council before retiring in 1965. Slaney had also been present at the autopsy Dr. Pepper had performed in 1952.

Slaney's brief described working conditions from the start of mining in St. Lawrence and the impact of industrial disease on miners and their families. The submission included a list of names of 84 dead miners, more than 70 of whom, Slaney claimed, had died from lung cancer and various respiratory diseases. Slaney claimed that in only about 25 of these cases had dependents received any compensation. He also listed thirteen cases of former miners living but too sick from cancer and respiratory diseases to work, only six of whom were being compensated (Winter 1966, pp. 42-43).

Information that the Review Committee requested from the WCB in an effort to corroborate Slaney's claims, however, indicated that the first death from industrial disease associated with the St. Lawrence mines occurred in 1952, and that from then until 1965 there were 34 deaths from lung cancer in St. Lawrence miners, as well as 4 deaths from silicosis/tuberculosis. In addition, the WCB's records showed just 7 cases of silicotic miners still living, with varying degrees of disability (Winter 1966, p. 50). Regarding the discrepancy between Slaney's figures and those provided by the WCB, the Review Committee concluded that the explanation was a simple one: many cases, especially in the pre-1951 period, simply had not been compensated and therefore had not been counted. The Review Committee concluded, therefore, that the figures provided by Slaney were "much nearer the truly ghastly total" than those in the WCB's files (Winter 1966, p. 51).

Slaney's submission highlights the vital role that the history of a community and the demographic traits of a workforce can play in shaping the recognition of industrial disasters. One of the oldest settlements on the island of Newfoundland, by the early 20th century St. Lawrence had a population of nearly 1,000 people, mostly the descendants of Irish and English settlers who had come there to work in the cod fishery. That Slaney was able to keep such close track of victims over the years illustrates the importance of the fact that, because St. Lawrence was an old, established community when the mining industry was founded, and because the vast majority of the workforce was drawn from the local population, the situation was not marked by the high labor turnover and workforce migration characteristic of other resource communities. Thus, the impacts of work upon health were easier to monitor, since workers tended to stay in or near the community after becoming ill and/or leaving work. In addition, because they were local men, most workers tended not to move frequently from one mining community to another and worked only in the St. Lawrence mines, which removed much of the uncertainty that arises when workers develop illnesses after working in many different places and environments (Burke 1985; Derickson 1998).

The wide variation between Slaney's figures and those supplied by the WCB also points to the danger in using workers' compensation statistics as a source of information about industrial diseases, and to the necessity of bearing in mind the distinction between actual diseases and *recognized* diseases. The St. Lawrence case is a clear illustration of the fact that workers' compensation statistics can conceal more than they reveal, and often represent, as Weindling puts it, "only the tip of the submerged mass of illness" (1985, p. 11). Such statistics must be understood as having been produced within certain parameters and for certain ends, the gathering of knowledge about industrial disease not necessarily among them (Müller 1985, p. 134). Calling the situation at St. Lawrence a "national disaster" (Tragedy, *St. John's Evening Telegram*, March 31, 1967), the Review Committee recommended that an inquiry be held to investigate the situation "in the utmost detail" and to uncover not only the medical and scientific aspects of the case but also "the sociological and human side" (Winter 1966, p. 51). The decisive conclusions and recommendations of the Review Committee forced the government to finally undertake a detailed study of the St. Lawrence situation. In March 1967, the government appointed a Royal Commission to investigate and make recommendations upon radiation, compensation, and safety at the St. Lawrence mines.

While public and media interest had quickly faded after the initial flurry generated by the revelations about radiation and cancer in 1960, the conclusions of the Workmen's Compensation Review Committee and the subsequent establishment of the Royal Commission rekindled attention on the St. Lawrence situation and touched off yet another public relations skirmish. The story even briefly regained national notice, with articles appearing in such popular magazines as *Maclean's* and the *Star Weekly* (Adams 1967; Bernard 1967).

Government authorities moved quickly to counter this most recent flood of negative press, and objected strenuously to the Review Committee's description of the St. Lawrence situation as a "national disaster." A Department of Health official pointed to the Review Committee's use of this phrase as an example of how the situation had been "blown out of proportion" (Tragedy, *St. John's Evening Telegram*, March 31, 1967), while Newfoundland Premier Joseph Smallwood himself criticized the media's coverage of the issue as "greatly exaggerated," and dismissed much of it as "history."[20] The company took similar measures. Shortly after establishment of the Royal Commission, for instance, Wiseman issued a press release to present what was, in his view, a more balanced view of the situation. By his account, the publicity given the St. Lawrence situation had been "very much one-sided, with the grim side of the picture being highlighted and exaggerated, and the brighter side of the picture being entirely eliminated,"[21] with the result that the general public, especially outside the St. Lawrence area, had been "grossly misinformed"[22] about the dimensions of the problem. The company also brought in professional help, transferring Harry Ethridge from the Public Relations Department of its national office to St. Lawrence to combat the negative publicity and to assist Newfluor in its dealings with the Royal Commission.

Despite the best efforts of the government and the company, however, the "grim side of the picture" continued to be displayed. A television special that aired in March 1967, for instance, explored the history of mining and industrial disease in the community. Shortly after, a lengthy and scathing newspaper article by Rennie Slaney described the toll the mines had taken and the government's mishandling of the situation (*St. John's Evening Telegram,* Compensation should be paid, 1967, March 31).

In September 1967, on the eve of the Royal Commission's first public hearing scheduled to take place in St. Lawrence in November, a fatal accident at Director mine provided yet another occasion for a war of words in the press. Three men were buried under several tons of fallen rock, an incident that provoked outrage from the union, community residents, and the media. In a newspaper article that described Director as the "Killer Mine," activist Rennie Slaney noted that the three recent deaths had brought to 27 the number of miners who had lived within a 250-foot radius of his house and been killed by industrial diseases or accidents over the years (*St. John's Evening Telegram,* Killer mine, 1967, September 18). Newfluor management responded to this outpouring of negative publicity by correcting what it called inaccuracies in the media's coverage. Wiseman pointed out, for instance, that "just seven" miners had been killed by accidents over the entire life of the Director mine. He did not mention the number killed by industrial diseases (*St. John's Evening Telegram,* Mine fatalities, 1967, September 29).

The attention garnered by this accident highlights the marked difference in the recognition of and response to industrial disasters involving accidents as opposed to diseases. Accidents, especially those involving multiple fatalities, tend to be immediately recognized as disasters and treated as such by authorities, the media, academics, and the general public (e.g., Bercuson 1978; McCormick 1992; McKay 1983; Palmer and Lunn 1997). On the other hand, as one historian has observed with respect to health hazards in the mines of Ontario, when workers are killed slowly, one at a time, as they are by industrial disease, it tends to provoke little public interest or outrage (Baldwin 1977). While the deaths of these three miners was certainly no less tragic than the deaths of others from industrial disease, and the outrage expressed at the incident was entirely appropriate, it nonetheless serves as a clear illustration of this phenomenon.

Newfluor's contribution to the Royal Commission consisted largely of defending its record with respect to workplace hazards and industrial disease. At the November 1967 hearing, for instance, Newfluor representatives insisted that the company had always cooperated with government and medical officials in detecting, uncovering, and responding to health hazards. Alcan's Industrial

Health Officer Frank Brent declared, for example, "Everyone was most anxious to find out what was the cause of this great misfortune," and to "do everything we could to keep the Company's skirts as clean as possible."[23]

Not surprisingly, the SLWPU/CNTU presented a different version of events, claiming, among other things, that bitterness and mistrust harbored by workers and others in the community resulted not from of a lack of understanding or from distortion of the facts by the media, but from people's knowledge of the actual dimensions of the disaster, which had never been fully recognized by the government or the employer.[24]

Regarding actions, or lack of same, with respect to detecting industrial diseases over the years, the Royal Commission criticized the provincial Department of Health for being "slow in its acknowledgment of serious occupational health hazards" in the mines at St. Lawrence. The Commission's report also charged that the federal Department of Health and Welfare had been "unwarrantedly bureaucratic" in its response to the requests for intervention during the 1950s (Aylward 1969, pp. 42-43).

To decide the extent to which compensation coverage should be extended, the Royal Commission sought to find out as much as possible about the causes and incidence of illness and mortality among miners over the years. This study determined that, of the 240 deaths from all causes known to have occurred by 1967, among those who had worked for either company since 1933, 25 were caused by silicosis and tuberculosis, 9 by other diseases of the respiratory system, 53 by cancer of the lungs, 21 from cancer of the stomach and digestive system, 10 by other cancers, and 61 by diseases of the heart and cardiovascular system. Of the 53 deaths from cancer of the lungs, 24 had occurred in the period 1963-67 alone, 35 of the victims had been under 55 years old, and all but 2 had worked underground for one or both companies (Aylward 1969, pp. 178-179).

The Commission's report drew special attention to the issue of cancer of the digestive system, noting that while the rate of death from cancer of the stomach and digestive system among miners was not markedly higher than the provincial rate, and was roughly the same among surface and underground employees, there was a striking difference in their average age at death. For surface employees with this type of cancer, the average age at death was 71.2 years, while for underground employees it was just 52.6 years, suggesting "an as yet unrecognized effect of occupational exposure," which might have been related to the ingestion of water in the mines (Aylward 1969, pp. 136-137).

Against this backdrop of the statistics on mortality and illness, the Royal Commission examined those workers' compensation claims that had been accepted, the potential claims that had never been filed, those that had been filed but rejected, and the grounds for rejection in such cases. It found that claims had usually been rejected because they arose from deaths or disabilities occurring prior to 1951, or because the worker was suffering or had died from an illness other than lung cancer or silicosis, including a large number who had died from bowel cancer, stomach cancer, kidney cancer, tuberculosis, and chronic bronchitis (Aylward 1969, pp. 260-261).

Based on these findings, the Royal Commission concluded that of the 99 claims which had either been rejected or had never been filed, 47 were entitled to compensation (Aylward 1969, pp. 266-272). The 52 claims judged to be not entitled fell into two groups: deaths not considered related to underground employment, including deaths from cardiovascular diseases, gastrointestinal and urinary system diseases, and cancers other than those of the respiratory system and lungs; and deaths of individuals with no record of underground employment or with a record of underground employment incompatible with the disease that had caused disability or death. Note that while the Royal Commission had indicated its suspicion that the ingestion of water was responsible for gastrointestinal cancers, it did not recommend compensation in such cases. It is also worth noting that while the dust study of 1957 had confirmed dust levels well above allowable limits in surface operations, underground employment was still a prerequisite to qualifying. The Royal Commission was careful to point out that it could not ensure that any claim would be accepted or rejected: that hinged on which of its recommendations, if any, the government accepted and acted upon.

The government's initial response to the Commission's recommendations signaled little willingness to break with the status quo. The government refused to institute many of the Commission's key recommendations primarily because it was unwilling to retroactively apply the Act to the pre-1951 period and to diseases other than silicosis and lung cancer. The Royal Commission had recommended, for instance, that since the medical evidence regarding loss of pulmonary function was in some cases complicated by the interaction of several conditions, including bronchitis, silicosis, tuberculosis, and tumors, loss of pulmonary function itself should be taken into account when considering claims regarding those employed in the mines before 1960. To this the government replied that any such consideration would be limited to cases where the worker had ceased employment after 1 April 1951. Similarly, the government agreed with the recommendation that all cases involving disablement or death from lung cancer or silicosis should be compensated, but stipulated that these cases would also be subject to the limit on retroactivity to 1 April 1951 (Newfoundland 1970, pp. 6-7).

In addition to extending compensation coverage to pre-1951 claims, the Royal Commission also recommended extending coverage to diseases other than lung cancer and silicosis, including to tuberculosis, any chronic obstructive pulmonary disease, and respiratory cancers other than lung cancers, such as those affecting the nose and throat. The government agreed only to recognize silico-tuberculosis as a compensable disease, which had minimal impact given the very small number of cases where a worker had developed silico-tuberculosis *and* had terminated employment after 1951. Ultimately, because of the government's refusal to enact most of the recommendations that would have extended compensation coverage, only 7 of the 47 claims the Royal Commission had identified as worthy of acceptance were initially approved.[25]

By making more explicit the boundary between what would and would not be considered and treated as an industrial disease, the government's initial reaction to the Royal Commission's recommendations brought into sharp relief the polarization between the minimalist and maximalist positions. In doing so, it deepened the atmosphere of grievance and mistrust in the community and workplace, which would be a key factor in drawing increased public and media attention to the disaster during subsequent years.

That the union and others in the community intended to use whatever channels at their disposal to draw attention to their plight became apparent during a labor dispute in April 1971. Though the strike was ostensibly over wages, at one point during the strike several women in the community took over the picket lines while miners marched through the town to the cemetery carrying a coffin and a cancer symbol, an event that captured the attention of the media and provided a forum for airing complaints over such issues as the government's refusal to extend compensation coverage (*St. John's Evening Telegram,* St. Lawrence strike, 1971, May 10).

Developments in provincial politics also began to play a more prominent role in the St. Lawrence situation in 1971 and brought increased pressure to bear on the government. The ruling Liberals under Joseph Smallwood were losing the grip they had held on Newfoundland politics since confederation with Canada in 1949. The government was under intense pressure from a highly vocal group of Progressive Conservatives that included Alex Hickman, representative for the district in which St. Lawrence was located, who missed no opportunity to raise the St. Lawrence issue in the media and in the House of Assembly (Newfoundland, 8 June 1970, pp. 6431-6433).

As the strike, the political squabbling and the media attention they generated continued through the spring and summer of 1971, the government made several attempts to stem the tide of criticism. In May the government introduced a moderate increase in monthly payments to widows (*St. John's Evening Telegram,* St. Lawrence strike, 1971, May 10) and in July it announced the establishment of the "St. Lawrence Special Fund." This scheme was one of Alcan's recommendations to the Royal Commission and was meant to provide support to compensation recipients whose benefits were considered inadequate to their needs. Initially, about 50 cases qualified for the $30.86 a month per disabled miner or widow and $7.72 per month for dependent children paid under the Special Fund, which was jointly financed by Alcan and the provincial government.[26] After several years of operating on a limited basis at several of its smaller sites during the late 1950s and early 1960s, the St. Lawrence Corporation had ceased operations altogether and left town in 1962. It never contributed anything to the Special Fund and, apart from some moderate increase in workers' compensation premiums as a result of the few silicosis claims that had been accepted up to that time, escaped all liability for its role in the disaster.

While such concessions may have contributed to the union's willingness to settle the strike and return to work in September 1971, and temporarily alleviated some of the criticism being directed at the government, they did little to address the more fundamental issue of the continued refusal to recognize and compensate many cases of industrial disease. Some change in that direction came after the Liberal government was defeated in the election of March 1972. Shortly after taking office, the new Tory government passed an amendment to the *Workmen's Compensation Act* that extended coverage to two types of cases previously excluded. The first was those cases of chronic obstructive pulmonary diseases where the exact causal connection between the disease and working conditions was unclear, but where "rational observation indicates the probability of such a connection." This coverage was limited, however, to cases were the worker had been employed underground in a St. Lawrence mine between 1 January 1951 and 31 December 1960. A second group to which coverage was extended under the 1972 amendment was the workers listed in the Report of the Royal Commission as being entitled to compensation (Newfoundland 1973).

The union, however, was still not satisfied and continued to press for coverage of what it believed to be deserving cases still excluded from the Act. This included those cases where workers had been employed in such places as the mill and crushing plant and had developed pulmonary diseases but were not covered because they had not worked underground. The union also rejected the assumption underlying the 1972 amendment that the danger from radiation and dust ceased to exist after 1960 and therefore no justifiable claims could arise after that date. Furthermore, the union argued that the decision to accept claims in cases where the worker had ceased employment before April 1951 because they were deemed worthy of acceptance by the Royal Commission, while denying other claims where the worker had ceased employment before April 1951 simply because they had not been named in the Commission's report, was an indication of the continuing arbitrariness of how the Act was applied. The union urged the government to abandon this capricious and piecemeal approach and simply recognize illnesses as industry-related, regardless of when workers left the job, and compensate such cases accordingly.[27]

The government only took action on some of the union's demands in the context of yet another labor dispute. In April 1973, workers again went on strike after failing to reach a settlement on wages (*St. John's Evening Telegram*, St. Lawrence miners strike, 1973, April 2). In a move that illustrated the government's strategy of extending compensation coverage as a way of securing labor peace, one month into the strike the government passed further amendments to the *Workmen's Compensation Act,* this time allowing for claims arising from underground employment "at any time, before or after 1951, and for claims arising in cases where the worker was not employed underground at the time of the disability" (Newfoundland, 1974). These changes were made public on 2 May 1973, and the next day the SLWPU accepted the company's wage offer and returned to work (Workmen's compensation, 1973, May 2, and Fluorspar miners, 1973, May 4).

Because it extended coverage to cases where a worker had been employed in a surface occupation and to pre-1951 claims, the 1973 amendment represented an important victory. The amendment led to an immediate increase in the number of claims filed and accepted, and to a reversal of previous decisions in some cases. Claims continued to be denied, however, for various reasons, usually because of a lack of evidence that an illness or death was attributable to working conditions.

The catalyst for a new battle in the war over recognition and compensation was another labor dispute that began in June 1975, when the union rejected what the company claimed was its final wage offer (*St. John's Evening Telegram,* Alcan labor dispute, 1975, June 27). About a week into the ensuing standoff, some 200 women came out in support of the union and blocked the ore carrier from taking on fluorspar at the loading dock. Twelve days into the blockade, the company suspended all mining operations and imposed a lockout.

As with previous labor disputes, the 1975 strike became a forum for airing complaints over industrial disease and inadequate compensation coverage, prompting the government to amend the legislation yet again. In response to the union's continuing complaints that previous amendments had been based on the assumption that there was no risk of contracting silicosis or cancer among those workers who began work after 1960, a new amendment passed in June 1975 extended coverage to such cases (Newfoundland 1976).

This did little, however, to combat the hostility and mistrust that had built up over the years, and as the strike continued through the summer of 1975 it became a flashpoint for many long-festering grievances. Peter Curtis of the CNTU pointed out that the dispute was fueled largely by the history of disease and death in the community and by the government's refusal to adequately recognize and respond to the disaster. The Newfluor manager himself noted: "There's an emotional feeling of bitterness against Alcan which exists all the time below the surface" (*St. John's Evening Telegram,* St. Lawrence miners, 1975, June 12). This bitterness was no doubt increased by the mounting death toll: during 1974 and the first half of 1975, five miners, all under 50 years old, died of lung cancer (*St. John's Evening Telegram,* New contract, 1975, June 21).

At a crucial time in the escalating conflict, the St. Lawrence disaster began to gain national attention with the publication of Elliot Leyton's *Dying Hard: The Ravages of Industrial Carnage.* Published in May 1975, *Dying Hard* was based on a series of interviews Leyton had conducted with widows and sick miners, and detailed from their perspective the physical, emotional and psychological pain inflicted by industrial disease and the frustrating and often humiliating ordeal of seeking workers' compensation benefits (Leyton 1975a).

While the unrest that marked the situation at St. Lawrence during the 1970s was instrumental in generating the kind of interest that led to the publication of *Dying Hard*, the book in turn brought unprecedented public and media attention to the St. Lawrence disaster. Leyton went on a national publicity tour and appeared on national radio and television programs (Leyton 1977a). Because the book was designed as social advocacy rather than an academic exercise, it also generated many book reviews and coverage in the popular press (e.g., Leyton 1975b). A Newfoundland theater troupe, "The Mummers," which used theater as a vehicle for social advocacy, toured a play called "Dying Hard," and the CBC produced an hour-long feature based on the book (Leyton, 1977a). Leyton also used his work in St. Lawrence as the basis for a submission to the government and the WCB critiquing their response to the St. Lawrence disaster and making a number of recommendations (Leyton 1977b), which was apparently completely ignored (Leyton 1977a).

In December 1975, actors and musicians staged a benefit concert in St. John's for the miners and widows at St. Lawrence that was sponsored by the New Democratic Party of Newfoundland and several activist groups (*St. John's Evening Telegram,* Miners in St. Lawrence, 1975, December 12). Despite the attention and the assistance, by February 1976, after nine months off the job, workers could no longer hold out against the company. They accepted a new wage offer and returned to work (*St. John's Evening Telegram,* Alcan miners, 1976, February 7).

Though the St. Lawrence dispute was over, labor unrest among Alcan workers in Quebec combined with the availability of cheaper fluorspar on the open market hampered the revival of the St. Lawrence operation. In July 1976, Newfluor began laying off the 250 men it had re-hired to that point, and shortly after announced that it was shutting down the St. Lawrence mine effective 1 February 1978 (*St. John's Evening Telegram,* Alcan will close, 1977, July 25).

When the Newfluor gates were locked for the last time in February 1978, 78 miners were dead from lung cancer alone, in addition to the many who had died from other cancers and from silicosis, various pulmonary diseases, and accidents. A further 120 who had worked during the pre-1960 period were deemed to be at risk (Wright and Couves 1977). In 1983, a British-based company known as Minworth took advantage of generous provincial government tax breaks and other concessions to establish a subsidiary called St. Lawrence Fluorspar Inc. and revived one of the old mine sites. Four hundred men signed up for the 100 available jobs, and one applicant depicted in stark terms the dilemma in which many found themselves when he remarked that, "It's just as well to die with money as live without" (Story 1987, p. 186). The first shipment of fluorspar in ten years left St. Lawrence in 1987, but just four years later, in 1991, Minworth declared bankruptcy and left town. The population of the community currently stands at about 1,500, and the main source of employment is a shellfish processing plant.

While little is known about any possible health impacts of the Minworth enterprise, the toll from the earlier phase of mining continued long after Alcan left town. By 1988, 116 miners were dead from lung cancer and 28 from silicosis and other obstructive lung diseases (Morrison 1988, p. 45). In addition, 72 others had died from other types of cancer, including 22 from stomach and other gastrointestinal cancers (Morrison 1988, p. 52). Many were never compensated.

Just as media and public interest in the St. Lawrence disaster had over the years been fueled by such events as labor unrest and public protests, attention faded quickly once such actions ceased in the wake of industry closure. These developments, especially during the 1970s, had nonetheless served to draw widespread attention to the true dimensions of the St. Lawrence disaster and were instrumental in having what might have otherwise been regarded as an unfortunate but limited incidence of industrial disease recognized *as* a disaster. As the St. Lawrence case illustrates, the recognition of and response to an industrial disaster can be shaped by a host of conflicting perspectives and interests, including those of victims and their advocates, medical experts, employers, the state, and the media. Central to this process is what Graebner (1988, p. 17) calls the "political economy of knowledge," which refers to the process by which information and opinions about an industrial disaster are suppressed or disseminated by the various forces and parties involved. The political economy of knowledge therefore includes not only medical and scientific information, but also a wide range of social, economic and political factors. The St. Lawrence case highlights the fact that, especially with respect to industrial diseases, the very recognition of the existence of a disaster is as much a social as a clinical process, shaped by elements of power, inequality, and conflict.

ACKNOWLEDGMENTS

The author would like to thank the Social Sciences and Humanities Research Council of Canada (SSHRC), the Institute of Social and Economic Research (Memorial University of Newfoundland), and the J. R. Smallwood Centre for Newfoundland Studies (Memorial University of Newfoundland) for their financial support of this research. Thanks also to Ingrid Botting, the Town Council of St. Lawrence, the St. Lawrence Memorial Miners' Museum, and the former miners who welcomed me into their homes and shared their stories and their knowledge with me.

ENDNOTES

1. For example: A. E. Cave, Report on mines inspection of Newfoundland, November 6, 1936, and A. E. Cave, Inspection report on the mining operations in Newfoundland, 1940, Archival Collection of the Newfoundland and Labrador Department of Mines and Energy.

2. Report of the Ranger, St. Lawrence Detachment, for July to December, 1945, Provincial Archives of Newfoundland and Labrador (PANL), Records of the Commission of Government (GN38), File S2-5-2.

3. In keeping with the policy of the Social Sciences and Humanities Research Council of Canada regarding research involving human subjects, the names of interviewees are pseudonyms.

4. In the interest of historical accuracy, the term "workmen" is used throughout to refer to specific pieces of legislation and government agencies, as this was the term used during the period under study. In more generic contexts, "worker" is used.

5. BCG Testing and Vaccination, July 1954, PANL, Records of the Newfoundland Department of Health (GN78), File 1/B/51.

6. Irving Fogwill, Chairman, Workmen's Compensation Board of Newfoundland, to Donald Poynter, Manager, St. Lawrence Corporation of Newfoundland, November 13, 1954, PANL, GN78, File1/B/51.

7. Proceedings of meeting on the subject of detection and handling of silicosis held in the office of the Chief Inspector of Mines, 30 October 1953, PANL, GN78, File 1/B/51.

8. Leonard Miller, Deputy Minister of Health, Government of Newfoundland, to G. C. Brink, Department of Health and Welfare, Ottawa, November 10, 1953, PANL, GN78, File 1/B/51.

9. F. Lukins, Chief Inspector of Mines, Government of Newfoundland, to Leonard Miller, Deputy Minister of Health, Government of Newfoundland, February 27, 1957, PANL, GN78, File 1/B/51.

10. F. Lukins, Chief Inspector of Mines, Government of Newfoundland, to Leonard Miller, Deputy Minister of Health, Government of Newfoundland, and to Irving Fogwill, Chairman, Workmen's Compensation Board of Newfoundland February 27, 1957, PANL, GN78, File 1/B/51.

11. Aloysius Turpin, St. Lawrence Workers' Protective Union, to Chairman of the Cancer Convention, St. John's, 28 January 1958, Archival Collection of the St. Lawrence Memorial Miners' Museum (SLMMM).

12. Leonard Miller, Deputy Minister of Health, Government of Newfoundland, to G. C. Brink, Department of Health and Welfare, Ottawa, 14 July 1958, PANL, GN78, File 1/B/51.

13. F. D. Brent, Chief Industrial Medical Officer, Alcan, to Leonard Miller, Deputy Minister of Health, Government of Newfoundland, July 18, 1958, PANL, GN78, File 1/B/51.

14. James McGrath, Minister of Health, Government of Newfoundland, to Aloysius Turpin, President, St. Lawrence Workers' Protective Union, March 4, 1960, SLMMM.

15. F. D. Brent, Chief Industrial Medical Officer, Alcan, to James McGrath, Minister of Health, Government of Newfoundland, 22 January 1960, PANL, GN78, File 1/B/51.

16. Donald Poynter, Manager, St. Lawrence Corporation of Newfoundland, to N. S. Batten, Unemployment Insurance Commission, St. John's, Newfoundland, March 28, 1960, National Archives of Canada, Record Group 27 (Labor Canada), Volume 540, Reel T-3401, Strike 39.

17. J. P. Windish, Department of National Health and Welfare, Occupational Health Division, to St. Lawrence Workers' Protective Union, April 3, 1960, PANL, GN78, File 1/B/51.

18. R. Wiseman, General Manager, Newfoundland Fluorspar Limited, to Leonard Miller, Deputy Minister of Health, Government of Newfoundland, March 25, 1960, PANL, GN78, File 1/B/51.
19. Leonard Miller, Deputy Minister of Health, Government of Newfoundland, to R. Wiseman, General Manager, Newfoundland Fluorspar Limited, March 31, 1960, PANL, GN78, File 1/B/51.
20. L. G. Vey, Senior Administrative Assistant, Department of Health, Government of Newfoundland, to de A. J. de Villiers, Occupational Health Division, National Department Health and Welfare, 17 February 1967, PANL, GN78, File 1/B/220.
21. Press Release Issued by Mr. R. Wiseman, General Manager, Newfoundland Fluorspar Limited, 17 February 1967, Records of Royal Commission on Radiation, Compensation and Safety at the Fluorspar Mines, St. Lawrence, Newfoundland, PANL, GN6.
22. Press Release Issued by Mr. R. Wiseman, General Manager, Newfoundland Fluorspar Limited, 17 February 1967, PANL, GN6.
23. Transcript of a public hearing held at St. Lawrence, 27 November 1967, PANL, GN6.
24. St. Lawrence Workers' Protective Union submission to the Royal Commission on Radiation, Compensation and Safety at the Fluorspar Mines, St. Lawrence, Newfoundland, PANL, GN6.
25. W. J. Keough, Deputy Minister of Mines, to J. R. Smallwood, Premier of Newfoundland, November 17, 1970, Centre for Newfoundland Studies Archive, Collection 075, File 3.27.037.
26. Memorandum regarding St. Lawrence Special Fund, Collection 075, File 3.21.048, Centre for Newfoundland Studies Archive, Memorial University of Newfoundland.
27. George Doyle, President, St. Lawrence Workers' Protective Union, to T. Alex Hickman, Minister of Justice, November 27, 1972, SLMMM.

REFERENCES

Secondary Sources

Adams, I. (1967, June) The Forgotten Miners. *Maclean's, 80*: 21-23, 40-43, 46.
Aylward, F. (1969) *Report of the Royal Commission on Radiation, Compensation, and Safety at the Fluorspar Mines, St. Lawrence, Newfoundland.* St. John's, Newfoundland: Office of the Queen's Printer.
Baldwin, D. (1977) A Study in Social Control: The Life of the Silver Miner in Northern Ontario. *Labor/Le Travailleur, 2*: 79-107.
Bayer, R. (1988) Introduction. In R. Bayer (ed.), *The Health and Safety of Workers: Case Studies in the Politics of Professional Responsibility.* Oxford: Oxford University Press.
Bercuson, D. J. (1978) Tragedy at Bellevue: Anatomy of a Mine Disaster. *Labor/Le Travailleur, 3*: 221-232.
Bernard, M. (1967) The Flesh Just Melts—Then the End. *Star Weekly Magazine,* July 8, 1967: 10-15.
Brown, C. (1979) *Standing into Danger: A Dramatic Story of Shipwreck and Rescue.* Garden City, New York: Doubleday.

Bryder, L. (1985) Tuberculosis, Silicosis, and the Slate Industry in North Wales, 1927-1939. In P. Weindling (ed.), *The Social History of Occupational Health* (pp. 108-126). London: Croom Helm.

Burke, G. (1985) Disease, Labor Migration and Technological Change: The Case of the Cornish Miners. In P. Weindling (ed.), *The Social History of Occupational Health* (pp. 78-88). London: Croom Helm.

de Villiers, A. J., and Windish, J. P. (1964) Lung Cancer in a Fluorspar Mining Community: Radiation, Dust and Mortality Experience. *British Journal of Industrial Medicine, 21*: 94-109.

Derickson, A. (1988) *Workers' Health, Workers' Democracy: The Western Miners' Struggle, 1891-1925.* Ithaca: Cornell University Press.

Derickson, A. (1998) Industrial Refugees: The Migration of Silicotics from the Mines of North America and South Africa in the Early 20th Century. *Labor History, 29*(1): 66-89.

Farrell, E. E. (1983) *Notes toward a History of St. Lawrence.* St. John's: Breakwater.

Fellman, C. M. (1926) The Mining of Fluorspar and Its Uses. *Proceedings of the Lake Superior Mining Institute, 25*: 197-211.

Fogwill, I. (1950) *Report of the Workmen's Compensation Committee of Newfoundland on the Organization and Administration of a Workmen's Compensation Board for Newfoundland.* Unpublished, Center for Newfoundland Studies, Memorial University of Newfoundland.

Gibbs, G. H., and Pintus, P. (1978) *Health and Safety in the Canadian Mining Industry.* Kingston: Queen's University Press.

Graebner, W. (1988) Private Power, Private Knowledge, and Public Health: Science, Engineering, and Lead Poisoning, 1900-1970. In R. Bayer (ed.), *The Health and Safety of Workers: Case Studies in the Politics of Professional Responsibility* (pp. 15-71). Oxford: Oxford University Press.

Howse C. K., and Fischer, R. P. (1939) Newfoundland Ships Fluorspar: Production from St. Lawrence Region, Begun in 1932, has Increased Steadily. *Engineering and Mining Journal, 140*: 7.

Ison, T. (1978) *The Dimensions of Industrial Disease.* Kingston: Industrial Relations Center, Queen's University.

Leyton, E. (1975a) *Dying Hard: The Ravages of Industrial Carnage.* Toronto: McClelland and Stewart.

Leyton, E. (1975b) The Bad Death. *Maclean's, 88*: 6, 42-43, 46, 48, 50.

Leyton, E. (1977a) *Public Consciousness and Public Policy.* Unpublished, Center for Newfoundland Studies, Memorial University of Newfoundland.

Leyton, E. (1977b) *The Bureaucratization of Anguish: The Workmen's Compensation Board in an Industrial Disaster.* Unpublished, Center for Newfoundland Studies, Memorial University of Newfoundland.

McArthur, J. (1960) Cancer Tragedy Deadly Mystery in Newfoundland. *Financial Post, 54*: 41.

McCormick, C. (1992) *The Westray Chronicles: A Case Study in Corporate Crime.* Halifax: Fernwood.

McKay, I. (1984) Springhill 1958. *New Maritimes, 2*: 4-16.

Martin, W. (1985) *Once Upon a Mine: Story of Pre-Confederation Mines on the Island of Newfoundland.* Montreal: Canadian Institute of Mining and Metallurgy.

Morrison, H., and Canada, Atomic Energy Control Board (1988). *The Mortality Experience of a Group of Newfoundland Fluorspar Miners Exposed to the Rn Progeny*. Ottawa: Atomic Energy Control Board.

Müller, R. (1985) A Patient in Need of Care: German Occupational Health Statistics. In P. Weindling (ed.), *Linking Self Help and Medical Science: The Social History of Occupational Health* (pp. 127-136). London: Croom Helm.

Murray, A., and Howley J. P. (1881) *Geological Survey of Newfoundland*. London: Edward Stanford.

Neary, P. (1988) *Newfoundland in the North Atlantic World, 1929-1949*. Kingston: McGill-Queen's University Press.

Newfoundland (1909) An Act with Respect to Compensation to Workmen for Injuries Suffered in the Course of Their Employment. In *Acts of the General Assembly of Newfoundland: Passed in the Eighth Year of the Reign of His Majesty King Edward VII* (pp. 10-27). St. John's: Office of the King's Printer.

Newfoundland (1942) *Settlement of Trade Dispute Board Appointed for the Settlement of a Dispute between the St. Lawrence Corporation of Newfoundland and the St. Lawrence Workers' Protective Union*. St. John's: Office of the King's Printer.

Newfoundland (1952) An Act Respecting the Safety of Workmen in Mines, 1951. In *Statutes of Newfoundland*. St. John's: Office of the Queen's Printer. no pagination.

Newfoundland (1959, 29 September) The Mines (Safety of Workmen) (Amendment) Regulations. In *Newfoundland Gazette* (pp. 1-2). St. John's: Office of the Queen's Printer.

Newfoundland (1960, March 29) The Mines (Safety of Workmen) (Amendment) Regulations. In *Newfoundland Gazette* (p. 1). St. John's: Office of the Queen's Printer.

Newfoundland (1961) An Act to Further Amend the Workmen's Compensation Act, 1960. In *Statutes of Newfoundland* (pp. 315-318). St. John's: Office of the Queen's Printer.

Newfoundland (1970) *Decisions of the Government on the Report of the Royal Commission Respecting Radiation, Compensation, and Safety at the Fluorspar Mines, St. Lawrence*. Unpublished, Center for Newfoundland Studies, Memorial University of Newfoundland.

Newfoundland (1970, June 8) *Journal of the House of Assembly of Newfoundland* (pp. 6431-6433). St. John's: Office of the Queen's Printer.

Newfoundland (1973) Workmen's Compensation (Amendment) Act, 1972. In *Statutes of Newfoundland* (pp. 537-539). St. John's: Office of the Queen's Printer.

Newfoundland (1974) Workmen's Compensation (Amendment) Act, 1973. In *Statutes of Newfoundland* (pp. 1073-1082). St. John's: Office of the Queen's Printer.

Newfoundland (1976) Workmen's Compensation (Amendment) Act, 1975. In *Statutes of Newfoundland* (pp. 193-201). St. John's: Office of the Queen's Printer.

Overton, J. (1990) Economic Crisis and the End of Democracy: Politics in Newfoundland during the Great Depression. *Labor/Le Travail, 26*: 85-124.

Palmer, B. D., and Lunn, R. L. (1997) The Big Sleep: The Malartic Mine Fire of 1947. *Labor/Le Travail, 39*: 225-240.

Raffle, P. A. B. (ed.). (1994) *Hunter's Diseases of Occupations*. London: Edward Arnold.

Rosen, G. (1943) *The History of Miners' Diseases: A Medical and Social Interpretation*. New York: Schuman's.

Rosner, D., and Markowitz, G. (1992) *Deadly Dust: Silicosis and the Politics of Occupational Disease in Twentieth Century America*. New Jersey: Princeton University Press.

Ryan, E. (2000, February 7) Personal interview, St. Lawrence, Newfoundland.

Schepers. G. W. H. (1964, June) Silicosis and Tuberculosis. *Industrial Medicine and Surgery,* pp. 381-399.

Slaney, R. (1975) *More Incredible than Fiction: The True Story of the Indomitable Men and Women of St. Lawrence from the Time of Settlement to 1965.* Montreal: La Confédération des Syndicats Nationeaux.

Spencer, H. (2000, October 13) Personal interview, St. Lawrence, Newfoundland.

St. John's Daily News (2 March 1960) Government officials meet to discuss radiation hazard in fluorspar mines. 3, 16.

St. John's Daily News (18 March 1960) Radiation picture at St. Lawrence overemphasized says Wiseman. 2.

St. John's Evening Telegram (2 March 1960) Miners get more cancer. 2.

St. John's Evening Telegram (3 March 1960) Miners "wait and see" as cancer cause checked. 3

St. John's Evening Telegram (11 March 1960) Miners back request as walkout endorsed. 2.

St. John's Evening Telegram (24 March 1960) Miners stay out, seek jobless aid. 3.

St. John's Evening Telegram (1 April 1960) Ventilation system is installed. 3.

St. John's Evening Telegram (31 March 1967) Compensation should be paid says St. Lawrence miner. 7.

St. John's Evening Telegram (31 March 1967) Tragedy termed "National Disaster." 1.

St. John's Evening Telegram (18 September 1967) Killer mine snuffs out three more lives. 1.

St. John's Evening Telegram (19 September 1967) Most dangerous sections of deadly mine closed. 3.

St. John's Evening Telegram (29 September 1967) Mine fatalities. 1.

St. John's Evening Telegram (10 May 1971) St. Lawrence strike could be a long one. 3.

St. John's Evening Telegram (2 April 1973) St. Lawrence miners strike. 1.

St. John's Evening Telegram (2 May 1973) Workmen's compensation payments increased. 2.

St. John's Evening Telegram (4 May 1973) Fluorspar miners back on job. 1.

St. John's Evening Telegram (12 June 1975) St. Lawrence miners charged with intimidation by violence. 3.

St. John's Evening Telegram (21 June 1975) New contract won't settle real issues. 5.

St. John's Evening Telegram (27 June 1975) Alcan labor dispute still at standstill. 3.

St. John's Evening Telegram (12 December 1975) Miners in St. Lawrence prepared to go to prison. 3.

St. John's Evening Telegram (7 February 1976) Alcan miners going back to work. 3.

St. John's Evening Telegram (25 July 1977) Alcan will close down mine at St. Lawrence. 2.

Story, A. (1987) Old Wounds: Reopening the Mines of St. Lawrence. In G. Burrill and I. Mckay (eds.), *People, Resources, and Power: Critical Perspectives on Underdevelopment and Primary Industries in Atlantic Canada* (pp. 186-190). Fredericton.

Thompkins, R. W. (1944) Radioactivity and Lung Cancer: A Critical Review of Lung Cancer in the Miners of Schneeberg and Joachimsthal. *Journal of the National Cancer Institute,* 5: 23-34.

Weindling, P. (1985) Linking Self Help and Medical Science: The Social History of Occupational Health. In P. Weindling (ed.), *The Social History of Occupational Health* (pp. 2-31). London: Croom Helm.

Windish, J. P., Sanderson, H. P., and Newfoundland Fluorspar Limited (1958) *Dust Hazards in the Mines of Newfoundland: I. Newfoundland Fluorspar Limited, St. Lawrence, Newfoundland.* Ottawa: Laboratory Services, Occupational Health Division, Dept. of National Health and Welfare.

Windish, J. P., Canada. Occupational Health Division, and Newfoundland Fluorspar Limited (1960) *Health Hazards in the Mines of Newfoundland: III. Radiation Levels in the Workings of Newfoundland Fluorspar Limited, St. Lawrence, Newfoundland.* Ottawa: Occupational Health Division, Dept. of National Health and Welfare.

Winter, H. A. (1966) *Report of the Review Committee Appointed to Review, Consider, Report Upon, and Make Recommendations Respecting the Workmen's Compensation Act.* Unpublished, Center for Newfoundland Studies, Memorial University of Newfoundland.

Workmen's Compensation Board of Newfoundland (1953-1960) *Annual Reports.* 1953-1960.

Wright, E. S., and Couves, C. M. (1977) Radiation-Induced Carcinoma of the Lung: The St. Lawrence Tragedy. *Journal of Thoracic and Cardiovascular Surgery, 74*(4): 495-498.

CHAPTER 5

The Long Road to Action: The Silicosis Problem and Swedish Occupational Health and Safety Policy in the 20th Century

Annette Thörnquist

THE HEAVY STEPS

It was an evening in late autumn 1948. It was snowing and a biting wind blew. Lundh, a moulder, passed the foundry around nine o'clock on his way home from a meeting, when he caught sight of his former workmate Nilsson walking uphill toward the village. Nilsson was moving slowly and—strangely enough— backwards. Lundh hurried up to him to ask how he was feeling, but in reply he got only gasps. Nilsson was totally exhausted. He simply didn't have the strength to walk against the wind. Lundh took his friend by the arm to help him home. Slowly, and in involuntary silence, the two men walked the kilometer to Nilsson's house. It almost took an hour to get there.

The scene is from Österbybruk, an old Walloon ironworks community located in the province of Uppland, in Central Sweden. Workers here were among those most affected by silicosis in the country. In the mid-1920s the ironworks was merged with the leading Swedish iron and steel industrial concern, *Fagerstakoncernen*. The ironworks in Österbybruk became one of Sweden's most highly reputed for the manufacture of high quality steel products, especially castings in high-alloy steel for machine parts and tools. In his youth, Nilsson had worked at the Martin furnace and, after that, in the foundry as a cleaner of castings. Each of his jobs entailed heavy exposure to quartz dust from the lining in the furnaces and the sand in the moulds. In 1942, at the age of 47, Nilsson was diagnosed with silicosis. He was then transferred to the construction department, but this work became too heavy for him. As his silicosis progressed rapidly, he became gatekeeper at the ironworks, the last resort for many disabled workers, and it was coming home from one of his shifts that Lundh caught up with him on the hill (Thörnquist 1993).

Silicosis is a non-reversible lung disease caused by the inhalation of dust from crystalline silica (SiO_2). Silica exists mainly in quartz, which is one of the most common components in the earth's crust. Silicosis develops slowly, normally only after decades of over-exposure to silica dust. Particles less than 0.005 mm damage the lung tissue, and the resulting build-up of connective tissue successively reduces breathing capacity. Heart problems and tuberculosis often set in during advanced stages of the disease. Silica mixed with other dust may cause mixed-dust silicosis (Ahlmark 1967, pp. 21-28). In recent decades, the relationship between silica dust and cancer has been widely discussed.

From the first recorded case of silicosis in Österbybruk in 1933 and up to the mid-1950, 54 workers were reported to have contracted the disease. At the end of this period the disease had progressed for 20 workers, nine of whom had died from silicosis or silicosis complicated by tuberculosis. The ironworks community, where much of the paternalistic old order prevailed during the first part of the 20th century, was socially traumatized by the problem of silicosis. The workers lived in houses owned by the company and received other benefits as well. The relative social security of this arrangement created a strong dependence on the employer and on the community, which was heightened in an era characterized by mass unemployment, lack of housing, and wartime. Thus, most workers stayed in the ironworks community despite of the risk of silicosis.

The labor inspectors took little action on the silicosis problem in Österbybruk until the mid-1940s. Thus, protecting workers from this danger became mainly a question for management and the trade unions. In this paternalistic milieu, it was not until 1920 that the trade union movement were established, but once the workers were organized, they became politically radical and active. The local departments of the Moulders' Union and the Metal Workers' Union demanded technical measures to protect workers from the hazardous dust. In addition, the company doctor oversaw the dusty settings and even suggested measures for dust suppression. Although some improvements were made, the dust hazard remained, especially for the unskilled workers who had been most exposed from the beginning. It was only after the Second World War, when there was a large labor shortage, that the company significantly improved the work environment. In the early 1950s, when the company underwent a major rationalization including a rebuilding of the foundry, it radically reduced the indoor dust hazard. However, as the castings varied greatly in size and shape, much of the dusty and dangerous work still was manually performed. As in many other steel foundries with a similar type of production, the solution was to move the dustiest parts of the process, such as the shake-out of moulds, sandblasting, and other heavy cleaning of the castings outdoors, thereby creating a new work site with both old and new health risks. The site was named "Karelia," after the Finnish province on the Russian (Soviet) border, because not only it was cold and windy, but also for the Finnish immigrants who worked there. In the 1960s and 1970s, the workplace became involved in nationwide governmental projects that targeted silica dust and other air pollutants, and even later, it was the subject of state-supported efforts to improve the work environment in the foundries (Thörnquist 1993; 2001, pp. 91-96).

THE PROBLEM

In 1931 silicosis was acknowledged in Sweden as an occupational disease, for which compensation might be awarded (SFS 1931:31). Since then, approximately 4,900 established cases of silicosis have been recorded. Over the decades, the share of cases of silicosis in advanced stages has decreased, and the disease has generally been diagnosed at older age. From the mid-1970s, the number of diagnosed new cases began to decline, and today, new cases are rare (Ahlmark and Gerhardsson 1981, p. 12; ISA 2001; Riksförsäkringsverket 1931-1979). According to Torsten Bruce, Axel Ahlmark and Åke Nyström, the most prominent silicosis experts in Sweden, a great many people must have contracted silicosis before the effects of pneumatic tools were fully realized. Even after 1931, it is most unlikely that all cases were discovered and reported, especially among retired workers (Ahlmark et al. 1956). Silicosis and illness caused by lead were the most common occupational diseases in the 1930s and early 1940s, and silicosis was the leading disease causing work-related disabilities and deaths. Consequently, silicosis generated the highest insurance costs as well (Lundh and Gunnarsson 1987, pp. 67-69; Nordin 1947). In the 1920s and 1930s silicosis emerged as a great problem in many industrial countries. Although the silicosis problem in Sweden did not develop as dramatically as it did, for example, in the United States, it became a longstanding threat to workers' health in many trades, such as the mining and stone industry and the iron and steel industry (cf. Rosenberg and Levenstein 1999; Rosner and Markowitz 1991). For afflicted individuals, as well as for communities, such as Österbybruk, where working life was strongly dependent on a "dusty trade," silicosis was indeed a disaster.

As the Österbybruk story indicates, there was a long delay between the initial recognition of silicosis as a problem and the taking of effective action. The reasons for this delay, however, are not immediately obvious, considering that seemingly favorable conditions existed to address the danger. During the period from 1932 to 1976, the Social Democratic Party was uninterruptedly in power. Moreover, the "Swedish model" of cooperation between strong and well-organized labor market parties and between them and the state dominated this period, and industrial safety was one of its main issues. Furthermore, the post-war period was a time of technical and economic progress and the building up of the Swedish welfare state, the "People's Home" *(Folkhemmet)*. Some companies considerably reduced the dust hazard, for example, through automation and encapsulation of dangerous work processes. Yet, as a whole, it was not until the 1970s that the silica dust hazard was brought under control.

The main purpose of this chapter is to explore the reasons for this delay. As such, it engages with the politics of both recognition and response. The handling of the silicosis problem during this period reflects in many ways the general development of occupational health and safety (OHS) policy in Sweden. It illustrates the historical pattern of interactions between scientists, doctors, the government, employers, unions, and workers over a specific hazard (silicosis), but situates those interactions within a broader political, economic, and institutional context.

Regarded as a social issue, the silicosis problem can best be understood from a political economy perspective that takes into account the conflicting economic interests between the parties involved in production and in society as a whole. Thus, from this vantage point, occupational health and safety is not a technical, neutral issue between the labor market parties, as has often been claimed in both the political and scholarly debate, but to a large extent depends on attitudes and interests (see also Levenstein and Woskie, 2002; Navarro 1983; Nichols and Tucker 2000; Thörnquist 1993, 2001).

Employers have been more sensitive to economic incentives to reduce accidents than to prevent diseases, as occupational accidents, unlike disease, cause direct disruption in production, raise labor turnover, and increase insurance costs in the short term. Moreover, management strategies to abate accidents have often implied that the workers' behavior is the main cause of accidents. This approach, propagated by for example the Tayloristic Safety Movement, has been highly influential in other industrial countries, and has been revitalized in modern OHS management strategies as well (cf. Nichols and Tucker 2000).

The prevention of industrial diseases, on the other hand, has generally required more radical and expensive investments. In addition, since such diseases develop usually after a long time has elapsed the question of their origin, as well as the problem of responsibility, has generally been a complicated matter. Therefore, occupational diseases have often been an even greater source of conflict between the parties in the labor market, and between the actors in the political arena than have accidents. Silicosis provides a good example.

Silica dust is one of the oldest occupational health risks and exposure to it has increased with industrialization, particularly during the inter-war years, due to the growth in mechanization and rationalization of production that had started some decades earlier. The use of pneumatic machines and tools, in particular, immensely increased dust levels. As silicosis is a disease of protracted latency, it took some time before its effects became visible on a larger scale (Ahlmark et al. 1960; Rosner and Markowitz 1991, ch. 1).

The concrete examples in this chapter are mainly from the iron and steel and mining industries. In iron and steel, quartz was used for the linings of furnaces, in the manufacturing of silicon alloys, and for the sand in the moulds.

When heated to the extremely high temperatures needed in the steel production processes, quartz could develop into other forms of crystalline silica (tridymite and cristobalite) as well, producing dust even more hazardous to inhale (Ahlmark et al. 1960, pp. 144-152). In addition, the production of steel castings generally needed dry moulding sand with a higher percentage of quartz than was used for the manufacture of iron castings. Moreover, the higher temperatures caused sand to stick to the surface, which made the steel castings difficult to clean, and thus forced the use of sandblasters and other pneumatic tools. As the example of Österbybruk illustrates, the production of castings could be strongly diversified, making it nearly impossible to automate or encapsulate all of the dangerous work operations.

In the mining industry, the growth in underground mining and the use of pneumatic drills were the main sources of silicosis risk. The risk varied considerably according to the sort of ore extracted and the composition of the enclosing rock. In all trades the risks varied also between different categories of workers, depending on their actual exposure to dust and its specific content, amount, and intensity. Thus, the timeframe for the development of disease varied greatly as well. Silicosis developed in moulders, often only after decades of exposure and the disease generally progressed slowly. For workers exposed to large amounts of dust with a high content of crystalline silica, for example, quartz crushers and sandblasters, or those who cleaned steel castings with pneumatic tools, silicosis could develop after a considerably shorter time, in extreme cases within a couple of years. Tuberculosis was a common complication in cases of intense exposure to dust of high quartz content, and in these cases, the disease generally progressed rapidly as well (Ahlmark et al. 1960, part I).

RECOGNITION OF SILICOSIS IN SWEDEN

As mentioned, silicosis is not a new disease. It has been known since antiquity that stone dust may cause lung illness. In the 17th and 18th centuries, scientists began to document more systematically their observations of such disease in, for example, mines, quarries, and knife factories. The Italian physician Bernardino Ramazzini (1633-1714), known as the father of occupational medicine, is perhaps the most noted but, in the international context, the Swedish scientist Carl von Linné (1707-1778) should also be mentioned. In the 1730s, he observed that farmers in the village of Orsa generally died young of lung disease. The reason, he surmised, was that the men quarried and manufactured sandstone grinding wheels during the winter season, and it was the heavy stone dust, particularly in the confines of the small sheds where manufacturing took place, that caused the disease. In the following century, other physicians made the same observations in Orsa, which was called "the village of widows and unsupported children" (Bruce 1942, pp. 14-32; Mascher 1930, pp. 145-147).

Pneumoconiosis (lung disease caused by the inhalation inorganic of dust) was widely discussed in the international medical literature in the late 19th and early 20th centuries. The long-term effects of the inhalation of stone dust were successively recognized through studies of workers in, for example, the British and German coalmines and stone industry and, not least, in the extremely quartz-rich South African gold mines. In the 1910s, the injurious effects of silica on lung tissue were finally confirmed, and "silicosis" was acknowledged in the medical literature as a non-infectious, work-related disease (Bruce 1942, pp. 14-32; Katz 1994; Nordin 1943, pp. 128-137).

Despite the early international and Swedish observations on the dangers of stone dust, there was little debate on the problem in the Swedish medical literature during the late 19th and early 20th centuries (Bruce 1942; Mascher 1930). Sweden lagged behind in the development of occupational medicine and occupational hygiene compared to several other countries that had been industrialized earlier and where the rationalization process proceeded more rapidly (Lundh and Gunnarsson 1987, pp. 66-72). Nor was the problem of stone dust a much-discussed subject within the trade unions until the 1930s (Thörnquist 1993, pp. 51-60; 2001, pp. 86-91). Protective labor legislation, as well as voluntary initiatives in this area, mainly concerned the problem of accidents. Moreover, in Sweden, as in many other countries, tuberculosis "camouflaged industrial dust as a source of disease" for a long time (Rosner and Markowitz 1991, p. 9). This meant that lung disease of any kind was generally attributed to workers' hereditary disposition, hygienic standard, and living conditions rather than to their working conditions (Ahlmark et al. 1960).

On the other hand, the fear of tuberculosis also helped the recognition of silicosis (cf. Rosenberg and Levenstein 1999). Observations made by company doctors and district medical officers on the relationship between stone dust and tuberculosis—or rather, what they thought was tuberculosis—were important early steps in the process of gaining recognition for silicosis. For example, at the beginning of the 20th century the company doctor Karl Edvard Hällsjö at the Domnarvet Ironworks, one of the largest in Sweden, found a very high death rate in tuberculosis among workers in the steel foundry who had been engaged in quartz crushing and cleaning of castings, and he thought that the dust helped to cause, or worsen tuberculosis. In line with his recommendation, the management therefore transferred workers in these settings to other jobs after one or two years (Pontén 1953, pp. 31-32).

In 1911, Dr. Nils Holmin published a comprehensive study of the frequency of tuberculosis among over 4,000 workers in the steel manufacturing industry in Eskilstuna. He found that the rate of tuberculosis, which in many cases was most likely silicosis or silicosis in combination with tuberculosis, was five times higher among the grinders, who used grinding wheels of sandstone, than among other workers. Once Holmin realized it was the dust that was the main cause of disease, he made detailed suggestions for protection against dust through watering of the grinding wheels, ventilation, and protective masks (Ahlmark et al. 1960, pp. 300-301; Holmin 1911).

Moreover, the results of a local study provided the basis for the legal recognition of silicosis as an occupational disease in Sweden. The first *Insurance Act for Certain Occupational Diseases*, passed in 1929, included, among other things, injuries caused by arsenic, lead, mercury, and phosphorous, and their compounds, but not silicosis (SFS 1929, no. 131-133). That same year the Swedish Parliament (*Riksdagen*) had rejected a bill to include silicosis in the act, mainly because medical experts did not consider it possible to clearly distinguish silicosis from other lung diseases. Nor did the ILO Convention issued in 1925 on compensation for occupational diseases include silicosis. Then in 1930, Willy Mascher, a physician at a sanatorium in the west of Sweden, conducted a medical investigation of about 30 workers in a silica brick factory, including a quartz quarry and quartz mill in the region. He showed that almost all workers who had worked with quartz for more than two years had contracted silicosis, and he claimed that silicosis could be distinctively diagnosed through x-rays. In his report, Mascher also made concrete suggestions on medical prophylaxis of silicosis based on methods being used in, for example, South African gold mines and the German stone industry (Mascher 1930). Mascher's results forced an amendment to the Swedish *Insurance Act for Certain Occupational Diseases*, which from 1931 included silicosis (SFS 1931:31). In 1934, silicosis was also inscribed in the revised ILO Convention on Workmen's Compensation for Occupational Diseases (ILO 1934).

However, the existence of legislation covering silicosis, or any other occupational disease, did not mean that it was easy for workers to receive compensation. Originally, the law only applied to cases of silicosis diagnosed after the act had come into force in 1931, and where the worker's exposure to silica dust occurred within one year of the diagnosis. In 1937, this period was extended to 10 years because of the protracted latency of silicosis. In addition, applications had to be submitted to the insurance companies or to the superior governmental authority, the National Insurance Institute *(Riksförsäkringsanstalten)*, within two years of silicosis being diagnosed. Compensation could be awarded in cases where working capacity was considered reduced by 10% or more, but the Institute was very restrictive in their assessment of silicosis and other occupational diseases (Nordin 1943, ch. 5).

The formal acknowledgment of silicosis as an occupational disease did not immediately result in the workplace parties becoming commonly aware of the silicosis problem, although it had been known for a long time in some industries, for example, in the pottery industry and in the sandstone industry, that dust caused lung injuries. Tuberculosis still overshadowed silicosis as the major pulmonary disease. In companies which mechanized late, such as in many foundries, the parties and the company doctors seemed almost not to have heard of silicosis until some workers were diagnosed with it. According to Johan Pontén, a district medical officer and a well-known forerunner in the field of silicosis prevention, the situation was the same in the mining industry (Ahlmark et al. 1960, pp. 55-57, 245-250; Pontén 1975, pp. 11-12).

When the first case of silicosis appeared in Österbybruk in 1933, it was a surprise not only for the workers but obviously also for the company doctor, Ola Oredsson. The afflicted worker was a 43-year-old sandblaster who had contracted silicosis after a very short and intense exposure to quartz dust. Initially, Oredsson suspected tuberculosis, but in late autumn 1935 silicosis complicated by tuberculosis was finally confirmed. According to the insurance company, the diagnosis came too late for compensation, since silicosis in this cases must have been already evident to the doctor in summer 1933. However, Oredsson claimed that at that time he had had no experience of silicosis. It was only after the sandblaster's death in 1936 that he was granted compensation, which his widow received. The public labor inspector was later sent for to examine the working conditions in the shed where the sandblasting had been carried out. However, he did not consider the worksite as particularly hazardous if the workers wore protection masks. Thus, he emphasized the workers' responsibility rather than the employers' and he paid no attention to the fact that the masks often provided weak protection and were uncomfortable to wear. This case was not unique in the history of silicosis in Sweden (Thörnquist 1993, pp. 116-121; cf. Nordin 1943, pp. 274-305; Pontén 1975, pp. 11-12).

The sandblaster's illness and death became the start of the identification of dusty and hazardous settings in Österbybruk, with the left-wing trade unions and Dr. Oredsson as the driving forces. In addition to the furnaces and the steel foundry, there was a quartz crushing shop, a knife factory, and an associated factory that produced sandstone grinding wheels, which all generated large quantities of dangerous dust. The local departments of the Moulders' Union in the region cooperated unofficially to inform themselves about silicosis and its prevention and, nationally the central board began to collect information on the prevalence of silicosis among the members. However, in many workplaces, especially those without an active union presence or without company doctors committed to the problem of silicosis, the problem remained unknown or neglected for many years (Thörnquist 1993, pp. 51-60, 117-119; 2001, p. 81).

The disease only became more commonly known in Sweden as a result of a nationwide study on silicosis conducted in the 1930s. The first ILO conference on silicosis held in Johannesburg in 1930 recommended international cooperation in research (ILO 1930). The Swedish government supported the idea, but provided no special grants for the purpose. Instead, the investigation, consisting of a pilot study and a nationwide study, had to depend on external grants. Among those organizations supporting it were the National Association against Tuberculosis (Nationalföreningen mot tuberkulos), the Swedish Trade Union Confederation (Landsorganisationen, LO), the Swedish Iron Works' Association, (Järnbruksförbundet), the employers' trade organization, and a couple of major companies. The large-scale study was conducted at the request of the Employers' Mutual Accident Insurance Company *(Arbetsgivarnas Ömsesidiga Olycksfallsförsäkringsbolag)*, which also had a clear economic interest in gaining knowledge on the spread of the disease (Bruce 1942, pp. 7-13).

Torsten Bruce, a physician at the Serafimer Hospital in Stockholm, carried out the investigations between 1934 and 1939. The project comprised about 2,500 of the estimated 6,500 workers exposed to silica dust in different trades, but only a few retired workers were examined. According to the final report published in 1942, about 600 or 24% of the examined workers had silicosis. Bruce's investigation showed that silicosis appeared frequently among workers in the quartz mines and quartz crushing works. All of the examined workers who had worked below ground for 10 years or more had contracted silicosis. The disease was also a great problem in the iron ore mines, especially in the north of Sweden where around 40% of the examined workers were afflicted. In the steelworks and steel foundries, 20-40% had silicosis among the examined furnace masons, moulders, cleaners of the castings, and sandblasters. Among the examined ceramic workers, the rate was around 23%. The most serious cases appeared among quartz crushers, drillers below ground, sandblasters, and other cleaners of steel castings, who could develop end stage silicosis after 15 years of exposure. Bruce concluded that silicosis had never been as prevalent and serious in Sweden as it was in the 1930s, and he assumed that the disease might progress even after exposure to dust was discontinued (Bruce 1942). In many countries, such as Britain, Germany, and the United States, silicosis was a great problem in the granite industry (Rosenberg and Levenstein 1999). In Sweden, however, no cases had been reported to the authorities at the time of Bruce's investigations. Later, silicosis experts supposed that variation in the level of mechanization mainly explained the great international differences in the recorded cases (Ahlmark et al. 1960, pp. 126-127). However, in this context, it is also worth mentioning that the granite industry was declining rapidly in the 1930s, as well as during the world wars (SOU 1949:44).

REGULATING WORKERS OR REGULATING WORKING CONDITIONS?

How, then, did the government respond to the alarming reports of the prevalence of silicosis, and what were the consequences for the workers involved and for the general development of silicosis prevention? In light of Mascher's and Bruce's results and concrete recommendations on medical prophylaxis, and influenced by international experiences, the government issued a regulation concerning medical supervision in 1938 (SFS 1938:711). It included medical examination and surveillance of workers in settings with "extremely high risk" *(synnerlig fara)* for silicosis, both when they signed on for jobs and periodically thereafter. According to the regulation, workers who had some kind of illness or infirmity that could make them more predisposed to silicosis—particularly those with tuberculosis or an hereditary disposition for the disease, chronic bronchitis, heart problems, deformations of the chest, and nasal breathing problems—should not start work in dusty settings. Even deficient personal care was reason enough for the exclusion of workers from dusty jobs, since these persons were supposed to be careless in general and not able to follow safety instructions. In cases where silicosis was established or suspected, workers were to be transferred to dust-free jobs. The National Insurance Institute, which at the time supervised the Labor Inspectorate (*Yrkeinspketionen*), decided, in consultation with the medical authorities which trades and workplaces should be subject to medical supervision, as well as the intervals for the examinations. The examinations were to be organized and financed by employers and by governmental grants (Nordin 1943, pp. 250-265). Hence, an important aim was to limit insurance costs as well.

The purpose of medical supervision was also to provide information on the effectiveness of technical dust prevention measures undertaken by the companies. The physicians, who the medical authorities authorized to give the physical examinations, were required to report deficiencies to the public labor inspectors (SFS 1938:711). However, this assumed that they had a certain amount of knowledge about technical conditions, and that they acted independently from business interests. Moreover, the results of the examinations generally reflected the risks that had existed decades before, rather than current conditions (Ahlmark 1960, pp. 148-149). The regulations concerning dust prevention were mainly formulated in general terms, making them difficult to enforce. It was only in the early 1970s that the National Board of Occupational Safety and Health (*Arbetarskyddsstyrelsen*), established in 1949 as the supervising government authority for workers' protection and working hours, began to issue directions on annual dust measurement and technical preventive measures aimed at the prevention of silicosis specifically (Ekman 1997, pp. 2-3). As well, although the ambitions and attitudes of the governmental labor inspectors could vary, they traditionally pursued a cooperative policy of advising and persuading (Arbetarskyddsstyrelsen 1999).

The government regulation on medical prevention reflected the predominant policy of prevention in OHS, which implied that the individual worker's physical and mental disposition and behavior were the crucial factors determining the risk of workplace injury. This policy, which has been called "disposition prevention" (*dispositionsprevention*), aimed to create "safe persons," rather than "safe places" (cf. Gallagher 1997). The opposite, "exposure prevention" (*expositionsprevention*), was based on the conception that the work environment may cause illness and accidents, and it implied that preventive measures should focus more on the creation of "safe places" (Didrichsen and Jahnlert 1981; Gustafsson 1994, pp. 265-266; Thörnquist 2001, pp. 79-82).

The formulation "extremely high risk" meant that the regulation on medical supervision applied only to settings where there was a documented risk that silicosis progressed and caused disability among employees and insurance costs. In other settings, "mild silicosis" could develop after long-term exposure. Thus, in trades and workplaces that were not covered by the regulation, as well as in trades where the first periodical examination was to be carried out after 10, 15, or even 20 years, there was a great risk that dust prevention measures were delayed. For example, until the late 1960s, the regulation did not include workers in iron foundries or in the granite industry because of the few cases reported there. Yet, the dust hazard increased with continuous mechanization and, in the 1950s and 1960s, these trades developed serious problems with silicosis.

The focus on medical prophylaxis mainly benefitted employers. Although it was important to discover silicosis as early as possible, and stop exposure to dust for these workers, silicosis in an initial stage has a tendency to progress even after exposure ends. Since it generally takes decades to develop silicosis, symptoms were often discovered very late, and thus the regulation did not *prevent* silicosis. Worse still, the regulation legitimized worker exposure to silica dust and the possibility that they would contract silicosis, not least, in settings where the silicosis risk was not regarded as "extremely high." Since silicosis in an initial stage normally did not affect working capacity, and the disease often appeared only after the worker had been retired, the silicosis risk in these settings caused little problem for the employers related to production and insurance costs. For the workers, however, there was always a risk that the disease would progress.

The regulation on medical supervision remained essentially unchanged until 1963, when its provisions were extended to workplaces with "special risk" (*särskild fara*) for silicosis. This revision, however, produced little change. Now the regulation was also made to apply to other kinds of pneumoconiosis—asbestosis, aluminosis, talcosis, siderosis, berylliosis, anthracosis, and hard-metal pneumoconiosis—that since 1950 were covered by the law on industrial injury insurance. From the beginning, the main principles of the regulation also applied to diseases caused by lead and, from 1949, benzene (Ahlmark 1967, ch. 8; SFS 1963: 660). Until the late 1960s, the authorities prescribed medical supervision of workers exposed to silica dust at about 100 companies and workplaces; mainly within the mining industry and the steelworks and steel foundries, but also within the sandstone and quartz industries, the ceramic industry, and some workplaces where sandblasting was conducted. Many larger companies provided voluntary physical examinations through the company health service. Yet, the extent of this control should not be overestimated. Most companies were small ones, for example, the iron foundries and those within the stone industry. In the mid-1960s, approximately 120 companies conducted voluntary examinations periodically (Ahlmark 1967, pp. 142-146). It was only in the 1970s that the system of company health services spread more generally (Lundh and Gunnarsson 1987, pp. 105-108).

Overall, the regulation concerning medical supervision was problematic. It was still difficult to diagnose silicosis, especially in an early stage, and it was not always easy to recruit competent physicians for the task, particularly in remote places in the country. Moreover, transfer of workers caused difficulties. For example, for workers like moulders, who had received many years of training and who had great professional pride, the transfer itself could be a tragedy, even in cases where they suffered no wage reduction. In Österbybruk, most of the proud craftsmen in the foundry refused to leave their regular jobs. However, for moulders, silicosis generally progressed very slowly. For the many afflicted unskilled workers who were exposed to dust at higher levels, the only option was often to accept a transfer to less well-paid jobs, which weakened their position in the labor market even more, and caused conflicts between the local parties (Thörnquist 1993, pp. 121-129).

Female workers were not mentioned explicitly in the regulation on medical supervision. However, women were often excluded by law or by social practice from many of the workplaces where exposure to silica was common. For example, the *Workers' Protection Act*, passed in 1900, prohibited women from working below ground, in mines and in quarries (Karlsson 1997). According to the statistics, comparatively few women contracted silicosis. Of course, many women could have been afflicted before the statistics on silicosis began in 1931, and even later, but during the period 1931-1975, slightly more than 50 of the recorded cases of silicosis in Sweden were attributable to women workers, who had worked mainly in the pottery industry. In most cases, however, the disease progressed to advanced stages (Ahlmark and Gerhardsson 1981, pp. 32-35).

The silicosis problem provided new potential arguments for the policy of protecting women by excluding them from certain jobs. In the international medical literature in 1930s and 1940s, it was often claimed that silicosis progressed more rapidly for women than for men. In a comment on the governmental regulation of 1938, John Nordin, one of the main experts on labor legislation in Sweden, wrote that women should not work in such settings at all (Nordin 1943, pp. 243-250). It is unknown, however, to what extent women were excluded from jobs due to the silicosis risk specifically.

There are interesting parallels between gendered exclusionary laws and practices and the regulation on medical supervision. In both cases, the focus is on the worker rather than the environment, and the logic of disposition prevention is clearly illustrated. In the matter of gendered protective regulations, the exclusion of women from certain jobs not only weakened their position in the labor market, but also potentially harmed the health of men by allowing them to be exposed to high levels of risk. Once a female norm was adopted, exposures for all workers might be reduced. The *Work Environment Act* of 1977 ended formal restriction on women's work. Yet, as Karlsson has shown, remnants of gender-based protection still remain. According to the new provision for work with lead, issued by the National Board of Occupational Safety and Health in 1992, the limit permitted for lead in the bloodstream of female workers under age 50 was half of the limit allowed for male workers. The reason for changing the regulations, which earlier had been the same for women and men, was the injurious effects of lead on foetuses (Karlsson 2001).

The guiding principle of the government's regulation on medical supervision to prevent silicosis was the same as that of gendered protective labor legislation; it protected certain groups of workers by excluding them from the dustiest settings, while the other workers continued to be exposed and ran the risk of being diseased, perhaps only after they retired. Hence, rather than regulating the working conditions, for which the employers had the ultimate responsibility, the government regulated the workers. This policy contributed to the delay of the general development of effective silicosis prevention. In the 1970s, mandatory as well as voluntary medical supervision of workers in dusty settings was radically extended, at the same time as the governmental control of the dust situation in the companies increased (Arbetarskyddsstyrelsen 1982, pp. 129-130; Ekman 1997, pp. 4-5).

Hence, for a long time, the governmental policy concerning silicosis prevention weakly protected workers. The tardy progress toward an OHS policy that focused more on the creation "safe places," which implied increased governmental control of the dust situation in companies, was complicated by the Swedish model's policy of cooperation between the state, capital, and labor, since it was difficult to force stricter government regulation and control of the work environment in opposition to the employers' interests. To explain these further developments, however, it is necessary to provide a short overview of the organization of OHS within the Swedish industrial relations system.

THE OHS SYSTEM IN POST-WAR SWEDEN

In the 1930s and 1940s the interest of labor market parties and the state in industrial safety increased considerably. The main driving force was the increase in accidents that came about in the wake of greater mechanization and rationalization in industry. As mentioned earlier, OHS was one of the main issues addressed in the so-called Swedish model of industrial relations. This institutional framework, which included both a welfare model and a negotiation model, was built on long tradition, but had its breakthrough in the progressive industrial era after World War II. Its purpose was to promote peaceful labor relations, economic development, full employment, and social reforms (Johansson and Magnusson 1998, ch. 5; Kjellberg 1998).

At the core of the Swedish model was the principle of centralized self-regulation. This meant that the labor market parties should handle labor market issues as far as possible without governmental interference, which employers especially wanted to avoid. In 1942, the Swedish Employers' Confederation (*Svenska Arbetsgivareföreningen, SAF*) and its counterpart, the LO, concluded a central agreement in which the main principles for the local organization of industrial safety were laid down. At the same time, the LO and the SAF established the Joint Industrial Safety Council (*Arbetarskyddsnämnden*) as the central body for cooperation, information, and training in this field (Ekström 1992). The OHS agreement was the first peak level agreement for cooperation that followed in the wake of the general agreement for the "Swedish model" of cooperation and self-regulation settled in Saltsjöbaden in 1938. Other central agreements concluded in the 1940s concerned works councils, apprentice education, and time-and-motion studies. These agreements were all mainly recommendations. As regards industrial safety, the LO had preferred binding collective agreements at the industry level and, therefore, the LO also advocated stricter protective labor legislation. Thus, the reinforced *Workers' Protection Act*, which came into force in 1949, codified the main regulations laid down in the central agreement, including the principles of cooperation between the parties. In that way, the system of safety representatives and joint safety committees, which had spread rapidly in the 1940s, became legally mandated as well (SFS 1949:1, 1949:108).

Another keystone in the Swedish model was tripartite cooperation between the state and the main labor market parties. This corporatist system included the parties' representation on the boards and commissions of government OHS authorities, such as the National Board of Occupational Safety and Health and the National Institute of Occupational Medicine (*Arbetsmedicinska Institutet*), as well as in temporary committees and projects.

The *Workers' Protection Act* of 1949 strengthened the Labor Inspectorate, which was empowered to issue injunctions, in addition to prohibitions (a power it had issue since 1938). In practice, however, the Inspectorate seldom used these measures. For example, in 1953 the labor inspectors made over 42,000 visits and issued more than 12,000 improvement notices, many of which were neglected. Yet, only 26 injunctions and 33 prohibitions were issued that year (Arbetarskyddsstyrelsen 1999, pp. 17-18). The trade unions often criticized the Labor Inspectorate for pursuing a non-interventionist policy toward the employers, which led to a governmental overhaul of the Inspectorate in the mid-1950s. The labor inspectors were ordered to be stricter and, if necessary, to use coercive measures. Furthermore, regional boards were instituted in the 11 inspectorate districts with representatives from labor market parties and local governments. The boards had an advising role, but they also allowed for greater public control of the inspectors' work. Overall, however, the policy of persuasion and cooperation prevailed, which also was in line with the general idea of the Swedish model of industrial relations (Arbetarskyddsstyrelsen 1999, pp. 24-25).

The problem of occupational accidents dominated OHS in Sweden even during the post-war period. The Joint Industrial Safety Council's first nationwide campaign and mass training program "*Safety Pays*" (*Arbetarskydd lönar sig*), published in 1954, exemplified this orientation, which the employers in particular preferred. Influenced by the legacy of the Safety Movement and international research on the "human factor" (which theorized that a small number of persons cause a great number of accidents), it concentrated on the problem of accidents and pursued a policy of creating "safe persons." The Council's second campaign, *"Why does it happen?" (Varför händer det?)*, published in 1958, still focused on the problem of accidents, but the causes were discussed in a broader social and organizational context, which reflected a more analytical approach influenced by industrial psychology. Only later, in the 1960s, did the problem of diseases, including silicosis, gain more attention (Ekström 1992; Forssman 1958).

Yet, occupational medicine and occupational hygiene also developed steadily after World War II, albeit from a low starting point. One reason for this was that the number of diseases covered by the *Insurance Act for Certain Occupational Diseases* increased continuously. Since it took some time before these disciplines were established in the country, influences from abroad, in particular from Germany, Italy, Britain, and the United States, were important. With regard to occupational hygiene, developments in the United States served as the main model. In 1938, the National Institute of Public Health (*Statens Institut för Folkhälsan*) was established with considerable financial support from the American Rockefeller Foundation, which sponsored the development of public health in many countries (Gerhardsson 2002, pp. 12-14), also as part of an effort to consolidate American interests in Europe.

Like the American public health institutes, the purpose of the Swedish National Institute of Public Health was to carry out applied research, provide education, and conduct investigations at the request of industry, the authorities, unions, and others. The institute, established as a government authority, had four departments, one of which dealt with occupational medicine and occupational hygiene. During the first decades of its existence, the Department of Occupational Hygiene was mainly a small medical institution with a rapidly growing number of commissions and tasks. However, as in many other countries, occupational hygiene developed from a medical sub-discipline into an independent and interdisciplinary field for research and engineering. The Department continued its contacts with American institutions, not least through its head, Dr. Sven Forssman, and many Swedish professionals in occupational medicine and occupational hygiene trained at American universities and Public Health Institutes. In the 1950s and 1960s, the Department of Occupational Hygiene became strongly involved in nationwide investigations of silicosis, at the same time that the role of technical experts in the treatment of the silicosis problem increased (Gerhardsson 1992).

SILICOSIS IN EARLY POST-WAR SWEDEN

In the 1930s, the prevention of silicosis was primarily the concern of a few medical researchers, such as Mascher and Bruce, the authorities, the company doctors, and the local labor market actors, for which the trade unions usually were the driving force. During the post-war period, however, there was increasing professionalization in the field of OHS in Sweden as well as in many other industrial countries. The growth of occupational medicine and hygiene at the National Institute of Public Health, and the establishment of the National Board of Occupational Safety and Health in 1949, reflected this development, as did the hiring of safety engineers by bigger companies. The increasing involvement of experts in OHS seemed sometimes to decrease the dialogue on silicosis between the parties at the company level. In Österbybruk, for example, the workers were involved little in the decision to move the dustiest parts of the work process outdoors. Instead, it was a matter for the engineers and the labor inspector. Overall, however, the Swedish trade union movement grew stronger after the war and, at the industry level, the commitment to various aspects of the silicosis issue steadily increased. Since the unions did not manage to get any guarantees for silicosis prevention through negotiations, they put the question on their political agenda. Thus, they also needed more data on the development of silicosis in different trades. Some unions conducted their own investigations, but they also needed support, mainly from the medical experts, to legitimate their demands (Thörnquist 2001, pp. 89-90).

After Bruce's studies in the 1930s, however, it was not until the mid-1950s that silicosis again became the focus of a large-scale investigation, even though the number of cases increased. An exception was a separate study of dust problems in the mining industry conducted by the Swedish Steel Producers' Association (*Jernkontoret*) in the early 1940s (Pontén 1947). Why, then, was the problem not followed up earlier? Despite the formal establishment of the Department of Occupational Hygiene, the Joint Industrial Safety Council, and the settling of a central agreement, OHS was not a high-priority issue during the war, despite the fact that the exceptional war-time conditions in production and working life implied great risks for workers' health. The state planned and partly directed industry, often for the purpose of producing armaments. Untrained, temporary employees replaced those who were mobilized for military service. In addition, trade blockades forced reliance on hazardous substitute substances, such as producer gas and benzene. Thus, widespread fear of carbon monoxide and benzene poisoning risks dominated both public debate and the work of the Department of Occupational Hygiene at the National Institute of Public Health for many years after the war as well (Gerhardsson 1992, pp. 22-25).

Moreover, as the silicosis expert Axel Ahlmark later recapitulated the development, the implementation of the government regulation on medical supervision created a general feeling that the silicosis problem was under control (Ahlmark and Gerhardsson 1981, p. 49). Nevertheless, the trade unions concerned with silicosis called for a new nationwide investigation. The increasing number of silicosis cases worried not only the unions, but also the insurance institutes. Moreover, high insurance costs and labor shortages contributed to a rising interest among the employers, at least in the larger firms, to bring the silicosis problem under control (Thörnquist 2001, pp. 84-90). In the mid-1950s

Ahlmark, who had succeeded Forssman as the head of the Department of Occupational Hygiene at the National Institute of Public Health, started an epidemiological study together with Torsten Bruce and Åke Nyström, head of the Department of Industrial Medicine at the Södersjukhuset. Both the LO, several trade unions, and the SAF provided grants for this purpose, as did the state and the National Association against Tuberculosis (Ahlmark et al. 1960).

The epidemiological investigation included approximately 2,220 cases of silicosis and mixed dust silicosis registered at the insurance institutes during the period 1931-1956 (Ahlmark et al. 1960). The study also included other kinds of pneumoconiosis registered in the industrial injury insurance system. With regard to silicosis, the report showed about 1000 cases caused after 1930, which indicated that the measures taken to prevent silicosis were insufficient. Furthermore, the study identified new hazardous workplaces. It also confirmed that silicosis continued to develop even after exposure to silica dust was discontinued. The iron and steel industry represented almost 40% of the registered cases during the period 1931-1956. The mining, quarrying, and tunneling industries had a somewhat lower share of silicosis cases, while the ceramic industry represented around 13% of established cases, reflecting a clear improvement of the dust situation in these plants.

One of the most conspicuous results of the study was that the number of silicosis cases had increased sharply in iron foundries, while decreasing in the steel foundries, where preventive measures had been taken since the 1930s. Still there were comparatively few recorded cases in the granite industry, which had experienced economic recovery after World War II. However, the risk of silicosis increased considerably with the use of pneumatic tools and machines, and in enclosed workplaces. The study found that with regard to other forms of pneumoconiosis, asbestosis was a growing threat, since the industrial use of asbestos had increased rapidly. Ahlmark and his colleagues recommended that all kinds of pneumoconiosis should be included in the governmental regulation on medical supervision. They also recommended an extension of the regulation on medical supervision to workers in all settings with risks for pneumoconiosis (Ahlmark et al. 1960, pp. 379-380; SFS 1963:660). As mentioned, a radical extension did not occur until the 1970s.

THE LAISVALL TRAGEDY

The report's most striking example of the great dust hazard in the mining industry was the explosive development of silicosis in the Laisvall lead-mine in the 1940s. The mine was located in the province of Lappland in northwestern Sweden. Since the mid-1920s the owner, the Boliden Mining Company, had extracted gold and other kinds of sulphide ore, such as copper, arsenic, and cobalt in the vast Skellefte Ore Fields in the neighbor province of Västerbotten. Central management was situated in the mining community of Boliden, "the Swedish Klondike," 250 kilometers south east of Laisvall. The lead ore deposit in Laisvall was discovered in 1938, but was not regarded as profitable until the war, when there was a shortage of lead. The government became greatly interested in the extraction, and contracted with the company to produce a certain quantity annually from 1943-1946. As the extraction was meant to be a temporary project, little attention was paid to the hygienic conditions in the mine. Yet, the homogeneous ore in this mine contained 85 to 90% quartz. After the war, it was obvious that the ore deposit in Laisvall was much larger than expected, and the company expanded successively its highly profitable operation, becoming one of the largest lead mines in Europe until 2001, when it finally shut down. During its first years approximately 150 workers were employed, but as extraction increased the workforce was enlarged steadily in the 1940s, and labor turnover was high. Working conditions seem to have been about the same throughout the decade. The ventilation system was highly insufficient, and hardly any other effective dust prevention measures were undertaken. Until the late 1940s, when several cases of silicosis were discovered, blasting occurred in the daytime and dry-drilling was carried out in addition to the more commonly-used wet-drilling in the company's mines (Ahlmark et al. 1960, pp. 31-42, 338; Kavian-Lanjani 1999; Norviit 1959; Pontén 1975, pp. 48-56).

In Laisvall, silicosis appeared after very short exposure, on average after five-and a-half years, and was diagnosed at a very low average age, 37 years. Among the slightly more than 40 cases reported up to 1975 (comprising miners who mainly had worked in Laisvall), as many as 32 were diagnosed between 1949 and 1953. In the early 1950s considerable technical-preventive and medical control measures were eventually taken, and after 1960 only a few new cases appeared. By 1960, the disease had progressed for one-third of those diagnosed, and 15% had reached the final painful stage. By 1975 seven workers had died from silicosis or silicosis complicated by tuberculosis. Among the first 15 cases observed, 20 years later no less than 13 had progressed, and six had reached the final stage (Ahlmark et al. 1960, pp. 31-42; Ahlmark and Gerhardsson 1981, pp. 25-30).

Even though the mining operation was a result of the wartime crisis, and was located in a remote place, it is hard to understand why nothing was done about dust problems earlier. While the reported cases of silicosis had been relatively few in the lead mines, the extremely high quartz content in the Laisvall mine was known to the authorities, as well as to the local parties. According to the government regulation on medical supervision, the first periodical examinations of the miners in Laisvall, as well as in the company's mines in the Skellefte Ore Fields, were to be conducted after seven years of employment. Workers in quartz mines (below ground) and in quartz cross works were examined after one year, while workers in the iron ore mines normally were examined after 10 years (Pontén 1975, pp. 49-50).

Since the early 1940s, the Swedish Miners' Union, which had raised awareness of the silicosis problem in the trade, represented the Laisvall miners. Although not all miners were members of the union, and labor-management relations sometimes were strained, there existed a working joint safety committee and there were several safety representatives in the mine and associated facilities (minutes of the local department of the Miners' Union in Laisvall 1941-1950). Nevertheless, the dust problem was hardly discussed until 1949, when several cases were diagnosed. The union and the joint safety committee dealt mainly with great accident risks and with poor sanitary conditions in the mine (ibid; annual reports of the local department of the Miners' Union in Laisvall 1946-1950).

Even more remarkable in the Laisvall case was that the Boliden Mining Company had been a leader in silicosis prevention in Sweden in the 1930s. During this decade, Johan Pontén was employed as a district medical officer and mining physician in Boliden. As mentioned, he became a well-known expert on silicosis prevention in Sweden. Pontén, who previously had worked in the province of Dalsland, had become interested in the silicosis problem through his colleague, the pioneer Willi Mascher, so when the first case appeared in Boliden in 1933 he was already familiar with the disease. In cooperation with the management and the workers, Pontén immediately started an ambitious program for medical and technical preventive measures. The neo-paternalistic welfare system of the Boliden Mining Company meant, among other things, that the workers in these young and remote mining communities were entitled to free medical treatment. In accordance with Mascher's recommendations on medical supervision, the workers were examined when they were employed and periodically thereafter. Hence, the main principles for examinations were the same as those stated in the governmental regulation that came into force about 10 years later, but Pontén made the examinations more frequently. In addition, medical supervision was supplemented by considerable technical measures to prevent dust development.

When the first case of silicosis was discovered, the company bought an X-ray apparatus and, after some years, Pontén started continuous dust measurements in the company's mines using a conimeter, which counted the number of dust grains in the air. Management reorganized the contract with Pontén so he could concentrate more on preventive health care, including surveillance of the hygienic conditions in the company's mines in the Skellefte Ore Field. He went down in the mines to carry out dust measurements and he provided concrete advice on dust prevention. Before extraction started in a new mine, he carefully examined the dust situation together with the engineers. The Boliden Mining Company was among the first companies in the country to take silicosis prevention measures to this extent. The company was also one of those that financially supported Bruce's investigations in the 1930s, and Pontén and some representatives from the company management in Boliden had a leading position on the committee that conducted the investigation on mineral dust at the Swedish Steel Producers' Association in the early 1940s. In short, the routines that had been established in Boliden in the 1930s served as a model for the introduction of dust measurements in other companies. However, in the 1940s, the approach of the Boliden Mining Company changed radically (Pontén 1947; 1975, pp. 9-13, 39-40).

Shortly after the extraction had begun in Laisvall in 1943, Pontén left the company for another position in central Sweden and, about the same time, a new company management team took over in Boliden. Prior to Laisvall, Pontén diagnosed slightly more than 10 workers with silicosis, but the National Insurance Institute acknowledged only five of them. Because they had worked mainly in other mines, they were not recorded as cases caused in the Boliden Mining Company's operations. The Institute felt that Pontén was far too ambitious in diagnosing silicosis. Probably this opinion also influenced the new management in Boliden and the local management in Laisvall. Moreover, it seems to have influenced the authorities' view of the risk for silicosis in Laisvall mine. The new management was not similarly committed to dust prevention and lacked the same practical knowledge of mining. After the regulation on medical supervision came into force in the mining industry in 1943, management dissolved the old voluntary routines for silicosis prevention. According to Pontén, the periodical dust measurements that had been carried out continuously since 1937 were discontinued as well, and no initial investigation of the dust situation was carried out in the Laisvall mine before extraction started (Pontén 1975, pp. 48-50).

In the early 1940s, the Boliden Mining Company began to dismantle its paternalist welfare system, including free medical care for wage workers. District medical officers located in the different mining communities replaced the central mining physician, and the doctors were contracted mainly to provide accident care and to conduct the silicosis examinations prescribed by government. The company employed a central safety engineer to supervise the hygienic conditions in the mines. However, the silicosis problem was no longer a high-priority issue. In Laisvall, the local management obviously neglected the serious dust hazard, as did the legendary doctor there, Einar Wallqvist. Being a provincial medical officer in a vast district of Lapland, and, in addition, a well-known folklorist, writer, and painter, his main interest was not occupational medicine (Pontén 1975, pp. 48-50; Annual reports from the local department of the Miners' Union no 110 in Laisvall, 1946-1951). This was symptomatic of the difficulties of recruiting medical experts to work in remote places.

When the extraction in Laisvall started in 1943, Pontén warned of the high silicosis risk. In 1945, when the company invited him to Boliden, Laisvall, and the other mining communities to talk about health risks in the mining industry, he repeated the warning. With regard to the extremely high quartz content in Laisvall mine, Pontén emphasized that the threshold limit for dust particles in the air should not exceed 200-300 dust grains per cm^3 air, which was half of the limit that he had recommended for the other mines (Pontén 1947). In the following year, after dust measurements had been carried out, some of the safety representatives in Skellefte Ore Fields required that medical examinations should be performed in the company's mines as soon as possible. However, the National Insurance Institute did not consider it necessary to hold the examinations earlier than prescribed, since no case of silicosis had been registered up to that time among workers who had only worked in the Boliden Mining Company's mines (Pontén 1975, pp. 49-51).

Thus, despite the high quartz content, especially in the Laisvall mine, the interval was not changed. The management, the safety engineer, and the doctors relied on the authorities' judgment. The decision not to change the time for the first periodic examination was important for the further development of the silicosis problem in Laisvall, because it confirmed the opinion that workers contracted silicosis only after very long exposure to silica dust (*Gruvarbetaren* November and December, 1969). This may also help to explain the silence of the union in Laisvall until the first cases of silicosis were confirmed.

In 1949, when the great silicosis risk in Laisvall was obvious to all parties, the Boliden Mining Company engaged Pontén as a consultant to carry out dust measurements in the mine and to organize silicosis prevention. By that time, both the local manager in Laisvall and the central safety engineer had left the company, and their successors were mandated to take vigorous measures to solve the dust problems. The results of the dust measurements confirmed the extremely high silicosis risk in the mine, as well as in the crush works and concentration plant. According to Pontén, the dense damp that developed through wet-drilling in such extremely hard ore was hazardous to inhale as well, since the small water drops contained particles of silica dust even less than 0,002 mm. These particles were difficult to discover through dust measurement with the help of the conimeter, but the phenomenon had long been known in knife factories which used wet grinding wheels of sandstone (Pontén 1975, pp. 49-57). Along with the enlargement of the mine, which mainly consisted of a vast underground room, the ventilation problem had grown worse. In some sites, the only supply of fresh air was the pipeline for compressed air (Pontén 1975; Norviit 1959, 1962). Now, the ventilation in the mine was radically improved, continuous dust measurements and dust suppression by watering was started, and a general prohibition was issued against dry drilling (minutes of the Joint Industrial Safety Committee in Laisvall, November 22, 1949). This meant that technically the silicosis problem in Laisvall was solved mainly through simple methods that had been known for a long time in the Boliden Mining Company.

The medical examinations were also intensified and, in the mid-1950s, the company employed a medical expert, Lembit Norviit, whose main task was preventive health care with special regard to the dust hazard. However, as the industrial welfare system was further specialized between the medical and technical experts, Norviit concentrated on the medical aspects, while the central safety engineer supervised safety and hygienic conditions in the mines. Norviit published several epidemiological articles on the silicosis problem in the Boliden Mining Company. He reflected on the fact that the cases of silicosis declined as rapidly as they did in the 1950s and that the rate of tuberculosis was high. He did not neglect the dust problems in the Laisvall mine in the 1940s, but he redefined the silicosis crisis as a problem not primarily related to the working conditions, but rather to the workers' individual disposition for silicosis. In this sense, he represented the still dominant policy of disposition prevention. His main idea was that primary stage tuberculosis significantly increased workers' susceptibility to silicosis. Even the BCG vaccination increased the risk, he claimed, and many of the miners in Laisvall were vaccinated in the 1940s. According to Norviit, this relationship between tuberculosis and silicosis explained almost half of the cases of silicosis in Laisvall, including those that had progressed (about one-third), and he viewed the other cases as mild, without a tendency to progress. Until the 1960s, about 70 cases were recorded in the company's other 9 mines in the region, most of them in the early 1950s. However, Norviit claimed that many cases had been over-diagnosed in the wake of the dramatic development of the silicosis problem in Laisvall (Norviit 1959, 1962).

Rosner and Markowitz have shown that the silicosis problem in the United States was redefined after World War II:

> The language of science and medicine replaced the language of politics and negotiations in discussion of silicosis. Silicosis was now defined as a disease of the past that could be adequately addressed by medical researchers, and engineers working with an enlightened business community. (Rosner and Markowitz 1991, p. 179)

In Sweden, there had been no broad public debate on silicosis before the war. Nevertheless, Norviit's analysis of the development in Laisvall mirrored that of many American professionals, since it implied that silicosis was a disease of the past, and, whether this was his intention or not, it relieved the Boliden Mining Company of much responsibility.

The silicosis problem in Laisvall occurred during a time of transition and unrest, not only at the international and national levels, but also on the local front. Wartime conditions, the expansion of the mining operations, the new company management, and the transformation of the system of industrial welfare meant big changes. The old system had worked well due to a unique commitment to the silicosis problem on the part of Pontén and the old company management. However, the new management that took over in Boliden in the 1940s, as well as the local management and doctor in Laisvall, relied more on the central experts and authorities than on Pontén's assessment of the silicosis risk, despite his well-reputed competence and long experience. Hence, the development in Laisvall also corresponded well with Ahlmark's opinion that the medical supervision regulation created a feeling that the silicosis problem was under control.

From a historical perspective, many aspects of the silicosis problem in Laisvall remain to be analyzed. One important question is how wartime conditions and the interests of the government in the production of lead affected labor relations and the attitudes of all involved toward the working conditions in the mine. For the purposes of this chapter, however, the most interesting fact is that this tragedy actually happened, about 15 years after the formal acknowledgment of silicosis as an occupational disease. The Laisvall case illustrates very clearly the limitation inherent in the regulation on medical supervision to prevent silicosis, even in "extremely high risk" settings. Further, it illustrates how the prevention of silicosis was highly dependent on the local actors' attitudes, interests, knowledge, and power to define the problem, and to force resolutions. Finally, it shows that the existence of a working local industrial safety organization of the sort the Swedish model implied did not necessarily put the risks of *industrial diseases* on the agenda.

THE BREAKTHROUGH IN SCIENTIFIC DUST MEASUREMENT

The results of the epidemiological silicosis investigation in the 1950s became a driving force for the development of nationwide projects on dust measurements in Sweden. In the final report, Ahlmark, Bruce and Nyström (1960) concluded:

> It cannot be too strongly stressed that it is the technical prophylactic measures which are decisive as regards risk of pneumoconiosis. Until such prophylaxis is perfected, however, it must be supplemented by medical examinations and limitation of working time in scheduled occupations. (p. 379)

The fact that leading medical silicosis experts so clearly stressed the need to reduce dust in the workplaces supported indirectly the unions' old demand for stricter governmental regulations on dust exposure. Until this time, the main agents for the prevention of silicosis had been physicians committed to the problem and the unions, especially the left-wing unions. The government had played a minor role. The Swedish Moulders' Union, the Swedish Metal Workers' Union and some other unions concerned with the silicosis problem had long criticized not only the employers, but also the LO and the Social Democratic Party, for not taking sufficient action on the problem of occupational diseases (Thörnquist 1993, pp. 59-60; 2001).

The 1961 LO Congress became the turning point for the LO's approach to the field of industrial safety and health risks, including silicosis (cf. Johansson and Magnusson 1998, pp. 154-156). After the Congress, LO delegates in the Social Democratic Party caucus submitted a bill to Parliament (Riksdagen), proposing that the authorities should thoroughly map out hazardous workplaces, elaborate indicators for the assessment of the risk of silicosis, and suggest measures for dust control. The government commissioned the Department of Occupational

Hygiene at the National Institute of Public Health to plan and conduct the investigation in cooperation with the National Board on Occupational Safety and Health. The investigation, which started in 1963, comprised approximately 170 workplaces with known or presumed silicosis risks, among them about 50 iron foundries. This initiative signaled the government's greater commitment to dust prevention. The project also received broad support from various groups and associations in society, such as insurance companies, medical authorities, and the SAF (Ahlmark 1967, ch. 1).

This study led to a breakthrough for scientific dust measurements in Sweden, now with strong influences from American ideas and methods. After World War II the leading American industrial hygienists, Philip Drinker and Theodore Hatch from the Harvard School of Public Health and the University of Pittsburgh became highly respected advisors to colleagues at Swedish National Institute of Public Health. They were pioneers in the field of engineering control of dust hazards and experts on the measurement and analysis of dust. In 1936, they had published *Industrial Dust*, which became a standard reference. They were consulted by the Department of Occupational Hygiene on the design of investigations on the risk of welding in the late 1940s and, in the mid-1950s, on the risk of carbon monoxide. These studies paved the way for the silicosis investigation (interview with Gideon Gerhardsson 9 February and 20 August 2004, 2003; Gerhardsson 1992, pp. 17-19; 2002, p. 14). Drinker and Hatch focused strictly on the technical aspects of the dust hazards. Hatch, who was involved in the scientific debate on silicosis, questioned the methods used by general practitioners to diagnose pneumoconiosis by x-rays and occupational histories, which, in his view, led to over-diagnoses. Instead, he argued that diagnosis should rely on measurement of the dust level at the work sites (Rosner and Markovitz 1991, pp. 185-190). Drinker, who among other things conducted the Harvard Cotton Dust Project in North and South Carolina in the United States in the 1940s, concluded that there were no significant health problems in the industry, without conducting medical examinations of workers (Levenstein and Woskie 2002). This technological view revealed a conflict between the industrial hygienists, who were technical and chemical experts, and the doctors committed to resolving the silicosis problem, as well as between the technicians and the workers, and their opinion of the working conditions.

The conflict also existed in Sweden. According to Gerhardsson, physicians and unions were often suspicious of the "new experts" and their measurements and analysis (interview with Gerhardsson 20 August 2004). However, the first Swedish nationwide occupational hygiene project on silicosis was pushed through by the trade union movement and carried out in cooperation with engineers and the main medical experts on silicosis, Ahlmark, Bruce and Nyström (1960). Thus, it caused little political controversy. A dust index was established to estimate the risk of silicosis at workplaces. Based on this index Ahlmark, who edited the final report, *Silicosis in Sweden* (1967), proposed a scale for technical preventive measures against silicosis in companies. The index was also meant to provide a better criterion for the authorities in deciding which workplaces should be submitted to medical supervision (Ahlmark 1967).

According to the report, the number of workers exposed to silica dust at that time was approximately 25,000. More than half of them had been exposed for 10 years or more, and about one-sixth of them had been at risk more than 30 years. The situation was worst in small enterprises, for example, in the many small iron foundries. Although the problem of silicosis had worsened in the iron foundries, government regulations on supervision still did not cover them. Dust problems were also great in the stone-crushing trade, in which many small companies operated during the construction boom in the 1960s. Still there was also the great risk for silicosis in the mines and in the quartz industry. In addition, the recorded cases had now increased considerably in the granite industry, where many workers were diagnosed with advanced stage silicosis. Along with the mechanization of the dressing processes, the amount of dust had increased considerably (Ahlmark 1967, pp. 71-99, 143-145, 169-171).

As a result of the study, the National Institute of Occupational Safety and Health established a tripartite committee, with representatives from the labor market parties and the government, to deal with the silicosis problem (Andra lagutskottets utlåtande no. 63, 1970). Thus, the first large-scaled occupational hygiene project on silicosis also led to a breakthrough in tripartite cooperation dealing with industrial dust. However, in the late 1960s the political climate changed in Sweden, as in many other countries and, at the same time, the debate on work environment issues intensified. Growing left-wing movements increasingly challenged the Swedish model of organized bipartite and tripartite cooperation, including the projects on industrial dust.

THE BIG SILICOSIS PROJECT

Nevertheless, the tripartite committee planned a new and more extensive silicosis project. The LO, in particular, advocated that all workplaces where workers were exposed to silica dust should be investigated, including small companies where the handling of quartz up to that time was less known to authorities. In 1966, the Department of Occupational Hygiene at the National Institute of Public Health was reorganized within the newly established National Institute of Occupational Medicine, and enlarged to include a separate technical department. Sven Forssman, who since the early 1950s had been a medical expert at the SAF, became the head of the institute and Gideon Gerhardsson was appointed as director of the technical department. Gerhardsson had worked as an engineer at the Department of Occupational Hygiene, but since 1957 he was employed by the SAF as an expert on occupational hygiene (Gerhardsson 1992, pp. 17-22). In 1968 the government commissioned Gerhardsson to conduct the engineering project. The Communist Party and other representatives of the left-wing movements regarded the project as a concession to business interests. Instead of new investigations, which they thought would only delay the solution of the silicosis problem, they wanted stricter legislative regulations. Those who best could assess the risks at the workplaces were the workers, they argued, not experts allied with the SAF (see for example Motion in Andra kammaren, no 449:1970; minutes of Andra kammaren, 15 January, 20 March, 4 November 1970; *Dagens Nyheter* 14 January 1969).

The new project comprised approximately 1,700 workplaces in 42 industries. Gerhardsson consulted Drinker and Hatch for the design of the field studies and, in line with their ideas, it aimed to measure and analyze the dust situation at the workplace as a way of estimating the risks of silicosis and devising concrete suggestions for dust prevention measures. The results of the company studies, including dust measurements and recommendations for both immediate and long-term preventive technical measures, were given to companies and the unions, as well as to the labor inspectors (Interview with Gideon Gerhardsson, 9 February, 2003).

Personal dose sampling showed that in 28 of the 42 industries studied, the dust index exceeded the recommended value 1.0; in nine the dust index exceeded 2.0. The general results showed that in most industries studied, at least half of the workers examined were exposed to unsatisfactory dust conditions. Since the foundries still had large problems with silica dust and other kinds of dust and smoke, the project dealt a lot with this trade (Gerhardsson 2002). In Österbybruk the results of the measurements showed that the dust level in the steel foundry was low. At the outdoor workplace, "Karelia," on the other hand, the dust index for the cleaners of the casting far exceeded the recommended dust index and was as high as 8.3. Due to the high percentage of cristobalite in the dust, the situation was even more alarming (Isaksson and Engman 1971, p. 47). Such was the dust situation at "Karelia" about 20 years after the "solution" of the silicosis problem in this company. During the 1950s and 1960s, the problem had lost its acuteness, since the silica dust risks were regarded as having been eliminated through the rebuilding of the foundry and the removal of the dustiest work operations outdoors with a subsequent decline in the number of silicosis cases. In that way, "Karelia" had been separated from the foundry both spatially and socially. On the whole, the silicosis problem reinforced the social distinctions among workers in the foundries that had begun with the mechanization process, since the disease most afflicted those who occupied the weakest position in the labor market, and exercised the least control over their labor process. In Österbybruk, as in many other foundries, the first step had been to separate the dustiest processes from the forming shop, something that mainly benefitted the craftsmen. Finally the problem had been solved partly at the expense of creating a new hazardous workplace for workers who were ranked lowest socially, among them Finnish immigrants. Thus, the work environment at "Karelia" had been neglected (Thörnquist 1993, pp. 137-152; 2001, pp. 91-96).

The silicosis project also found very high risk for silicosis in many small enterprises, within the scouring powder industry, for example. The five enterprises investigated exceeded the recommended hygienic threshold limit for air-borne quartz dust (0.2 mg/m^3) by up to 60 times (Arbetarskyddsstyrelsen 1982, p. 97). In the case of one small family company in central Sweden, most of the workers contracted silicosis. Production was carried out in a barracks with no exhaust ventilation, and the workers wore no protective masks. Yet, the mixing of the powder, as well as the packaging, caused an extremely high level of dust with a quartz content of 95%. In 1966, the owner of the company died at the age of 38, after about 10 years' work in the factory. At that time, no one suspected silicosis, and the regulation on medical supervision did not cover the scouring powder industry. Two years later, his wife died at the same age, shortly after being diagnosed with the end-stage silicosis. The labor inspector found that the dust level in the air exceeded the recommended hygienic limit by 20 times. Their 17-year-old son, who worked in the factory at the time of the inspection, was immediately suspended from his job. When all five employees at the factory were examined, it was found that four of them had indications of silicosis. In some cases silicosis had developed after only two to three years. The labor inspector condemned the premises and the factory was forced to shut down. Four other small enterprises that manufactured scouring powder were also shut down in the 1970s because of silicosis risk (Arbetarskyddsstyrelsen 1982.; *Expressen* 4 September 1969). This was an illuminating example of the great environment problems that existed in some small enterprises, as well as the difficulties involved in controlling them.

The large silicosis investigation was, as mentioned, criticized from the beginning by left-wing movements for being a tripartite project conducted by persons connected to the SAF. Among other objections, the critics were concerned that the project involved cooperation with the companies, and that proposed solutions to the silicosis problem would be constrained by productivity concerns raised by consulting engineers (Gerhardsson 1992, 2002; cf. Levenstein and Woskie 2001).

In spite of the inborn political conflict, the silicosis project helped to put the silicosis problem on the national agenda. It provided data that was used by all parties in the work environment debate. The fact that one of the oldest and most serious industrial diseases still remained a real threat for about 25,000 workers became something of an anomaly in an otherwise advanced industrial and welfare society, particularly since the technical knowledge for dust elimination existed.

The silicosis debate in Sweden emerged in the broader context of a vast national and international debate on environmental and work environment issues. The general background was a strong reaction against the social and human costs of the hard exploitation of nature, the use of toxic chemical substances, and rapid rationalization and structural transformation in industry. During the post-war period the well organized and strong labor market parties, the stable Social

Democratic government, and the good state of the market had been the basic pre-requisites for successful cooperation on issues concerning wages, as well as OHS—albeit for a long time mainly concerning accidents. At the end of the 1960s, however, the general negotiating climate got tougher. In 1969/1970, a three-month wildcat miners' strike occurred in the State-owned company LKAB in the ore-fields in northern Sweden. The strike was, largely, provoked by dissatisfaction with the physical and psycho-social working conditions, and it became the start of the broader work environment debate. In the following years—like in many other countries as well—a broad and radical public opinion demanded improvements in the work environment (Johansson and Magnusson 1998, pp. 155-167). The problem was discussed not only in the media and in political arenas, but also addressed in art, music, literature, film, and theater. Hence, the lively public discourse on work environment issues in general provided more fuel for the debate on silicosis. One might say that silicosis finally occupied center stage, 40 years after its legal recognition.

NEW PRECONDITIONS FOR SILICOSIS PREVENTION

In 1969, an alarming report from a study made by the LO concerning members' experiences of their working conditions was published. About 80% reported that, to various degrees, they suffered from problems in the work environment. Approximately 40% reported their problems were great. Noise, ergonomic problems, and climate were the most common concerns, but industrial dust, gas, and smoke bothered many workers as well. Against this background, the LO and the Social Democratic Party presented a joint work environment program, which demanded a radical revision of the *Workers' Protection Act* (SFS 1973:834; SFS 1977:1160). Fundamental to this program was a considerable widening of the work environment concept, and the principle that workplaces should be more adapted to workers' capacities and needs. The program included aspects of chemical risks, ergonomics, climate, and work organization, and thus specifically addressed occupational diseases. The program was basically codified in revisions to the *Workers' Protection Act* in 1973, and in the new *Work Environment Act* passed in 1977. It was further institutionalized in the new, binding central *Work Environment Agreement* settled in 1976, and in the Joint Industrial Safety Council's new big campaign and mass-training program, "Better Work Environment" (*"Bättre Arbetsmiljö"*, *BAM*), launched in the early 1970s (Ekström 1992, pp. 71-75; Oscarsson 1997, pp. 27-32). Moreover, economic support for research, information dissemination, and mass training in OHS radically improved through the establishment of the Work Environment Fund (*Arbetsmiljöfonden*) in 1972, financed by payroll taxes (Oscarsson 1997). In addition, the labor market reforms reinforced the position of the union representatives. Among other things, safety representatives were allowed to stop hazardous work while waiting for the Labor Inspectorate's decision (Oscarsson 1997; Tucker 1992, pp. 106-113).

Furthermore, in the early 1970s, there was a general reinforcement of the governmental work environment agencies. The National Board of Occupational Safety and Health now issued directions on hygienic threshold limits, technical preventive measures, and dust control in different trades, such as the foundries, the granite industry and the mines. The overhaul of the *Workers' Protection Act* in 1973, also reinforced the Labor Inspectorate, among other things, giving it the right to issue fines. As mentioned, medical supervision was radically extended as well; now, the aim was to encompass all exposed workers. Hence, state control increased, but in line with the old tradition of cooperation, the governmental OHS agencies and officials, including those involved in the silicosis project, also worked actively to support companies in implementing the regulations. Despite this, in many workplaces the problems of dust, gas, and smoke remained (Arbetarskyddsstyrelsen 1982, pp. 52-53, 129-130; Ekman 1997, p. 5).

The general reinforcement and extension of labor legislation, especially the new act on job security that passed in 1974, and the act on co-determination in 1976, was a radical departure from the classical Swedish Model of self-regulation between the labor market parties. In the wake of the new labor legislation, the energy crisis, and the growing international structural crisis in industry in the mid-1970s, the political climate deteriorated, and in the autumn of 1976, the Social Democratic government was defeated after more than 40 years in office. Yet, the previous working life reforms in the 1970s, and public opinion on OHS issues paved the way for the new *Work Environment Act* in 1977. Although it was passed during the bourgeois regime (1976-1982), it mainly followed the original proposals elaborated under the Social Democratic regime.

Chemical risks and air pollutants attracted special attention in the work environment debate in the 1970s. For example, the number of chemical and technical personnel at the National Board of Occupational Safety and Health increased considerably. In the early 1970s, the National Institute of Occupational Medicine had been reorganized and made part of the National Board of Occupational Safety and Health. By then, however, the former management of the Institute had left for other positions (Gerhardsson 1992, pp. 54-56). Between 1974 and 1980, the Board carried out a follow-up study of silicosis including a minor study on asbestos. A former study showed that the recommended threshold limit (2 fibers per cm^3 air) was often exceeded. The development of the response to the problem of asbestos had many similarities with that of silicosis. According to the revised regulation of 1963, medical surveillance was conducted in the most hazardous workplaces, but preventive measures were often not taken. However, in this case, the road to action was somewhat shorter.

In the early 1970s the asbestos debate intensified. The Communist Party demanded that asbestos be prohibited because of the risk of cancer. The authorities, however, disagreed, but suggested stricter dust prevention regulations.

The situation became even more alarming in 1975, when the results of an epidemiological study confirmed a clear connection between exposure to asbestos and mesothelioma, an uncommon type of cancer. Workers in the construction industry, the shipyards, the engineering industry, and many other settings were highly exposed to asbestos. In addition, the problem concerned people generally, since asbestos and asbestos cement was commonly used as building material. Even the new parliament building (*Riksdagshuset*) in Stockholm was insulated with asbestos (Arbetarskyddsstyrelsen 1999, pp. 99-104).

The alarming report led to an intense public debate, which put great pressure on the government and the work environment authorities to take action. The Communist Party, LO and several unions were important driving forces in this process. In 1976 the use of several products containing asbestos, including new installations of products with asbestos cement, was prohibited. This was an uncommon work environment policy, and in some places, it caused controversy, since it forced factories to shut down in a time of growing unemployment. Nevertheless, the restrictions were successively extended, leading to a general prohibition in the 1980s of the use of asbestos (Arbetarskyddsstyrelsen 1999; Sund and Åmark 1990, ch. 3).

The asbestos alarm in the mid-1970s highlighted the need for stricter protective regulations against industrial dust in general. According to the results of the follow-up silicosis project, the situation in many plants was still not acceptable in the mid-1970s. In most of the about 2,000 workplaces investigated, the measures taken to prevent dust were insufficient or defective. At "Karelia" in Österbybruk, the level of silica dust was not alarming, but other kinds of metal dust, especially nickel dust, which developed in the process of cleaning high-alloyed steel castings, caused great problems, as did smoke from new, thermal work processes. Although the company improved the ventilation system and made some changes in the way work was organized, many problems remained unsolved at this outdoor worksite in the early 1990s (Thörnquist 1993, p. 147).

Nevertheless, the general conclusion reached by the National Board of Occupational Safety and Health in the follow-up project was that considerable improvement had been achieved during the decade (Arbetarskyddsstyrelsen 1982). Several medical researchers questioned this conclusion, and pointed to the fact that measuring dust was problematic as a method for estimating change in environmental risk factors. Furthermore, their calculations indicated that the problem would remain unsolved for the remainder of the century or even longer (Ahlmark and Gerhardsson 1981, pp. 48-49; Westerholm 1980, pp. 52-53, 57). However, the cases of silicosis decreased significantly in 1980s and 1990s.

Through the passing of the *Work Environment Act* in 1977, the National Board of Occupational Safety and Health was empowered to issue binding provisions. In 1979, the hygienic limit for quartz was reduced from 0.2 to 0.1 mg/m^3 and for tridymite and cristobalite from 0.1 to 0.05 mg/m^3. Then, in 1981, the Board issued a binding and general provision on quartz, which applied to all kinds of work with quartz or material containing over 3% quartz (by weight). In addition, dust measurements became mandatory at these workplaces (Ekman 1997). By then, however, a vast structural transformation had radically reduced the number firms and workers in the traditionally dusty trades, such as in the foundries, the mines, and the stone industry. In addition, olivine sand had replaced quartz sand in many companies and, along with the technical rationalization and automation, many dusty works operations had disappeared. Hence, stricter legislation and state control appeared at a late stage in the history of the actual health risks. The silicosis risk was not the only example.

CONCLUDING REMARKS

The main question of this chapter was why there was such a long delay between the time silicosis was first acknowledged as an occupational disease in Sweden (in 1931), and the time that effective action was taken. Until the 1930s, the problem of stone dust was little discussed in Sweden. The general background was the comparatively late rationalization of industry, and the late development of occupational medicine and hygiene. It was only through doctor Bruce's nationwide investigations on the prevalence of silicosis in the 1930s that the problem of silica dust in plants became more commonly recognized.

The government responded to the alarming results by prescribing medical supervision of the workers, but not stricter regulations to reduce hazardous exposure to silica dust. This reflected the predominant policy of prevention, which for a long time focused more on the worker's individual *disposition* for contracting diseases or suffering injuries than on the problem of the worker's *exposure* to hazards in the work environment. Thus, the government regulated the workers rather than the working conditions. The policy to exclude workers who were regarded as predisposed for silicosis, and to transfer those who were diagnosed with silicosis in an early stage to dust free jobs, did not actually *prevent* silicosis. The disease could develop even after exposure to dust was discontinued. In addition, the regulation on medical supervision legitimized exposure to silica dust with the risk of contracting silicosis for those workers who remained in dusty settings. This especially concerned those who worked in trades and workplaces where the risk of silicosis was not regarded as "extremely high" and therefore were not included in the regulation. Thus, the prevention of silicosis was delayed. The development of silicosis in the iron foundries and in the granite industry exemplified this, while the Laisvall case illustrated very clearly that the governmental regulation concerning medical supervision provided weak protection against silicosis even in settings with an "extremely high" risk for the disease. Moreover, the regulation on medical supervision created a feeling that the silicosis problem had been brought under control.

The *Workers' Protection Act* included general regulations concerning the prevention of dust, but it was not until the early 1970s that the National Board of

Occupational Safety and Health issued stricter directions that specifically addressed the danger of exposure to silica dust. In addition, the Labor Inspectorate pursued an enforcement policy of persuasion and cooperation, rather than one of strict control. Hence, for a long time the state had a liberal attitude toward employers concerning the problem of silicosis prevention. Like other matters of OHS, the silicosis problem was to be solved primarily through self-regulation between the labor market parties. However, cooperation in OHS under the "Swedish model" concerned for a long time mainly the problem of accidents, which the employers more readily dealt with. As well, the cooperation policy made it difficult for the LO and government to force stricter state control against the employers' interests. Yet, this should not conceal the fact that until the 1960s, when a broader interest in the problem of industrial dust emerged, the unions, together with the physicians committed to the problem, were the main driving forces for the prevention of silicosis in Sweden.

The development of occupational hygiene, and the increasing professionalization in the field of OHS, meant that advanced technical, and organizational measures could be taken to solve the silicosis problem. However, since technical solutions to ventilation problems were often complicated and expensive, especially small companies lagged behind in the development of dust prevention. Yet, as the development in Österbybruk and Laisvall showed, good potential technical and economical prerequisites for the prevention of silicosis—or even knowledge and established OHS routines—were not a guarantee for action. As long as the authorities' control of the dust problems in workplaces was comparatively weak, the prevention of silicosis depended mainly on local actors' interest, competence, and power to define the problem and force a resolution. Ultimately it was a matter of attitudes and interests. In the 1960s, the leading medical experts strongly emphasized that technical prophylactics were decisive for resolution of the silicosis problem. This legitimized the unions' old demands for stricter regulations requiring technical preventive measures to control exposure to dangerous dust.

The government responded to these demands by providing grants for occupational hygienic projects on silicosis and setting up tripartite committees. However, tripartite cooperation, as well as the fact that leading persons at the National Institute of Occupational Medicine had established contacts with the SAF, made the big silicosis project conducted in the late 1960s and the early 1970s politically controversial at a time of growing left-wing opinion. Yet, in the long run, this project, as well as the other silicosis projects, contributed to increased governmental supervision of the dust situation in the plants, which forced voluntary solutions as well. The work environment reforms in the 1970s, enforced by old trade union demands and the strong public support for improvements in the work environment, codified a widening of the work environment concept, and a reorientation toward an OHS policy that focused more on the creation of "safe places." This provided new and better preconditions for the resolution of the silicosis problem.

REFERENCES

Ahlmark, A. (1967) *Silikos i Sverige. Redogörelse för Arbetsmedicinska Institutets och Arbetarskyddsstyrelsens utredning om silikos.* Studia Laboris & Salutis. Stockholm: Arbetsmedicinska Institutet. Vetenskaplig skriftserie 1967:1.

Ahlmark, A., Bruce, T., and Nyström, Å. (1960) *Silicosis and Other Pneumoconiosis in Sweden.* Stockholm: Svenska Bokförlaget (Norstedts).

Ahlmark, A., Bruce, T., and Nyström, Å. (1956) Silicosen som yrkessjukdom i Sverige. *Nordisk Medicin, 8*: 252-257.

Ahlmark, A., and Gerhardsson, L. (1981) *Silikosen i Sverige sedan 1930.* Arbete och Hälsa. 1981:15. Stockholm: Arbetarskyddsverket.

Andra kammaren motion 449 1970.

Andra kammarens protokoll: 15 januari, 20 mars, 4 November 1970.

Andra lagutskottets utlåtande nr. 63, 1970.

Arbetarskyddsstyrelsen (1982) *Silikosuppföljningsprojektet 1974-1980,* Undersöknings-rapport 1982:31. Stockholm: Arbetarskyddsstyrelsen.

Arbetarskyddsstyrelsen (1999) *Arbetsmiljön. En grundsten i välfärdsbygget.* Solna: Arbetarskyddsstyrelsen.

Bruce, T. (1942) *Die Silikose als Berufskrankheit in Schweden: Eine klinische und gewerbemedizinische Studie.* Stockholm: Tryckeriaktiebolaget Tule.

Dagens Nyheter (11 January 1970) Kritik mot institutet minskar budgetanslag.

Didrichsen, F., and Jahnlert, U. (1981) Preventionens historia. *Socialmedicinsk tidskrift, 1*: 5-9.

Drinker, P., and Hatch, T. (1936) *Industrial Dust: Hygienic Significance, Measurement and Control.* New York: McGraw-Hill.

Ekman, N. (1997) *Kvarts i arbetsmiljön. Historik, regler, åtgärder och uppföljning.* Stockholm: Arbetarskyddsstyrelsen. Enheten för kemi.

Ekström, Ö. (1992) *50 år i samverkan. Arbetarskyddsnämnden 1942-1992.* Stockholm: Arbetarskyddsnämnden.

Expressen (4 September 1969) Hon är ensam kvar i dödsfabriken.

Forssman, S. (1958) Den mänskliga faktorn vid olycksfall på arbetsplatsen. *Nordisk Hygienisk Tidskrift.*

Gallagher, C. (1997) *Health and Safety Management Systems: An Analysis of System Types and Effectiveness.* National Key Centre in Industrial Relations. Melbourne Monash University.

Gerhardsson, G. (1992) *Arbetsgivare synar arbetsmiljön.* Stockholm: Svenska Arbets-givarföreningen.

Gerhardsson, G. (2002) The End of Silicosis in Sweden—A Triumph for Occupational Hygiene Engineering. *OHS and Development, 4*:13-25.

Gruvarbetaren (November 1969) Laisvallgruvan 30 år.

Gruvarbetaren Laisvall (December 1969) Laisvallgruvan 30 år.

Gustafsson, R. Å. (1994) Traditionernas ok inom arbetsmiljöpreventionen. In G. Carlsson and O. Arvidsson (eds.), *Kampen för folkhälsan. Prevention i historia och nutid* (pp. 263-319). Borås: Natur och Kultur.

Holmin, N. (1911) *Förekomsten av tuberkulos bland järn- och metallarbetare i Eskilstuna.* Meddelanden från Svenska Nationalföreningen mot Tuberkulos. 6. Stockholm: Nationalföreningen mot tuberkulos.

ILO (1930) *Silicosis: Records of the International Conference Held in Johannesburg.* London: King & Son for the International Labor Office.

ILO (1934) *International Labor Conference: Eighteenth Session, Geneva.* Report V. Workmen's Compensation for Occupational Diseases. Partial Revision of the Convention Concerning Workmen's Compensation for Occupational Diseases. VIII. Geneva.

ISA (2001) *Arbetsskadestatistiken, silikosfall 1979-2000.* Stockholm: Arbetsmiljöverket.

Interview with Gideon Gerhardsson, Professor of technical occupational medicine, 15 September 2002 and 9 February 2003; 20 August 2004.

Isaksson, G., and Engman, L. (1971) *Dammsituationen vid Fagersta Bruks AB, Österbyverken, Österbybruk, 8-10 December 1970.* T 802/70. Stockholm: Arbetsmedicinska Institutet.

Johansson, A. L., and Magnusson, L. (1998) *LO andra halvseklet. Fackföreningsrörelsen och samhället.* Stockholm: Atlas.

Karlsson, L. (1997) I gruva och på kontor—genusstämpling av arbete. In I. Hagman (ed.), SOU 1997:113. *Mot halva makten—elva historiska essäer om kvinnors strategier och mäns motstånd. Rapport till utredning om fördelning av ekonomiska resurser mellan kvinnor och män* (pp. 79-96). SOU 1997:113. Stockholm: Fritzes.

Karlsson, L. (2001) Perspectives on Gendered Labor Legislation in Sweden during the 20th Century. In A. Thörnquist (ed.), *Work Life, Work Environment and Work Safety in Transition. Historical and Sociological Perspectives on the Development in Sweden during the 20th Century* (pp. 127-167). Arbetsliv i Omvandling/Work Life in Transition 2001:9. Stockholm: National Institute for Working Life.

Katz, E. (1994) *The White Death: Silicosis on the Witwatersrand Gold Mines 1886-1910.* Johannesburg: Witwatersrand University Press.

Kavian-Lanjani, Y. (1999) *Learning from Miners' Risk Management. A Case Study from the Swedish Mining Industry.* Department of Human Work Sciences, Division of Technical Psychology. 1999:07. Luleå: University of Technology.

Kjellberg, A. (1998) Sweden: Restoring the Model? In A. Ferner and R. Hyman (eds.), *Changing Industrial Relations in Europe* (pp. 74-117). Oxford: Blackwell.

Levenstein, C., and Woskie, S. (2002) The Cotton Dust Project. In C. Levenstein, G. F. DeLaurier, and M. Lee Dunn (eds.), *The Cotton Dust Papers: Science, Politics, and Power in the "Discovery" of Byssinosis in the U.S.* (pp. 53-72). New York: Baywood.

Lundh, C., and Gunnarsson, C. (1987) *Arbetsmiljö, arbetarskydd och utvärderingsforskning. Ett historiskt perspektiv.* Lund: Skrifter utgivna av Ekonomisk-historisksa föreningen. Wilber.

Mascher, W. (1930) Om dammlungesjukdom (Pneumokoniosis) med särskild hänsyn till silikos. *Hygiea, 92*:145-220, 232-272.

Miners' Union, Department no 110 in Laisvall (Swedish Metal Workers' Union Department no 65, Piteå).

Miners' Union, Department no 110 in Laisvall. Annual reports 1943-1955.

Miners' Union, Department no 110 in Laisvall. Minutes of the local meetings 1941-1955.

Miners' Union, Department no 110 in Laisvall. Minutes of the joint industrial safety committee in Laisvall 1946-1955.

Navarro, V. (1983) The Determinants of Social Policy: A Case Study: Regulating Health and Safety at the Workplace in Sweden. *International Journal of Health Services, 4*: 517-561.

Nichols, T., and Tucker, E. (2000) OHS Management in UK and Ontario, Canada: A Political Economy Perspective. In K. Frick, P. Langa-Jensen, M. Quinlan and T. Wilthagen (eds.), *Systematic OHS Management Perspectives on an International Development* (pp. 285-309). Oxford: Elsevier.

Nordin, J. (1943) *Yrkessjukdomar I.* Uppsala.: Almqvist & Wiksell Boktryckeri AB.

Nordin, J. (1947) *Yrkessjukdomar II.* Uppsala.: Almqvist & Wiksell Boktryckeri AB.

Norviit, L. (1959) Silikos i Laisvall. *Nordisk Medicin, 16,* VII. 1076-1081.

Norviit, L. (1962) Silikos vid Bolidens gruvor. Statistik. Analys av väsentliga faktorer. *Svenska Läkartidningen. Organ för Sveriges läkareförbund, 1:* 144-148.

Oscarsson, B. (1997) *25 år för arbetslivets förnyelse. Forskning och utveckling på arbetslivets område 1972-1997.* Stockholm: Rådet för Arbetslivsforskning.

Pontén, J. (1947) Om silikos. *Jernkontorets annaler, 2:* 31-39.

Pontén, J. (1953) Stålgjutgodstillverkningens problem ur medicinsk och yrkeshygienisk synpunkt I-II. *Verkstäderna. Organ för Sveriges Verkstadsförening, 2:* 31-33, *3:* 69-73.

Pontén, J. (1975) *Hälso—och sjukvård vid Bolidens Gruvaktiebolag 1930-1950.* (Unpublished paper).

Riksförsäkringsverket. Yrkesskadesstatestiken, silikosfall 1931-1979.

Rosenberg, B., and Levenstein, C. (1999) Social determinants of silicosis control in the Vermont granite industry 1938-1960. In A. Grieco, S. Iavicoli, and G. Berlinguer (eds.), *Contributions to the History of Occupational and Environmental Prevention* (pp. 195-210). Amsterdam: Elsevier.

Rosner, D., and Markowitz, G. (1991) *Deadly Dust: Silicosis and the Politics of Occupational Disease in the Twentieth-Century America.* Princeton: Princeton University Press.

SFS 1929:131-133 Lag om försäkringar för vissa yrkessjukdomar.

SFS 1931:31 Lag om ändring i kungörelsen den 22 nov 1929 med särskilda föreskrifter i anledning av lagen den 14 juni 1929 om försäkring av vissa yrkessjukdomar.

SFS 1938:711 Kungl. Maj:ts kungörelse om läkarundersökning och läkarbesiktning till förebyggande av vissa yrkessjukdomar.

SFS 1949:1 Arbetarskyddslagen.

SFS 1949:108 Kungl-Maj:ts kungörelse med föreskrifter angående tillämpningen av arbetarskyddslagen.

SFS 1963:660 Kungl. Maj:ts kungörelse angående ändring i kungörelsen av den 6 maj 1949 (nr 211) om läkarundersökning och läkarbesiktning till förebyggande av vissa yrkessjukdomar.

SFS 1973:834 Lag om ändring i Arbetarskyddslagen.

SFS 1977:1160 Arbetsmiljölagen.

SOU 1949:44. *Betänkande med förslag till rationalisering av gat- och kantstensindustrien. Avgivet av 1946 års stenindustriutredning.* Stockholm: Handelsdepartementet.

Sund, B., and Åmark, K. (1990) *Makt och arbetsskador.* Maktutredningen. Stockholm: Carlssons.

Thörnquist, A. (1993) *Silikosproblemet i Österbybruk 1920-1980. Skyddsarbetet—facklig kamp eller partssamarbete.* Stockholm: Arbetarskyddsnämnden.

Thörnquist, A. (2001) The Silicosis Problem in the Swedish Iron and Steel Industry during the 20th Century. In A. Thörnquist (ed.), *Work Life, Work Environment and Work Safety in Transition. Historical and Sociological Perspectives on the Development in Sweden during the 20th Century* (pp. 70-101). Arbetsliv i Omvandling/Work Life in Transition 2001:9. Stockholm: National Institute for Working Life.

Tucker, E. (1992) Worker Participation in Health and Safety Regulation: Lessons from Sweden. *Studies in Political Economy, 37*: 95-127.

Westerholm, P. (1980) Silicosis. Observation on a Case Register. *Scandinavian Journal of Work, Environment & Health, 2.*

CHAPTER 6

Disaster, Meaning Making, and Reform in Antebellum Massachusetts

Patricia Reeve*

At 4:47 P.M. on January 10, 1860 the five-story Pemberton Mill in Lawrence, Massachusetts collapsed into rubble in 60 seconds, burying the living and dead alike in oil-soaked timber, stone, and machinery. Throughout the evening more than a thousand rescuers searched for survivors in the ruins, hastening from one location to another as voices from below groaned, prayed, and cried out for help (Poirier 1990, p. 77). At 9 P.M. the day's horrors intensified when two men botched the transfer of a lantern and dropped it into the debris.[1] Fire ripped through the wreckage and roared in the ears of those above and in it. Rescue teams retreated unwillingly, lamenting the grievous cost of their impotence (Haskell and Mason 1860, pp. 10-11).

Witnesses to the mill's collapse described it as an appalling disaster.[2] Six hundred and seventy workers—the majority Irish immigrant women and girls—went down with the seven-year-old mill.[3] Of these 200 were traumatized but otherwise uninjured.[4] More than 300 workers suffered injuries of varying severity. One hundred or more died on January 10 or in the days that followed.[5] Thirteen of the dead were unrecognizable due to their injuries and were buried nameless.[6] City fathers estimated that "nearly a thousand families" lost their "subsistence."[7]

*I am grateful to the American Textile History Museum in Lowell, Massachusetts for the Sullivan Fellowship that funded the research for this chapter. I especially wish to thank Clare Sheridan, Librarian at the Museum's Osborne Library, who directed me to critical sources even as she prepared for the Museum's move to its current quarters. I also owe a debt to Allison Hepler and Kathleen Banks Nutter who commented on an earlier version of this chapter. Finally, I am obliged to Alvin Oickle who generously provided me with good counsel, corrections to my factual errors, and critical sources. I look forward to the publication of his manuscript, "The Fall of the Pemberton Mill."

According to Theodore Parker, the Transcendentalist preacher and labor reformer, the disaster had visited the carnage of warfare on Lawrence and its operatives.[8]

Nineteenth-century author Elizabeth Stuart Phelps recalled that news of the catastrophe "flashed over the telegraph wires, sprang into large type in the newspapers, [and] passed from lip to lip . . ." (Phelps 1869, p. 80). Scores of journalists streamed into Lawrence and twice daily filed stories with their publishers. Through March, the press captivated readers throughout the nation with dramatic accounts of the disaster's horrors, the victims' injuries and emotionalism, and the gritty realities of working-class life and labor.[9] Phelps recollected that "we were forced to think about the mills with the attending horror that no one living in that time . . . will forget" (Cameron 1993, p. 19). Throughout the winter and spring months Americans invoked Lawrence and its tragedy interchangeably.[10]

During a period of accelerating social change and conflict in the Northeastern United States, the Pemberton Mill disaster was a bellwether of political and social conflicts that were to follow in the next half-century. The factory had come to symbolize the nation's hopes for and misgivings about the trajectory of manufactures in a democratic republic.[11] The Lawrence calamity intensified national unease over the factory system. Moreover, disaster reportage confronted Americans with the previously unthinkable: a permanent working-class was forming in the United States. Swelling its ranks were wage-dependent women and children, many of them immigrants, who toiled in unsafe conditions and at their employers' pleasure.[12] The catastrophe provided incontrovertible proof that laboring Americans were dependent and susceptible to bodily injury and likely to remain so, the nation's idealization of producers as self-governing notwithstanding.[13]

In addition to increasing public awareness of the vulnerability of industrial workers, the tragedy engendered representations of laboring people that challenged their self-conceptions. For example, journalists immediately implicated the disaster and its victims in the nation's sectional crisis. On January 12, 1860, the *New York Herald* ignited a firestorm of protest by opining that factory work compared unfavorably to slavery.[14] The "Wife of a Worker" rejected the *Herald's* critique of northern manufactures in a scathing letter to the *Lawrence Sentinel:*

> We repel with *scorn* the assertion that we labor under 'tyrants' and 'task-masters!' [Would] we, well educated and respectable American men and women, voluntarily subject ourselves to such a life? It is false . . . let them blush at their unpardonable ignorance and misrepresentations. . . .[15]

Unquestionably, the "Wife" and her counterparts in New England's textile centers had a proprietary interest in depictions of their lives and characters. Moreover, her insistence on workers' attainments and respectability attests to the importance of these attributes as social capital in that era. Thus, not only did the fall of the Pemberton Mill gainsay civic idealism and the integrity of northern manufactures, but commentary on the tragedy made a spectacle of working-class labor and selfhood.

Although antiquarians and scholars have narrated the collapse of the Pemberton Mill, for the most part, they have described the tragedy without reference to its social and cultural moorings. Nor have they analyzed the breadth of its political effects. Clarisse A. Poirier—author of the single best history of the Pemberton Mill—is a notable exception to this characterization. Among other things, she has demonstrated that the insurance industry accomplished through fiat what the state would not through statute. In the wake of the disaster, insurers required policyholders to adhere to stipulated building codes or forfeit coverage (1990, pp. 93-99). It would seem that the catastrophe's significance inhered mainly in its aberrant and climactic occurrence.[16]

This chapter recognizes the greater historical roles of the Pemberton catastrophe by examining the resonance of the mill's collapse with antebellum Americans and the political effects of these reverberations. The Commonwealth's failure to enact corrective legislation after the tragedy bears scrutiny, but political response did not end here. After January 10, 1860, Americans were awash in private and public writings on the meanings and implications of the disaster. Imprinted by the era's social relations, these narratives mediated between the Mill's collapse and contemporaries' readings of it.[17] The result was the re-figuring of popular ideas about wage-earning people and their capacity for bodily defense and autonomy, the fruit of which would animate and constrain postbellum campaigns for labor law reform.

ENTERPRISING MEN, INDIGENT WOMEN, AND TEXTILE PRODUCTION

Lawrence, Massachusetts developed in the shadow of Lowell, built 25 years earlier, but soon exceeded it in scale of production and output.[18] Incorporated as a town in 1845 and then chartered as a city in 1853 (Dorgan 1918, pp. 31, 38), Lawrence was the brainchild of Lowell industrialists desiring to experiment with large-scale manufacturing. After the downturn of the 1830s and early '40s, demand for textiles grew even as intensification of production drove costs downward.[19] Lowell manufacturers and their financial backers were eager to capitalize on this opportunity but recognized that local waterpower was insufficient to the task. At the recommendation of Daniel Saunders, an agent of the Merrimack Water Power Association, Lowell entrepreneurs inspected Deer Jump Falls on the Merrimack River and determined to harness its motive power.[20] Negotiation over the purchase of adjoining lands ensued and then, in 1845, the Massachusetts General Court chartered the Essex Company to develop the proposed textile center (Josephson 1967, p. 303).

Company principals were men of means and, with one exception, seasoned manufacturers of textiles for profit. Nathan Appleton had earlier revolutionized U.S. textile production in partnership with Francis Cabot Lowell (Dalzell 1987; Rothenberg 2000). Abbott Lawrence had prospered in commerce and the railway industry before immersing himself in development of the state's textile industry.[21] Patrick T. Jackson, a risk-taker in business and director of the Boston Company, was the brother-in-law of Francis Cabot Lowell and joint developer of the city bearing his kinsman's name.[22] Rounding out their number was Charles S. Storrow, whom Lawrence recruited to serve as the Essex Company's agent and treasurer (or chief executive officer). Under Storrow's direction, the Essex Company undertook construction of a granite dam at Deer Jump Falls and began mapping out the town of Lawrence, named for the family of mill magnates.[23]

Lawrence was a "raw boom town" when John Amory Lowell contracted with Charles S. Storrow for construction of the Pemberton Mill.[24] Lowell, the great-nephew of Francis Cabot Lowell, assiduously nurtured the growth of manufactures in Massachusetts. Like his uncle, the younger Lowell had invested heavily in the Boston Manufacturing Company and its building of the city of Lowell, eventually becoming Company treasurer. Ever heedful of the main chance, Lowell invested in the Essex Company when it incorporated and then enlisted its principals to build his landmark mill.[25]

John Amory Lowell resolved to build a "fancy Mill" in Lawrence while touring British enterprises that manufactured high-end cotton goods. During the summer of 1851, Lowell wrote from Europe to John Pickering Putnam,[26] his brother-in-law and business partner, arguing for the merits of this plan. "I have no doubt," Lowell averred, "that a very good chance of making money and of showing what can be done would be afforded in Colored and fancy cambricks [sic]." Lowell was especially eager to incorporate British design elements and technologies suited to large-scale production, as evidenced by his specifications for the mill's construction.[27] While still in Europe, Lowell instructed Putnam to establish the factory.[28]

With Putnam's approval, in 1852 the Essex Company purchased land and water rights along Lawrence's North Canal and began mill construction in late January 1853. Captain Charles Henry Bigelow, the Company's chief engineer,[29] was charged with oversight of its construction. Bigelow had extensive experience building in Lawrence, having erected the dam at Deer Jump falls, the Lawrence Machine Shop, and Bay State Mills (Poirier 1978, pp. 12, 14-17). But in a break with Company practice, Bigelow's superiors entrusted the purchase of all construction materials to J. Pickering Putnam, as requested by John Amory Lowell.[30]

Clarisse A. Poirier has maintained that "[e]very detail of the building's plans came under Putnam's careful scrutiny." Driving him were concerns for the construction timetable and the mill's structural integrity. Putnam was committed to launching operations on schedule, for then the mill would generate revenues needed to repay investors. He also worried a good deal about potential threats to the factory's soundness. These included, among other things, water seepage into the foundation, vibrating machinery, and the weight of snow on the factory roof.[31] Therefore, Putnam took care in hiring contractors for "the glass, the shafting and gearing, and the iron columns [intended to support the mill]."[32] Nevertheless, his purchase of a less expensive support system for the mill's iron beams would have dreadful consequences for mill occupants.[33]

The Pemberton Mill opened in 1853 to acclaim from contemporaries who hailed it as a harbinger of progress and an aesthetic and architectural "advance" on New England factories.[34] Though built of the traditional brick and granite, the structure was unique in three ways. First, its dimensions (284 feet long and 84 feet wide) exceeded those of the nearby Bay State Mill, then New England's largest textile factory. Second, the mill's windows were "ten feet high by five feet wide, nearly twice the size of most factory windows." Finally, a nearly flat roof "pierced at intervals by skylights" capped the building.[35] Outlying buildings included an office ell, boiler and wheel houses, dyehouse, weaving shed, cotton house, picker building, and repair shop (Dyer 1860, pp. 6-7; Poirier 1978, p. 16).

Practically speaking, the mill was more a metaphor for Lawrence's changing economic fortunes than it was a "model mill" in a city that aspired to be the nation's premiere textile center (Cole, 1960, p. 48). The financial panic of the late 1850s savaged the city and its textile concerns.[36] Management of the Pemberton Mill rode out the panic until October 1857, when the firm's over-dependence on credit brought it down.[37] On February 8, 1858 David Nevins and George Howe of Boston bought Pemberton Mill at auction for its original cost. Nevins, a banker, and Howe, an entrepreneur, reorganized as the Pemberton Manufacturing Company and resumed operations one month later, reaching full capacity in March 1859.[38] In the winter of 1859, it seemed to most, including the city's operatives, that the economic prospects of Lawrence and the Pemberton Mill were conjoined.[39]

Writing in 1860, the poet O. K. Vates imagined the Pemberton millhands as "blithe and gay" while laboring on January 10, each lost in his or her thoughts and unaware of the day's impending cataclysm:

It was on a Tuesday afternoon,
While all was busy, blithe, and gay,
Toiling briskly at the loom,
Thinking soon to get their pay.

What pleasing thoughts ran through their minds,
As the payment now drew near,
Some thinking on the gay—the fine,
Some o'er their pittance dropt a tear.[40]

The factory workers of Vates' invention are purposeful and spirited, even picturesque. However, as Vates reminded readers, that day as on every day, Pemberton millhands toiled out of need.

By 1860 textile operatives in the Commonwealth were ensnared in a political economy of speed and privation. As Ardis Cameron and Thomas Dublin have argued, U.S. textile prices plummeted during the 1830s and early '40s due to increasing international competition. Mill owners, alarmed by shrinking profit margins and expanding debt, lobbied Congress to enact protective tariffs. Manufacturers also sought to increase productivity and decrease labor costs by intensifying and accelerating production processes. Favored strategies included the stretch-out (an increase in the number of machines operated by individual workers) and a speed-up in the pace of work. The costs of these "efficiencies" for workers were the degradation of work and declining real wages (Cameron 1993, pp. xiii-xv; Dublin 1979, p. 109; Siracusa 1979, pp. 108-110, 160-161). A Fall River, Massachusetts textile agent put the matter baldly in 1855: "I regard my work-people just as I regard my machinery. So long as they can do my work for what I choose to pay them, I keep them, getting out of them all I can" (Brown and Tager 2000, p. 171). Thus, in the winter of 1859-1860, Pemberton operatives (like their New England counterparts) earned an average of $.60 per day while working twelve-hour days (Poirier 1971, p. 141; Dublin 1979, p. 201).

THE DISASTER AS POLITICAL EXIGENCY

On January 10, 1860 nearly a thousand textile operatives occupied the Pemberton Mill, each contributing to the daily output of basic and "fancy" cotton stuffs. Females constituted a clear majority of the workforce and were, on average, nineteen-and-a-half years old. The average age for male workers was twenty-four years. A significant minority was children. Twenty-two percent of Mill operatives were native born. Of these, most hailed in roughly equal numbers from Maine, Massachusetts, and New Hampshire. The greater number of their foreign counterparts were Irish, with English, Scottish, and German workers filling out their ranks.[41] Minutes before 5:00 P.M., the Mill's predominantly female and immigrant workforce felt the factory shudder and then there was bedlam.

City father Edgar Jay Sherman recalled the minutes following the mill's collapse in his memoir published in 1908.[42] On the afternoon of January 10, 1860, Sherman and his law partner, Daniel Saunders, Jr., recently elected Mayor of Lawrence, were working in their offices on Essex Street. Minutes before 5 P.M., the men "heard a loud noise, like snow sliding from the roof of a building." Moments later, a friend "rushed into the office," and divulged that Pemberton Mill had fallen "without . . . warning" and "while in 'full operation'."[43]

Saunders and Sherman hurried to the mill where, he wrote, they "witnessed a heart-rending scene."

> The cries of the wounded and dying were terrible. They came from all sides; from the unfortunate victims, coming out with limbs broken, from others confined and crushed by fallen timbers and machinery, from mothers looking

for their children, and children calling for their mothers, the wife for her husband and the husband for his wife.[44]

Pemberton Mill cashier Robert H. Tewksbury described the cascading events that brought down the mill. According to Tewksbury, the roof "first sank at the southerly end and the whole roof, freeing itself from the wall supports, [and] came crashing down upon the floor below." The weight of the "falling roof carried down the upper floor . . . with all the load of machinery. . . ." Tewksbury reckoned that the mill's collapse was inevitable, for "[e]very timber acted as a lever to tilt and crush the walls." The northerly wall of the main building "was thrown outward" across frozen canal waters and the ruined upper floors "overhung the lower at the north end. . . ."[45]

Fires at the mill site were not yet extinguished when Dr. William Lamb, the Essex County Coroner, convened an inquest into the fall of the Pemberton Mill.[46] A jury of six, the majority skilled tradesmen, heard testimony concerning the technical and human dimensions of the calamity.[47] Expert witnesses concurred that the mill's walls were too thin and that defective iron pillars used as floor supports had failed, causing the building to collapse.[48] Implicated in the purchase and installation of these columns were John Amory Lowell, J. Pickering Putnam, and Captain Charles H. Bigelow. On February 2, the jury issued a report reiterating this finding but affixed blame for the cataclysm more narrowly than had witnesses. The jury concluded that Bigelow was liable for every eventuality leading to the tragedy, including its fatalities. Earlier, Bigelow had testified that while it was his "duty to save unnecessary expense," he had built the mill according to the principles of sound construction. The panel thought otherwise, and though its members acknowledged that Bigelow had not hired the contractors for the columns, jurists concluded that he should have detected their irregularities. Hanging in the air was the implication that he had cut corners to cut costs.[49]

The Massachusetts General Court drew much the same conclusion but without benefit of an investigation. On January 11 Representative John C. Tucker of Boston moved that the House Committee on the Judiciary "consider the expediency of providing by law for the inspection of" manufacturing work sites. The Committee was so ordered. Tucker's avowed goal was the "better protection" of factory workers from "the dangers of fire and other casualties."[50] Implicit in his motion and the House order were four novel and inter-related ideas. First, workers had a right to bodily defense. Second, the state had an obligation to uphold that right. Third, parties to the employment contract lacked equivalent capacities for securing workers' bodily integrity. Fourth, state intervention in the wage relation was potentially sound public policy. The Lawrence catastrophe had impelled House members to contemplate a law that, if passed, would reverse established policy barring state interference in the wage relation.

By 1860 the Massachusetts judiciary and legislature had intervened in every sphere of life save that of industrial relations, with the notable exception of

Commonwealth v. Hunt (1842). With this opinion, written by Chief Justice Lemuel Shaw, the Supreme Judicial Court of Massachusetts had established workers' liberty of free association by ruling that trade unions did not constitute a conspiracy.[51] That same year, Shaw had established employers' non-liability at law in *Farwell v. Boston & Worcester Railroad.* Writing for the Court, Shaw reasoned that employers were not liable for injuries sustained by their employees. The idea that master and servant were *sui juris* (or having all social and civil rights) was central to Shaw's argument. It followed that parties to the wage relation were equally endowed with the capacities needed to evaluate the hazards of an occupation and to allocate their costs. Shaw's belief in the wage earner's unfettered agency was evident in his holding that the employee voluntarily assumed the risks of employment. Based on this reasoning, the Chief Justice concluded that state intervention in the wage relation did not conduce to sound public policy.[52] The court's reasoning was unchanged in 1860 and would remain so until 1887, the antebellum legislature having declined to enact law concerning this matter.[53] Consistent with this, the Massachusetts General Court repeatedly rebuffed popular demands for reforms such as the Ten Hour day.[54] As the nation moved toward fratricidal struggle, there were few precedents to suggest that the state would exert its powers on behalf of its laboring populace.

Nevertheless, on February 15, 1860 the Massachusetts House of Representatives began deliberations over a bill calling for state inspection of the industrial workplace and its operations. That Wednesday, Representative Wentworth of Lowell, a member of the House Committee on the Judiciary, reported out House Bill Number 83 "to Provide for the Security of Public Buildings and Bridges." After due deliberation, House members recommitted the bill to the Committee on the Judiciary for refining. On March 23, Wentworth reported that the bill "ought to pass with . . . amendments." Six days later the House passed the revised bill for engrossment and sent it to the Senate for concurrence.[55]

The omnibus bill sent to the Senate called for public oversight of the most critical dimensions of the manufacturing worksite. Reacting to the fall of the Pemberton Mill, legislators mandated building codes for manufacturing enterprises and stipulated for their periodic inspection and maintenance. The bill also required machine guarding and the upkeep of public passageways and elevators. Penalties for failure to follow the law included fines (ranging from $100 to $2,000), the denial of certificates of inspection, injunctions against unapproved construction, and plant closings. The House vested authority for enforcement in local authorities rather than the state, but the bill also empowered the local citizenry to alert authorities to hazards. This provision was a critical first step toward the articulation of community standards for the industrial worksite.[56] The House bill was not only remarkably progressive in its scope, but also its provisions presaged reforms that postbellum lawmakers would enact incrementally.

Legislative records indicate that the Senate initially warmed to House Bill Number 83 before rejecting it. On March 30, Senate members referred the bill to the Committee on the Judiciary. Reporting for the Committee on April 3, Mr. Osgood stated that the bill should progress, whereupon his colleagues ordered the bill to second reading. The next day, Senate members refused the bill a third reading, effectively killing it.[57] Poirier has argued that legislative support for the bill lapsed when journalists stopped pressuring for its enactment, a reflection of their growing preoccupation with impending war. This explanation suffices insofar as it goes, but it fails to clarify the Senate Committee's April endorsement of House Bill Number 83. Neither does it adequately explain the main body's rejection of that bill just twenty-four hours later. Because extant records shed no light on the Senate's contradictory actions, we are left to conjecture that in the absence of constituent support for the bill, state industrialists successfully quashed it.

A labor movement capable of advancing a pro-worker legislative agenda had not yet materialized in Massachusetts. After 1820 and through 1860, waves of skilled tradesmen and unskilled and semi-skilled operatives protested the disassembling effects of industrial capitalism on their bodies and selfhood. Worker militancy spilled out of the work site and into the State House, but workingmen's associations and their champions failed to secure large-scale victories in either location. Various forces undercut the establishment of enduring labor bodies, the most important being the era's economic downturns. The collapse of the Pemberton Mill capped one such contraction, ensuring that labor would not play a meaningful role in legislative deliberations about this unprecedented social exigency.[58]

THE SOCIAL CONSTRUCTION OF ELIGIBILITY FOR RELIEF

Forty-eight hours after the collapse of the Pemberton Mill, the Massachusetts House of Representatives ordered its Committee on Finance to "inquire into the expediency" of appropriating one thousand dollars "for the relief of the sufferers in the recent calamity at Lawrence." The motion, made by Mr. Putnam of Danvers, and its approval testify to lawmakers' recognition of the catastrophe's effects on Pemberton millhands.[59] One day earlier, several legislators had traveled to Lawrence to view the mill site and consult with city fathers. It is likely that the delegation's report to House members moved them to sympathy and then action.[60] Two weeks later, however, Representative Henry K. Oliver of Lawrence moved that the Committee on Finance be "discharged from further consideration" of the proposed allocation. House records provide no explanation of Oliver's suppression of the appropriation.[61]

Henry K. Oliver may well have killed the appropriation after first consulting with the Pemberton Mill relief committee, of which he was a member, and his fellow lawmakers. Moreover, Oliver would have known of the committee's immediate success in fundraising. He and others may have reasoned that a subsidy by the Commonwealth was unnecessary so long as private donations were forth-coming. Oliver's motives aside, his elimination of the earmark was surprising but not exceptional in an era when government disaster aid was more a bestowal (or *ex gratia* payment) than a matter of right.

Had the legislature wanted to aid the disaster victims, it faced no legal prohibitions against doing so. According to the historian Michele Landis, the constitutionality of state-sponsored relief was "rarely contested" after 1827 when Congress approved relief for the fire-stricken Alexandria, Virginia. That said, there were no laws *mandating* state and federal disaster relief. Instead, state subsidies were contingent on investigations of the claimants' integrity and culpability for a given mishap.[62] When adjudged respectable and blameless, disaster victims were remade as "sufferers" and deemed worthy of empathy and relief. The term "sufferers"—evocative of Old Testament stoicism and fidelity—applied to persons of varying social and civic status. To suffer was to weather adversity while retaining a measure of personal dignity and sovereignty. According to Landis, the process of distinguishing the worthy from the unworthy engendered "narratives of blame and fate." These had the effect, in turn, of elevating certain "desperations" over others in the polity and at law. Thus, not all claims became grounds for redress and relief.[63] Absent a state-mandated welfare program, mill workers had no basis at law to make a claim on the state earmark that Representative Oliver deemed unnecessary. Ultimately, the question of whether the Commonwealth ought to relieve the Lawrence disaster victims was a historically constituted matter of conscience, not law.

Boston and Lawrence elites immediately undertook fundraising on behalf of the disaster victims, tacit acknowledgment that millhands' claims on charity were incontestable. On January 11, the New England Society for the Promotion of Manufactures and the Mechanical Arts launched a subscription for the "benefit of the sufferers." On the 13th, the Pemberton relief committee constituted itself for purposes of organizing "a system of inspection and relief. . . ."[64] Comprising it were Charles S. Storrow, Henry K. Oliver, William C. Chapin, and John C. Hoadley. Daniel Saunders, Jr., Mayor of Lawrence, served as chairman.[65] Each man was a recognized city leader; the surnames of three would eventually grace Lawrence schools.[66] Pardon Armington, the committee's hired Clerk, attended subsequent meetings, as did others involved in the relief effort.[67] The committee raised $65,834.67 in contributions and disbursed $51,834.67 to Lawrence opera-tives, their dependents, and individuals and businesses who incurred costs at their behest (Dorgan 1918, p. 57).

On January 16 and 28, the relief committee established both its purpose and method for achieving it. According to the minutes, those present concurred that the fund should be used for "relief of *extreme sufferers*" (emphasis added). The circumstances and conditions that constituted profound suffering were neither stated nor fixed. Instead, the committee relied on prima facie evidence of need to settle victims' claims.

Accordingly, committee members appointed six inspectors to canvass Lawrence's working-class enclaves and to assess operatives' needs and worthiness of aid. Daniel Saunders, Sr., the mayor's father, served as an inspector, as did five others.[68] The fruit of their labors was an extensive "list of the injured and the dead" and the victims' losses.[69] With this information, Chairman Saunders, Jr. and Treasurer Storrow "settle[d] all cases needing immediate aid according to their judgment both in kind and quantity of relief."[70]

Examination of the committee's Ledger of Assistance reveals that the committee took a businesslike approach to relief administration and distribution. For example, the committee accounted not only for monthly expenditures, including types of assistance rendered to operatives and their kin, but also gathered copious data on the victims' domiciles, family economies, and support networks. Working from inspectors' reports, the committee took particular care to tabulate all injured and killed workers, the number of their family members employed by the mill, and family dependence on operatives' wages.[71] The committee also sought to establish itself as the final authority for the collection and distribution of funds. On January 16 the body voted "that the public be cautioned against paying any monies to unknown solicitors . . . , excepting to those authorized by the Mayor."[72] Within a fortnight, committee members had rationalized citywide relief efforts, tempering compassion with efficiency.

Consistent with this the relief committee articulated four guidelines for the awarding of aid. Injured operatives and the families of the dead would receive "partial or final" relief. "Uninjured operatives" were ineligible for relief unless they were "extreme[ly]" destitute due to the loss of their clothing or employment. The committee also voted against replacing the lost clothing of victims who were not among the "naked destitute." Such claims, the committee proclaimed, were illegitimate.[73] The committee's anticipation of requests for apparel points to operatives' meager store of clothing and the costs for them of replacing it. Finally, the committee resolved that "well" persons who had lost their livelihood due to the mill's collapse were not entitled to compensation. The committee's reasoning was stark: "Loss of employment is an ordinary occurrence that we cannot remedy. . . ." Nonetheless, committee members willingly aided millhands seeking to return to a state of self-sufficiency, as evidenced by its facilitation of petitioners' search for employment or railway travel to family and friends.[74] Using these criteria, inspectors made recommendations orally and in writing concerning compensation.

Fund administrators took particular care to assuage the needs of families that had lost loved ones on January 10, but they did so with an eye to the marketplace. According to Storrow, "It was our wish that no family from whom a member had been taken by death, should be without some donation. . . ." These grants were "in addition to the payment of all expenses immediately consequent upon . . . bereavement." Practicality trumped empathy, however, for the committee allocated varying amounts of aid according to the centrality of the deceased to the household economy. Families that lost their primary or sole breadwinner received $200 to $500, while those families that had been "partially dependent" on the deceased received $100 to $200. Finally, families that had not relied on the deceased received $50 to $100.[75] In sum, the committee had established a hierarchy of need on market-based assessments of the value of working bodies and particularly the deceased as provider.

Three months later, Storrow again invoked the logic of the market in his denial of Edward O'Neil's appeal for $5 per week in board. Storrow observed that the Relief Committee deemed the request excessive on its face and in light of its "rapidly diminishing" fund. O'Neil had made his home available to Augusta Sampson, who had been grievously injured during the mill's collapse and required live-in nursing. The relief committee would eventually award her an annuity for life. O'Neil now sought an increase in the committee's payment of Sampson's board. Storrow firmly but tactfully denied the request, explaining that the sum exceeded what the Lawrence rental market would bear. Moreover, the committee had provided other resources for Sampson's care. As proof of the first point, Storrow cited the rates paid by the committee for the board of infirm workers. He informed O'Neil that the relief committee saw fit to pay him no more than $3 per week, an allocation its members described as generous when compared with market rates.[76]

In June 1860 Storrow confidently reported that the relief committee had been judicious in tendering relief. He averred that "in no single instance" did fund administrators provide relief without first engaging in "careful inquiry and deliberation." He then enumerated the criteria that informed decision-making: "1st, the number and age of the persons dependent, and their *bodily* & pecuniary condition; 2d, the former circumstances of the family, or the manner in which they had been accustomed to live"; and "3d, their ability to use the provision prudently" (*emphasis added*).[77] Adherence to the last principle led the committee to contravene antebellum gender relations. For example, Storrow and his fellows occasionally entrusted funds to female members of operatives' households rather than to male relations adjudged intemperate.[78] In effect, the committee prized fiscal prudence over maintenance of masculine authority in working-class households.

Successful though the committee was, it had its detractors. John Whitty, President of the Lowell Irish Benevolent Society, complained to Storrow about the latter's erroneous recounting of the Society's contribution. On December 7, 1860, Storrow wrote to Whitty, assuring him that the committee had not erred. Storrow hastened to add that he "that any seeming injustice should have been done to your excellent society."[79] In Storrow's *Final Report of the Treasurer of the Committee of Relief*, published in February 1861, he acknowledged that he *had* erred, but he did so obliquely.[80] Whitty's exchange with Storrow hints at the social tensions between Massachusetts Yankees and the state's Irish middle class. At stake, among other things, was the power to speak and act for the Commonwealth's largest ethnic minority. Evidently, Whitty did not intend to allow Storrow to misrepresent the Society's fundraising prowess, a measure of its capacity for caring for its own.

By January 21, 1860, several of the committee's benefactors sought to halt fundraising for the fund, an action that Charles S. Storrow opposed. In a letter to Amos A. Lawrence, Storrow argued against publication of a notice that would have left the public with the impression that there was a sufficiency of monies. He reasoned that "there is a stream coming in from New York, Philadelphia, & other places as well as [from] smaller town in New England which we do not wish to check as yet." Moreover, disaster victims and their dependents would conclude "from such a notice" that the committee was "overloaded with money, & would tend to increase their demands upon us beyond what is necessary. . . ." Worse still, the notice would "check" the victims' "readiness to help themselves & each other."[81] Fundraising was justified, Storrow reasoned, so long as victims had need of aid and were unable to provide for themselves.

Storrow buttressed his argument by reporting that the relief committee was especially taxed by "very numerous cases" of the permanently disabled and dependent children. The treasurer's anxiety was manifested in his halting prose:

> [P]ersons disabled for life, & . . . very young children whom we ~~do not feel should be~~ are unwilling to have left to the nursing of the poor house but who must for a long time be provided for—It is this ~~feature~~ which ~~shows to us~~ makes us realize the great extent of relief sooner or later to be needed.

Then, inexplicably, Storrow contradicted himself by stating that the New England Society, of which Amos A. Lawrence was a member, had "nobly" acquitted itself and need not "make any further effort."[82] Storrow's reasons for stemming the tide of relief from Boston elites are unknown. Given that the calamity was without precedent, Storrow lacked requisite data for calculating the long-term costs of maintaining large numbers of invalids and orphans. Writing in February 1861, Storrow acknowledged that it was far easier to accurately project the needs of those who were "in the enjoyment of ordinary health. . . ." By implication, tables of mortality were useless for any other purpose.[83] Nevertheless, he was disinclined to raise funds against unknown eventualities and instead urged the cessation of fundraising.[84] According to Storrow and his contemporaries, relief was temporary by definition.

For a time, the wants of Pemberton Mill operatives competed with those of their New Bedford counterparts, requiring negotiation by elites concerning outreach to private donors. In a letter dated January 24, Joseph Grinnell, Mayor of New Bedford, then a depressed shipping center, wrote Mayor Saunders to advance the claims of New Bedford's unemployed on public largesse. Grinnell reported that New Bedford leaders had collected funds to send to Lawrence, but having learned of the moratorium on collections, they would instead distribute the proceeds among the indigent in their own city.[85] In effect, the Pemberton relief committee had a duty to other distressed commercial centers in the Commonwealth. On January 26, Charles S. Storrow responded to Grinnell at the behest of Saunders. Storrow immediately explained that the Mayor would have written but for the "press of business devolving upon him." Next, Storrow addressed Grinnell's concern for New Bedford's "unemployed population," observing that the "aid afforded to us has been about as prompt and as ample as the disaster was sudden & extensive." He assured Grinnell, however, that the Pemberton relief committee would now step aside so that New Bedford could press its claims on public sympathy.[86]

Storrow's letters to Amos A. Lawrence and Mayor Grinnell illuminate the deficiencies of antebellum philanthropy in the northeastern United States, as well as the limits of public knowledge of industrial workers' economic distress. With the notable exception of fraternal organizations, neither a private nor a state-sponsored system of income maintenance was yet established. Consequently, the Pemberton relief committee relied on its own exertions to relieve the victims and their dependents. To be successful, committee members had to establish the primacy of their claims as against others. Thus, the committee emphasized the magnitude of the disaster, the gravity of its effects, and the millhands' suffering and worthiness of aid. Antebellum competition for public sympathy and charity bespoke the limits of each, especially in a society that had not yet articulated the right of injured workers to income maintenance.

On March 28, 1860, Storrow issued a public notice to Lawrence physicians, instructing them "to take no new cases under their charge without previously speaking to one of the Inspectors" or himself. He reported that during the weeks since the disaster, "a large number of the Sufferers by the Pemberton Mill had now been finally discharged from the care of the Committee of Relief."[87]

POPULAR PERCEPTIONS AND REPRESENTATIONS

Clarisse A. Poirier has demonstrated that the fall of the Pemberton Mill spawned voluminous private and public writings on the meanings and implications of the disaster.[88] Close reading of these materials reveals that American writers and readers were captivated by three main questions. First, who or what was to blame for the catastrophe? Second, who were the victims and how did they live and work? Third, were the ill-fated Pemberton millhands worthy of relief and if so, why?

Disaster reportage circulating in the weeks following the calamity unavoidably lacked the perspective of hindsight. Absent the coroner's verdict, widespread rumor-mongering and sensational press accounts had significant explanatory power.[89] Lawrence civic leaders had little time for corrective retrospection given the panorama of suffering and desolation surrounding them.[90] Instead, municipal authorities attended to the needs of a devastated citizenry. Thus, Charles

S. Storrow penned a laconic account of the Mill's collapse for the first committee's first report, issued in June.[91] Yet privately, Storrow informed Francis Cogswell, President of the Boston and Maine Railroad, that the "extent of the suffering cannot entirely be appreciated by you, it is hardly yet fully seen by us."[92] In contrast to Storrow's economy of detail and phlegmatic tone in his public writings, the greater number of disaster writings mimicked the era's cultural imaginings.

Popular narratives about the catastrophe and its victims were admixtures of fact, storytelling, and meaning-making.[93] Widely circulated texts included sermons, journalistic "ethnographies" of working-class life and culture, poetry, and correspondence to and from the relief committee. These retellings ranged from the didactic to the prurient according to their authors' divergent purposes.[94] Even so, disaster writings were more alike than different owing to their authors' use of narrative devices and literary tropes found in antebellum popular literature. Thus, writers moved and persuaded their readers by emplotting the calamity as allegory, melodrama, and sentimental tragedy.[95] Populating these accounts were iconic and grieving mothers, manly rescuers with "bleeding hearts," stereotypical Irish miscreants, suffering yet stoical victims, and pious orphans.[96] For example, one young woman lay in the ruins exhorting those trapped with her to appeal to God for redemption, all the while maintaining her spirits and those around her. The author dubbed her the "Christian heroine" (Haskell and Mason 1860, p. 19). As this suggests, fiction interposed between the tragedy and contemporaries' readings of it.[97]

Clerics in the textile center were among the first to explain the disaster. According to Clarisse A. Poirier, doctrinal differences mediated between the mill's collapse and the clergy's representations of the calamity (Poirier 1990, pp. 79-80). Evidence of this may be found in clerics' preferred "homiletic style." During the antebellum period, an increasing number of clerics discarded theological polemics and instead sought to edify and engage their congregations using illustrative stories and narration, or what David Reynolds has termed "religious fiction." In effect, "metaphysics" was giving way to disquisition on "the more tangible realm of moral behavior." According to Reynolds, the displacement of theology by "pulpit storytelling" occurred gradually and was never total.[98] Consistent with this, homilies delivered by Lawrence's clerics in the disaster's aftermath ran the gamut from treatises on the nature of sin and God's "'providential plan'" to spiritual entertainment. For example, the Reverends Henry F. Lane, a Baptist, and C. E. Fisher, a Congregationalist, spoke but little of the disaster and instead sermonized on its implications for humankind. In contrast, the Reverend E. M. Tappan at the Freewill Baptist Church began his homily with a "thrilling" account of the Mill's collapse; he then enumerated the tragedy's lessons for human beings and their social and political institutions (Haskell and Mason 1860, pp. 38, 40-43).

Doctrinal differences and rhetorical proclivities notwithstanding, the city's religious leaders also sounded many of the same chords. The sermon delivered by the Reverend E. M. Tappan captured sentiments expressed by the majority of his colleagues. Tappan repudiated the idea that God had struck down the victims in retribution for their sins. Instead he opined that the *"the inordinate love of money"* had caused the disaster. By Tappan's lights, the mill owners had knowingly imperiled their workers by capitulating to the laws of the marketplace. They had done so by purchasing defective building materials in defiance of what Tappan and others described as "physical law" or the law of gravity. Consequently, he reasoned, the mill owners had contravened God's law and failed to safeguard the operatives, whose right to bodily defense had then been abrogated.[99]

Theodore Parker shared Tappan's regard for the intertwined laws of God and nature, as evidenced by his private correspondence. Likening the mill's fall to "battles of industry," Parker wrote: "It is natural for us in our sorrow, as in our joy, to flee to the Infinite for consolation and hope. But, alas! How few ministers there are who can see and tell the causes of this disaster in human ignorance and cupidity. . . ." According to Parker, the telling of the tragedy was imperative if mankind was to learn from it.[100] He concluded with the observation that "Americans are careless, and must suffer until they learn prudence. Conform to natural law, and it shall be well with thee: that is the language of all 'accidents'" (Frothingham 1847, p. 470).

Parker, a Transcendentalist and liberal Unitarian, and Tappan, a Baptist, conceived of the Lawrence disaster as the manifestation of human failing and collective disequilibrium. Yet, had the two men crossed paths, good fellowship might well have foundered on the shoals of doctrinal differences. Still, Parker and Tappan agreed that personal rectitude and social stability flowed from introspection, reverence for nature and its laws, and assent to God's will. Each man reckoned that those responsible for the tragedy had foresworn mutuality, moderation, and altruism for the metaphysics of the marketplace. In so doing, they had imperiled Pemberton millhands—or as Boston's Transcendentalists had it, one thousand, infinitely valuable human souls. In the end, neither Parker nor Tappan explained how the imperatives of commerce might be harmonized with the requirements of mindfulness and forbearance. Instead, Parker prescribed prudence and Tappan called for factory inspection.[101]

Unlike Parker and Tappan, Charles S. Storrow conceived of the disaster as an act of God. That said, arguments and inferences that the operatives had suffered for their sins offended Storrow. He preferred to believe that the disaster made manifest "the works and glory of God" by bringing out "great traits of character" among the better and lesser denizens of Lawrence.[102] One month after the disaster's occurrence, Storrow reiterated this idea in his correspondence with a donor, pronouncing himself well pleased with the victims' disposition. The Committee Treasurer marveled that Pemberton operatives exhibited an "uncomplaining cheerfulness," a fact that Storrow characterized as "one of the most remarkable features in the most remarkable of events."[103]

In a letter dated January 25, 1860, Edwin Byrnes of Worcester, Massachusetts echoed Storrow's sentiments while reporting on local fundraising.[104] Byrnes averred that the mill's collapse was an "unparalleled misfortune" and "awful crisis," yet its occurrence had occasioned unprecedented generosity on the part of city fathers. Thus he called down God's blessings on the Committee, as well as "all those noble men whom this calamity seems to have joined so nobly together in a common effort to alleviate the woes so shocking, and so weighty, borne, as they are, by the weak and lowly. . . ."[105]

Byrnes' argument is suggestive for three reasons. First, Byrnes took it as an article of faith that society consisted of the better sort and their social inferiors. Second, he inferred that elites had a responsibility to their subordinates, in this case, the Lawrence "sufferers." Third, men who fulfilled their duty to social inferiors were the better for it. Yet, as was discussed, eighteen years earlier Chief Justice Lemuel Shaw had ruled that employers were not liable for injuries sustained by workers in their service. As he saw it, imperiled laborers could demand higher wages as compensation for their assumption of risk. If not forthcoming, they could decline employment. In short, occupational casualties were calculable costs of contract rather than "embodied experience."[106] Byrnes obviously did not share Shaw's analysis, nor did others who shared Byrnes' sense of noblesse oblige. The common law of employers' liability—an embodiment of the marketplace ethos—had not yet supplanted the pre-industrial ethos of mutuality.

Poetic and fictional treatments of operatives' grief and losses were frequently more allegoric and melodramatic than pious. Thus, poet O. K. Vates depicted the archetypal sorrowful mother in his poem, "Lines on the Great Calamity":

> The Mother comes, her child to find, —
> Closely she views the mangled pile;
> She sees! —she starts! —my God be kind!
> And closely clasps her dying child.[107]

Like Vates, journalists frequently depicted working-class women as unduly emotional. Female relatives of deceased operatives were supposedly overpowered by the "intensity of their grief" and given to "violent demonstrations of their wild despair" (Haskell and Mason 1860, p. 13). In contrast, narrators wrote glowingly of "fine-looking New England matrons, from the distant country towns" who were noble in their grief.[108]

POPULAR IMAGININGS OF THE IRISH

Journalistic treatments of Irish Mill victims frequently emphasized their irrationality. According to one account, the Irish mother of Mary Callahan refused to let the doctor remove her daughter's smashed leg despite appeals by the family physician and priest. Mrs. Callahan, who worked alongside her daughter in the mill's card-room, declared "Mary's condition in heaven would not be so happy if she were maimed." The narrator concluded by drawing out the tale's lesson: "[I]t seemed sad to sacrifice to dark superstition a life that had been spared in the perils of the falling building" (Haskell and Mason 1860, p. 132).

Relief committee inspectors were no less xenophobic in their representations of Irish claimants, as can be seen by H. Wood's report on Celia Connelly and her family. Connelly was an Irish woman who lived with her mother and a married sister who was also a mill operative. Those whom Wood consulted during his investigation described Celia's brother-in-law "as not doing much for the support of the family—wife and one child."[109] The Connelly family was, in short, the antithesis of respectable domesticity, the women providing for one another and their male kin.[110]

Wood scornfully enumerated Celia Connelly's claims on the Committee's largesse. The operative had informed Wood that she was injured and had "lost her clothes" during the mill's collapse. She also owed a substantial amount of back rent.[111] Yet, in his report to the relief committee, Wood opined:

As to how much she is really injured it is hard to tell—because of the exaggeration & much ado of the mother & the disposition on her part to make a mountain out of known trifles. She groans and sighs [and] looks all on the dark side, dwells & laments continually.[112]

Neither did Wood credit Celia Connelly's assertion that she was "much black & blue." He reported that "no serious injury can be discovered or is pretended." Yet by Wood's own admission, Connelly had recently been "out, but had a fainting fit & was taken home." Insensible to Connelly's trauma, Wood observed that the mill worker "broods over the calamity & talks so much about it, she can scarcely sleep. . . ."[113]

Wood's next statements reveal that even the most intimate details of operatives' lives were subject to investigation. Wood reported that Celia Connelly's "nervous system is still under much excitement, with occasional wandering of the mind." Moreover, "Her mother tells the Doctor, that the event has caused a disturbance to her monthly health [or menses]."[114] Because Connelly's doctor had not yet fully assessed her injuries, Wood refrained from advocating for or against aid to the factory operative. Instead, the inspector communicated his views obliquely, stating that the "facts of the case" would "enable" the Committee to make the proper judgment. However, he warned, "The case seems to be one requiring caution & some delay before much action."[115]

Not every account of the mill's Irish victims played to prevailing stereotypes. Ellen McCarthy was seriously injured on January 10, 1860 and she had not yet fully recovered by October of that year. John Fallon, whose relationship to McCarthy is undefined, wrote on Ellen's behalf to the relief committee, asking that her case be reconsidered if she "not be able to labor at the expiration of the year."[116] Fallon had previously consulted with Dr. William H. Burleigh,

Ellen McCarthy's physician. Burleigh informed Fallon that he desired "to call in an eminent Boston physician for consultation." Only then would Burleigh judge the "length of time" his patient "may be unable to labor." Ellen had already consented to travel to Boston in her doctor's "charge and care." According to Fallon, Burleigh expressed "the highest regard" for Ellen's respectability and stoicism in the face of acute "suffering." Burleigh had met Ellen after the disaster and as Fallon reported, he was much impressed by her "commendable patience" and "uprightness and . . . deportment."[117]

WORKING-CLASS PAIN

Female corporeality figured in disaster narratives to a lesser degree than evaluations of their character. Nevertheless, a compendium of disaster narratives served up salacious descriptions of the victims' mutilated, roasted, and promiscuously commingled corpses. For example, we learn that one girl

> had two fingers caught in the machinery. In an agony of despair she literally tore them off, and crawled through an opening in the ruins, stripping her clothes completely from her body. . . . A few days after, the fingers were found by the workmen and transmitted to the girl who had spared them for her life. (Haskell and Mason 1860, p. 20)

Why did the author emphasize the corporeality of a working-class girl? What effects did these extraordinarily raw images of a nude and dismembered girl have on the reader? Were they intended to titillate, thereby increasing the social and cultural distance between the reader and subject? Alternatively, were readers shocked into awareness by these accounts?

Elizabeth Clark has posed similar questions in her compelling analysis of anti-slavery fiction. As she has argued, abolitionist literature, "with its critique of interpersonal violence and sexual abuse, served as a vehicle for new arguments for a 'right' to bodily integrity" (Clark 1995, pp. 463-464). Likewise, Pemberton disaster narratives laid a foundation for the articulation and expansion of workers' rights to bodily defense and integrity by exposing the disjuncture between assaults on wage earners' bodies in the workplace and paeans to free labor.

Maurice Palmer's death made for equally ribald and "thrilling" copy, the result being that his story appeared in a variety of written media.[118] Palmer, a "second-hand in the spinning room," survived the mill's collapse but lay trapped in the ruins. According to the published chronicle of his demise entitled "Attempted Suicide of an Overseer," rescuers recognized Palmer's voice as he called out from below. The operative "implored his friends to save him quickly, or he should die." We are told that Palmer eventually felt the fire's heat and concluded that a "horrible death seemed inevitable." He withdrew his knife and reportedly declared "he should commit suicide rather than burn to death." Palmer then "drew his knife across his throat." Rescuers delivered Palmer from the wreckage, and after ascertaining that his self-inflicted injuries were not mortal, they carried him to City Hall, the site of a makeshift hospital and morgue. Palmer died soon after because of his internal injuries. As if to communicate the depth of this tragedy, Palmer's anonymous chronicler reported that he was "much beloved by his friends" (Haskell and Mason 1860, p. 15).[119]

WORKING-CLASS MANHOOD AND WOMANHOOD

Palmer and his extended family, residents of Rochester, New Hampshire, enjoyed the unconditional respect of that village's better men. From a letter written by John H. Fuller and later published, we learn that the overseer "was the sole hope of his aged parents." Moreover, Palmer left in their care "his three promising children (the oldest but nine years old)." Fuller thereupon requested that "this unfortunate family" be "remembered in their sore affliction." Fuller made his case for aid by establishing the worthiness of Palmer's family. According to Fuller, the deceased's father was "an excellent man, being highly respected by all who know him." Moreover, Maurice Palmer had been a "worthy and excellent son." Fuller concluded by conflating Palmer's role of provider with bodily capacity, asserting that the overseer's family's "only chance of support has gone *in the person of their . . . son*" (emphasis added) (Haskell and Mason 1860, p. 24). Using culturally resonant language, Fuller argued that the senior and junior Palmers were paragons of masculinity. Accordingly, Maurice Palmer's dependents deserved aid from the relief committee, Palmer's fellows in the era's fraternity of orthodox men.[120]

The publication from which Fuller's letter is excerpted is replete with comparable vignettes. Entitled *An Authentic History of the Lawrence Calamity* and compiled and published by E. G. Haskell and Samuel Mason in 1860, the collection recounted "thrilling incidents" previously written by journalists, sermons by Lawrence clerics, the coroner's report, and other writings. The sequencing and exposition of the compendium's sketches reflected the editors' intention to provide readers with well-paced, first-hand accounts of a disaster beyond their experience.

Palmer's attempted suicide notwithstanding, the Pemberton relief committee settled $857.61 on his next-of-kin, describing the sum as a "large special contribution."[121] Committee members did so after being persuaded by W. D. Joplin, their agent, that Palmer's dependents were worthy of assistance.[122] Joplin's report, a letter penned on January 31, 1860, survives as an ethnography of working-class family life and rural mores. Joplin reported that he had "visited the Parents and children of Morris H. Palmer at Rochester, N.H." Once there, Joplin learned that Palmer had two sons, Ralph B., born in 1848 in Lowell, and Walter M., born two years later in Biddeford. The locations of their births suggest that their parents sacrificed stability to the necessity of securing employment where they could find it. The boys lived with their grandparents, their mother having left for undisclosed reasons.[123] As Fuller had done with his readers, Joplin sought to move committee members by emphasizing the family's reduced circumstances and the manliness of Palmer's progeny.

Palmer's sons lived within an extended family whose members were susceptible to death and privation in the emerging industrial era. According to Joplin, the Palmer clan lived on a site originally deeded to the boys' great-aunt "who was killed on the Rail road about four years since—." The family consisted of the boys' grandparents, a 45-year-old aunt who "worked at tailoring," and "an aged maiden" great-aunt. Two months before Maurice Palmer's death, his parents suffered the loss of a daughter. She and her brother, Maurice, had been the family's financial mainstays. The boys' deceased aunt, nameless in Joplin's report, had earned "considerable money" and spent "all for the various members of the family," having paid for Morris's schooling at an academy. Maurice had paid for the boys' board with his parents. Joplin concluded that their deaths "seems to have so reduced the resources" of the family, "that unless some permanent relief is afforded, until the boys arrive at an age to be of pecuniary benefit, they must suffer for the necessities of life."[124] Joplin then itemized the family's indebtedness and the community aid at their disposal to buttress his recommendation that the relief committee come to the Palmer family's aid.

Pemberton mill operatives not only figured as subjects in the disaster writings, but also generated an extensive correspondence. Thomas Duffie's communication with Mary, his wife, is characteristically purposeful and unadorned by literary embellishment.[125] Duffie relocated to Fall River after the disaster and then wrote to his wife in Lawrence where she lived with their three children. Thomas reported that although work was scarce, he and their son James were earning enough to survive and anticipated finding steady work. Duffie sought to persuade his wife that she should relocate to Fall River immediately to reduce the family's cost of living. Reunification would make it unnecessary for the family to pay two rents. Thus, Duffie urged Mary to appeal to the Relief Committee. "[A]sk them if the[y] would be so kind as to give you [a] pass for your self [sic] and the furniture [so that you may come] to me and I will be ever thankful to them." It is evident that Duffie yearned for his wife, for he twice addressed her as "Dear wife" and signed himself as "your afectionate [sic] husband."[126]

Bitterness rather than tenderness infused a letter to the relief committee written by Ann McDonald on behalf of a Mrs. Mulineaux. The letter is intriguing because it hints at the possibility that Mulineaux held the mill responsible for the death of her daughter, Hannah Mulineaux, a spool worker. Hannah's mother came to Lawrence in search of Hannah after learning of the disaster. According to the elder Mulineaux, she then "found the murdered body of said Hannah in the dead House, and then procured a suitable coffin bringing her remains to Lowell."[127]

Family animosities percolate through the letter written for the elder Mulineaux. According to her characterization of her daughter, Hannah:

> Was a married woman at the time of her death having a husband and one child whom she had to work for from *dire* necessity as her husband from *dissipated* and *idle* habits was unable to give or render the deceased while living any assistance.[128]

Millhands at the NewMarket Manufacturing Company in New Hampshire evinced a keen understanding of the imperative of earning a living wage. After extending "their heartfelt sympathy" to the disaster victims, the Granite State operatives articulated the argument that would animate postbellum campaigns for employers' liability reform and workmen's compensation. They wrote, "Knowing that sympathy is of little avail, unless accompanied by substantial aid, . . . we enclose . . . the amount of one day's pay for the benefit of the Lawrence sufferers."[129]

DISASTER NARRATIVES AS SOCIAL INDICATORS AND POLITICAL FORCES

In an age when Americans were hungry to learn about the "other"—as evidenced by the popularity of abolitionist fiction such as Harriet Beecher Stowe's *Uncle Tom's Cabin* (1852)—writings about the Mill's collapse introduced wage earners to the reading public.[130] The stock characters that populated disaster narratives stood in for its victims and were, therefore, their ambassadors to inquiring Americans.

As rendered by others, Pemberton millhands were varied and massively contradictory beings. They were named and anonymous, singular and abstracted, conventional and disorderly. To the extent that factory operatives were conventional, they elicited readers' empathy and concern. When depicted as being nonconformist, operatives embodied the erosion of republican virtues and relations. Consequently, their portraits sustained and inverted antebellum ideas about respectable individuality and its measures.

Narrative portraits of Pemberton Mill workers derived explanatory power from five inter-related sources. First, authors fitted their working-class subjects with a "mask of realism" (Stoops 2002, p. 7) fashioned from actual and stereotypical behaviors and traits. Consistent with this, writers depicted a variety of working-class subjects, the particularities of which lent authenticity to workers' putative identities. Third, readers filtered these texts through their own perceptions and experiences. Fourth, the affordability and reproducibility of the popular press heightened its impact on antebellum Americans' "collective sense" of themselves and those "pictured."[131] Finally, the authors of disaster narratives "instructed readers as to how they should respond" to working-class pain and suffering (Barton 1998, p. 159).

In his study of disaster reportage in the *New York Times* after 1852, Michael Barton has concluded that American readers were told that accidents and disasters were "'sad'" and that disaster victims grieved. In effect, journalists served up stories along with their own feelings about a given "tragedy and its victims." Consequently, readers did not have to work at imagining the emotional impact of tragedy. Moreover, they were predisposed to emotionalism. According to Barton, this was "one of the defining characteristics of American public and private expressive life in the 1800s." Thus, not only did journalists engage in "emotional investigation and modeling," but also they spoke in terms that resonated with the reading public (1998, pp. 158-159).

Barton has also documented the popularity of accident and disaster reportage in the United States throughout the nineteenth century. *The New York Times* posted these stories on its first page under the byline "Latest Intelligence" and later, "News by Telegraph." Accounts of natural disasters and their effects appeared alongside sensational accounts of "railroad, steamship, and mining calamities" (1998, pp. 157, 162). According to Barton, journalists were equally preoccupied with the victims' emotional distress and injuries (1998, pp. 160-161). So pervasive were the stories that Edgar Allen Poe opined that journalistic sensationalism had effects "beyond all calculation," while Walt Whitman called it scurrilous.[132] Barton has concluded that, then as now, journalists paid "attention to disasters" and their readers paid "attention to disaster stories."[133]

It is striking that public consumption of Lawrence disaster reportage did not compel Massachusetts's readers to campaign for laws that might have prevented a recurrence of the disaster. A cursory reading of the antebellum *Journals* for the Massachusetts Senate and House of Representatives reveals that a civic culture of petition animated the polity through 1860. The ideals that engendered this political behavior originated in the Old World and were reinvigorated in the new by the War for Independence. At mid-century, white and African-American residents of Massachusetts still cherished this political legacy as their birthright. Neither civic nor social disabilities were barriers to political engagement with the state.[134]

Petitioners set out demands of varying scale and scope, each seeking state intervention in one or more spheres of public and private life. Individual appellants typically sought damages for property loss in which the state was implicated. Social reformers made use of petitioning to advance the amelioration of systemic ills and inequities. Petitioning was, then, a culturally sanctioned mode of claims-making and a living instrument for mobilizing state power. Thus, in 1860, state residents persisted in expressing their civic ideals and aspirations through petitioning, evidence of its cultural elasticity and congruence with stated political values.[135] Still, virtually no petitions were filed with the Massachusetts General Court during the disaster's aftermath.[136]

Public horror at the tragedy was considerable and extensive, but it did not bring forth a concerted political response on the part of Massachusetts citizens and non-citizens. A key barrier to citizen mobilization was the idea that employer and employee were social and civic equals. Abolitionists deplored the master's violations of the slave's right to bodily integrity, yet their critique did not encompass assaults on wage earners' bodies in the work place. Anti-slavery reformers argued that the mistreatment of slaves was especially heinous because they were unconditionally subordinated and therefore, defenseless. Like Chief Justice Lemuel Shaw, many abolitionists considered the rigors and risks of employment to be incident to employment and not a form of violence (Clark 1995, p. 490, fn. 68). Thus, abolitionists—the most prominent reformers in antebellum Massachusetts—failed to exert their political leverage on behalf of endangered industrial workers.

Adoption of the 13th and 15th Amendments (prohibiting slavery and disenfranchisement of African-American males, respectively) significantly altered the reform landscape in the Commonwealth.[137] By 1870, the fecund reform impulse of abolitionism had transmuted to concern for the terms and conditions of wage labor. The increasing density and political power of the postbellum labor movement provided the muscle needed to capitalize on this opportunity. These developments cleared the way to reevaluation of the worker's status and of employers' duties to industrial wage earners.

There are other measures of the social impact of disaster narratives on political thinking, including the adaptation of these texts to social policy making. Reform-minded authors such as Jennie Collins and Elizabeth Stuart Phelps made heavy use of the Pemberton disaster in their postbellum essays and fiction. Furthermore, their depictions of Pemberton Mill operatives mirrored earlier representations of Lawrence's working-class denizens. But unlike their antebellum counterparts, Collins and Phelps drove home the political lessons of the Lawrence tragedy for their readers.[138]

In all, public recognition of the Pemberton catastrophe presaged postbellum reform movements. After the Civil War, reformers inside and outside government lobbied for state-mandated shorter hours, factory safety, and employers' liability reform. Furthermore, by 1900 commentators increasingly described working-class casualties of industrial production as "victims" rather than "sufferers." Implicit in this discursive shift was acknowledgment that wage earners were subordinated at work and in the polity.[139] Henry K. Oliver, Pemberton relief committee member and Lawrence's Representative in 1860, led the way, having developed a reputation as a labor law reformer during the post-war decades. On November 13, 1869 Oliver assumed his duties as the head of the newly established Massachusetts Bureau of Statistics on Labor and quickly developed a reputation as an activist bureaucrat (Potter 1992, p. 23).

By 1900 the Commonwealth emerged as a national pacesetter in the development of labor law reform and the requisite state infrastructure.

CONCLUSION

Post-disaster writing about working-class life and loss had paradoxical effects on the social and civic status of industrial workers. Depictions of the social and physical vulnerabilities of Pemberton operatives generated widespread sympathy for them. That sympathy was manifest in public censure of mill owners' avarice and the disassembling effects of industrial capitalism on workers' bodies. Equally important, the fact of the mill owners' negligence exposed the "fiction of due care" integral to the common law of employers' liability.[140] Labor and its allies now had proof positive that the law of industrial accidents was insufficient to protect those most at risk for injury and death.

Conversely, narratives that emphasized workers' susceptibility to bodily ruin and employer dominion undermined wage earners' claim to equality with all other Americans. Critical to social respectability and civic equality were self-governance—including the maintenance of one's health—and free will.[141] The events of January 10, 1860 called into question workers' capacities for both. In short, workers' social and physical vulnerabilities were not only markers of mill owners' unbridled avarice, but also they diminished the respectability of those victimized by it.

Accordingly, many in the American reading public would enter the Civil War questioning the fitness of industrial workers for social and political life. Even the Civil War, which exposed Americans of all classes to premeditated injury and death, did not strip this idea from its social and cultural moorings. Arguably, the war reinforced it because of working-class men's disproportionate representation in northern and southern armies and the concomitant incidence of disabling injuries among them. For all these reasons, contradictory and entwined perceptions of working-class selfhood would endure in the postbellum era and condition its campaigns for labor law reform.

ENDNOTES

1. Historians seeking to reconstruct the Lawrence calamity must reconcile contradictory contemporary and scholarly accounts. Writing in 1900, Robert H. Tewksbury contended that a burning lantern "was broken by a chance blow from a pickaxe, wielded [sic] by another rescuer. . . ." The historian Donald Cole takes Tewksbury at face value, repeating the story. Clarisse A. Poirier provides a more persuasive account, which I have reported. Robert H. Tewksbury, "Historical Sketch. The Fall of the Pemberton Mill on the Tenth of January at Lawrence, Massachusetts" (1900), 6. American Textile History Museum, Lowell, Massachusetts: MSS 117 Pemberton Mill Relief Committee Series. Folder 1.59 The Fall of the Pemberton Mill by Robert H. Tewksbury 1900. Box 1: Papers, Reports, & Correspondence; re: Victims, etc; Cole (1960, pp. 51-52); and Poirier (1978).

2. According to one writer, Lawrence had "been the scene of the most terrible disaster on record. . ." Accounts of the collapse of the Pemberton Mill, whether penned in 1860 or later, depict it as an unprecedented disaster. See for example, Letter from [illegible] to J.C. Hoadley, Esq., January 16, 1860. American Textile History Museum, Lowell, Massachusetts: MSS 117, Pemberton Relief Committee, Box 1 Papers, Reports, and Correspondence, re: Victims, etc. Folder 1.5 To Relief Committee.

3. Clarisse A. Poirier has stated that the Irish constituted one-third of the Lawrence populace, but they comprised a disproportionate 75% of the Pemberton workforce (1990, p. 80; Dyer 1860, p. 6).

4. Charles S. Storrow, Treasurer of Pemberton Mill, reported that "some persons who appeared entirely uninjured were so affected mentally as to be for a long period wholly incapacitated for exertion. . ." Quoted in Poirier (1978, p. 106).

5. Most accounts put the number of dead at 88. See for example, Donald Cole's discussion of the dead and wounded. Alvin Oickle has revised that figure, putting the number of fatally wounded at 100 or more. He has asserted that the figure 88 was published within "a day or two of the collapse, even though several millhands died months later." Oickle has compiled a list of the 1,006 employees who labored at the Pemberton Mill between December 1, 1859 and January 10, 1860, and has "show[n] that more than 100 of them died because of the mill's collapse." Oickle's list is compiled from multiple sources, thus ensuring its accuracy. See Cole (1960, p. 53), and Alvin Oickle, correspondence with author, October 13, 2003.

6. A granite monument marked their burial site and bore the following inscription: "In memory of the unrecognized dead who were killed by the fall of the Pemberton Mill, January 10, 1860" (Dorgan 1918, p. 58).

7. During the previous five years, Lawrence's working-class populace had endured jingoistic attacks by the ascendant Know Nothing party, as well as work stoppages caused by the financial panic of the 1850s. For some operatives, especially veterans of these earlier reversals, the collapse of the Pemberton Mill proved too much. In the ensuing days and weeks, scores of factory workers quit Lawrence and sought their living elsewhere. Many had no choice but to leave family members behind until their debts and transport could be paid. See, for example, Thomas Duffie of Fall River to Mary Duffie of Lawrence, February 23, 1860. American Textile History Museum, Lowell, Massachusetts, MSS 117 Pemberton Mill Relief Committee Series. Box 1: Papers, Reports, & Correspondence; re: Victims, etc. Folder 1.18 Duffie, Thomas and Mary; and First Report of the Treasurer of the Committee of Relief (Lawrence, MA 1860), 11. Pemberton Mill Relief Committee, *First and Second Reports of the Treasurer of the Committee of Relief* (Lawrence, MA 1861), 77.08.32, Immigrant City Archives, Lawrence, Massachusetts.

8. Antebellum commentators such as Parker and Elizabeth Stuart Phelps used the metaphor of battle when writing about the Lawrence tragedy. Parker had already established himself as a critic of the excesses of industrial capitalism and its disassembling effects on workers' bodies (Phelps 1869, p. 80; Frothingham 1874, p. 470; Siracusa 1979, pp. 142-143).

9. In addition, news of the calamity drew thousands to the textile center by rail. Some visitors sought loved ones among the victims, while others were lured to the Mill ruins by the anticipated spectacle of devastation. Fascination with the disaster compelled many sightseers to take artifacts from the ruins, including the effects of the dead, until authorities put a stop to this macabre practice (Haskell and Mason 1860, p. 28; Poirier 1990, p. 78; Poirier 1978, pp. 182-184, 190).

10. Abraham Lincoln to Mary Todd Lincoln, March 4, 1860, Library of Congress, Rare Books and Special Collections Division.

11. An extensive literature analyzes the factory as a trope in antebellum U.S. political and cultural discourses (Marx 1964; Siracusa 1979; Zonderman 1992; Donegan 1984).

12. Ardis Cameron has made a comparable argument (1993, pp. 17, 19). This is not to say that wage labor was unknown. As David Gordon, et. al., has argued, "it was far from being a prevalent or even common way of organizing production." Various other forms of production predominated, including "[s]lave production, independent farming, craft and artisan production, household manufactures, trade and commerce, indentured servitude, family work, [and] petty commodity production. . . ." The authors have contended that "these were the chief relations of production within which the early-nineteenth century labor force operated" (1982, p. 55). Moreover, many antebellum Americans had already identified the chasm between the "factory in the garden" and the realities of industrial capitalism (Siracusa 1979, ch. 6).

13. The U.S. variant of republicanism, on which the nation was founded, held that civic virtue was contingent on the existence of free and independent producers. I examine the interplay between this ideal and the evolving law of industrial accidents in the larger study from which this chapter is taken. For background on this topic, see Kann (1991).

14. The *Boston Journal* and other northern papers responded to the *Herald* by arguing that industrial capitalism was a progressive social and economic force that benefitted employers and employees equally (Poirier 1990, pp. 84-87).

15. Poirier considers but rejects the possibility that these letters were plants (1990, p. 86 and fn. 24).

16. For example, there is little or no explanation of the reading public's preoccupation with the disaster and its political significance. Nor do these narratives probe the interplay between an industrial accident of the first magnitude and the developing law of employers' liability. Clarisse A. Poirier's analysis of the disaster is a notable exception. She has located popular discourse about the mill's collapse within the sectional crisis and pro-slavery critiques of wage labor. Moreover, she has asserted that the "fall of the Pemberton Mill elicited a variety of responses reflecting the attitudes and values of nineteenth century American society." Moreover, Poirier has argued that the "disaster had an impact on events and people beyond the boundaries of its own time and place. Some consequences were immediately apparent. . . . Other effects were slower to surface, though they eventually included positive building reforms and an increased awareness of working conditions in New England's textile factories" (1978, pp. 182, 186). I build on her excellent case study by asking how disaster narratives reflected, sustained, and altered popular ideas about work, workers, and the workplace and with what consequences for postbellum campaigns for labor law reform.

17. It is worth noting that the narratives themselves were mediated by the authors' judgments about their scope, content, aesthetics, and narrative forms and strategies. Michael Barton (1998) has argued much the same point in his analysis of disaster reportage featured in the *New York Times*.

18. Lawrence is located on the Merrimack River, midway between Lowell and Haverhill, Massachusetts. For a succinct summary of the development of Lowell, Massachusetts see Mitchell (1988, pp. 10-14).

19. For a discussion of the interrelated variables that produced these effects, see Rothenberg (2000) and Temins (2000, pp. 96, 122-124).

20. Deer Falls is approximately eleven miles from Lowell, Massachusetts (Cole 1991, pp. 18-19; Josephson 1967, p. 301).

21. Lawrence was also a committed philanthropist and aspirant to political office (Dalzell 1987, pp. 77-78, 148-151, 163, 165, 180).

22. Jackson's willingness to take business risks alarmed his brother-in-law, Francis Cabot Lowell, prompting the latter to write a letter urging Jackson to be enterprising but cautious (Dalzell 1987, pp. 9, 29).

23. It is likely that Storrow's skills as an engineer and his social standing appealed to Lawrence, for the railroad agent's lack of background in textiles would not have recommended him. Typically, the treasurer would rough out the building design and plans, and then consulted with a builder. Storrow had studied engineering at the Ponts et Chaussees in Paris and then served with distinction as chief engineer of the Boston & Lowell Railroad. He was also a Cabot in-law. He lacked the expertise, however, to design Pemberton Mill (Dalzell 1987, p. 150; Josephson 1967, pp. 304-305; Linter 1948).

24. According to Hannah Josephson, "Lawrence in its early years was noted for what Harriet Farley described as 'fomenters and nuclei of crime and iniquity': its hoodlums, its street fights, its gambling dens and saloons, its filth and squalor" (Josephson 1967, p. 305).

25. John A. Lowell invested in Merrimack Manufacturing Company, the first mill established in Lowell, Massachusetts. He then partnered with Abbott Lawrence to establish the Boott and Massachusetts Mills in Lowell. Not content to shape the Commonwealth's economy, he also lead an "offensive" by Boston elites against plebian culture. He did so as the first trustee of the Lowell Institute for public lectures (Poirier 1978, pp. 5-7; Hall 1997, pp. 406-407; Sellers 1991, pp. 364-365).

26. Hereafter I will refer to Putnam as J. Pickering Putnam, as his colleagues called him. His family knew him as John Putnam (Poirier 1978, p. 45).

27. For a comprehensive analysis of the mill's design and technologies, see Poirier (1978, ch. 1).

28. Lowell also proposed quintessentially British "plans for the financial organization" of the mill. Poirier has explained that large-scale American manufacturing enterprises were "most often joint-stock corporations," in contrast to English manufactures which "were owned privately or sometimes as partnerships." Lowell aspired to be free of "his old business colleagues, whom he described as 'inert' and 'fit for nothing but swallowing up the profits in good times and bullying the best men out of their service in bad.'" Lowell endeavored to underwrite all costs associated with the mill's establishment to control company management. John A. Lowell, "Journal of a Trip Abroad: April 3, 1850 to October 14, 1852," Houghton Library, Harvard University, and J. Pickering Putnam to John A. Lowell, [1858], Massachusetts Historical Society, Charles P. Putnam Papers, cited in Poirier (1978, pp. 10-11).

29. Bigelow was educated at West Point and served with the Army Corps of Engineers until 1846, when he retired as Captain and began working with Storrow (Poirier 1978, p. 14).

30. For an explanation of the Essex Company's accommodation of Lowell's wishes in this matter, see Poirier (1978, p. 17).

31. Despite Putnam's safety consciousness, the factory closed for short intervals due to structural problems (Poirier 1978, pp. 18, 22, 37-39).

32. Putnam also hired contractors for the carpentry and masonry work. Essex Company records provide ample evidence of his continuing involvement in what the architect

for the boardinghouses and tradesmen dubbed "Putnam's Mill." *Boston Journal,* January 19, 1860, cited in Poirier (1978, pp. 12, 14-17, 20) and elaborated on by Alvin Oickle, Correspondence with author, December 2003.

33. Bigelow had installed iron columns in the Lawrence Machine Shop and the Atlantic Mills using a clasp system. In the event of a fire, a structure's "upper floors would remain supported. . . ." Putnam instead subcontracted for a system of caps and pintles, a system of connective fittings that cost forty cents less per unit (Poirier 1978, pp. 22-23).

34. Poirier has noted that the mill's design anticipated "developments in factory construction that would become common only decades later" (Poirier 1978, p. 4).

35. Unlike the Pemberton Mill, New England mills typically featured dormers and "steeply pitched" roofs (Poirier 1978, pp. 28-31).

36. The regional economy was "sluggish" during the late 1840s and experienced an "upswing" in 1851 and 1852. In 1856 the national economy was strained by declining grain prices, leading to "bank failures and a general depression, particularly in the industrial Northeast, which relied on the lucrative Midwestern trade." According to Ardis Cameron, industrialists remained committed to large-scale manufacturing. In Massachusetts and elsewhere in New England, manufacturers and financiers launched "capital drives" to shore up corporations during the panic. Cameron reports that "[Abbott] Lawrence alone committed over one million dollars of his personal fortune" to this campaign (Poirier 1978, pp. 7, 39-40; Cameron 1993, p. xv).

37. The economic crash and failure of Pemberton Mill drove a wedge between John Amory Lowell and J. Pickering Putnam, thereby creating a fissure in their extended families. The mill's downfall also had its roots in Samuel Lawrence's disreputable and illegal business practices, which negatively affected other enterprises as well (Poirier 1978, pp. 41-43, 47-50).

38. Howe, who had been in the mill when it collapsed, recounted his purchase of the mill while presenting his testimony during the inquest into the disaster (Haskell and Mason 1860, p. 81; Poirier 1978, pp. 52-53, 57).

39. It was conventional wisdom among Boston businessmen that Pemberton Mill had proven a worthy investment. According to Donald Cole, Lawrence millhands also reaped the benefits of the economic upturn (Poirier 1978, pp. 55-57; Cole 1960, p. 47).

40. Vates wrote 19 stanzas commemorating the disaster, each more melodramatic than the next. O. K. Vates—Air Major's Only Son, "Lines on the Great Calamity at Lawrence, and Fall of the Pemberton Mills, Jan. 10, 1860," Library of Congress, Rare Books and Special Collections Division.

41. Using available data, Poirier has provided a detailed analysis of the demographics of the workforce; see Tables 7, 8, 9 (1978, pp. 125-128, 133-134).

42. After the calamity, Sherman served as Superior Court Judge. Edgar Jay Sherman, *Some Recollections of a Long Life* (Boston: Privately Printed, 1908). American Textile History Museum, Lowell, Massachusetts.

43. Edgar Jay Sherman, *Some Recollections of a Long Life* (Boston: Privately Printed, 1908), 28. American Textile History Museum, Lowell, Massachusetts.

44. Ibid.

45. Tewksbury recollected the disaster forty years after its occurrence in a didactic sketch based on firsthand testimony and archival records. The mill's collapse was, he wrote, "the most tragic event" in Lawrence history. By his lights, the calamity was "too profound, lasting and universal, in New England" and the nation "to be forgotten." Tewksbury allowed as his memorial might revive "recollections . . . that citizens, would, if possible, consign to oblivion; . . ." That possibility aside, Tewksbury declared himself committed to memorializing the catastrophe and its heroes for the edification of Lawrence's future generations. If the aging mill employee had private reasons for writing a definitive account of these events, he kept his own counsel. Robert H. Tewksbury, "Historical Sketch. The Fall of the Pemberton Mill on the Tenth of January, 1860, at Lawrence, Massachusetts." Pemberton Mill Relief Committee Series MS 117, Folder 1.59 The Fall of the Pemberton Mill by Robert H. Tewksbury 1900, Box 1: Papers, Reports and Correspondence; re: Victims, etc., American Textile History Museum, Lowell, Massachusetts.

46. Concurrent with the inquest, financiers and industrialists in Boston and Lawrence established relief funds to aid mill victims and their dependents. Contributors of all classes and from throughout the United States donated a total of $65,834.67. Accompanying these funds were letters expressing their writers' deeply felt sorrow over the mill's collapse.

47. According to Poirier, "The composition of the jury reflected its need to investigate the technical aspects of the mill's design and construction" (1978, p. 66). Lamb who served as judge and jurists included William P. Wright, an attorney and the chair of the jury; Edward Page, "a drive belt manufacturer; " James H. Dana, "an iron and tin smith"; Leonard Stoddard, "a carpenter and a general contractor"; Stephen P. Simons, a "master stone mason;" and Edward S. Creesey, a carpenter who participated in the building of Pemberton Mill. Caleb Saunders served as an appointed inquest Clerk (Alvin Oickle, Correspondence with author, December 2003). Testimony is recounted in Haskell and Mason (1860, pp. 57-96).

48. Robert H. Tewksbury observed that the "building was no stronger than its weakest part." Robert H. Tewksbury, "Historical Sketch. The Fall of the Pemberton Mill on the Tenth of January at Lawrence, Massachusetts" (Lawrence 1900, p. 5). American Textile History Museum, Lowell, Massachusetts, MSS 117 Pemberton Mill Relief Committee Series. Folder 1.59 The Fall of the Pemberton Mill by Robert H. Tewksbury 1900. Box 1: Papers, Reports, & Correspondence; re: Victims, etc. Donald Cole has explained that "to compensate for the unusual distance between walls and for the heavy machinery and floors, two rows of iron pillars ran the length of the Mill on every floor" (1960, p. 48; Dyer 1860, p. 91).

49. After the verdict was rendered, Bigelow vigorously defended his reputation while Lowell deflected blame from himself and Putnam to the Essex Company engineer (Haskell and Mason 1860, pp. 90, 92; Poirier 1990, pp. 90-93).

50. *Order 836/5* and *Report, 836/3,* Legislative packet for Bill No. 83, Senate—1860, Drawer 106, *Rejected; Journal of the House of Representatives (1860),* pp. 47, 284, 311-312, 457, 502, 534, 553-554, 571, and 618; and *Journal of the Senate* (1860), pp. 626, 661, and 679, Massachusetts State Archives.

51. *Commonwealth v. Hunt,* 45 Mass. 111 (Mass. 1842). Although the Commonwealth demurred from regulating the wage relation, the antebellum state inserted itself in other dimensions of life, eventually moving "inexorably into a position of greater

responsibility and greater control." For example, in 1837, Massachusetts surveyed its industries and after 1845, the state did so every ten years. The Commonwealth's involvement in the development of public improvements, growth of manufactures, public health, and the establishment of public schooling are well known (Handlin 1969). For a discussion of *Commonwealth v. Hunt,* see Levy (1957, ch. 11).

52. 45 Mass. 49 (SJC 1842). Shaw averred that the wage earner was thus empowered by virtue of his mental autonomy and acuity. See Reeve (1997).

53. According to Christopher L. Tomlins, the state legislature established a Committee to investigate accidents on the Western Railroad. Lawmakers concluded based on their inquiry that it was inexpedient to "censure" the railroad's directors. Moreover, they refrained from recommending that the legislature intervene in the railway industry for purposes of increasing its safety record. Instead, Committee members looked to industry leaders to regulate their own operations (1993, p. 361). On postbellum campaigns for employers' liability reform, see Reeve (1995).

54. On the Ten Hour movement, see Dublin (1979, pp. 109-116, 125-131, 200-202), and Murphy (1992).

55. *Order 836/4* and Legislative Packet for Bill No. 83, Senate—1860, Drawer 106, Rejected; *Journal of the House of Representatives (1860),* pp. 47, 284, 311-312, 457, 502, 534, 553-554, 571, and 618. Massachusetts State Archives.

56. Clarisse A. Poirier has rightly argued that lawmakers' decision to remand enforcement to localities rather than to the Commonwealth weakened the bill. Yet, it is also true that the Commonwealth lacked the requisite infrastructure to enforce its provisions and would not create it until after the Civil War (Potter 1992, ch. 3-4).

57. *Report 836/1* and Legislative Packet for Bill No. 83, Senate—1860, Drawer 106, Rejected; and *Journal of the Senate (1860),* pp. 626, 661, and 679. Massachusetts State Archives.

58. There is a rich and extensive literature about the storied history of nineteenth century Massachusetts labor militancy. Norman Ware's groundbreaking social analysis of nineteenth century industrialization addresses the multi-dimensionality of the antebellum U.S. labor movement, in which Massachusetts labor advocacy and mobilization figured prominently (1990). Numerous other historians have built on Ware's insights by emphasizing the importance of gender, ethnicity, and race for class formation and militancy (Blewett 1988, 2000; Cameron 1993; Dublin 1979, ch. 3-4).

59. Putnam made his motion on Thursday, January 12. *Journal of the House of Representatives (1860),* pp. 54-55.

60. *Boston Journal,* January 12, 1860 (Poirier 1990, p. 91 and fn. 41).

61. At my request, personnel at the State Archives of Massachusetts made a concerted but unsuccessful effort to locate the relevant legislative packet. Oliver made his motion on Thursday, January 26. *Journal of the House of Representatives (1860),* p. 147.

62. Debates over the appropriation to Alexandria turned on three clauses in the U.S. constitution: "the power to tax and spend for the general welfare, the power to make all laws necessary and proper, and the power to exercise exclusive legislation over the capital enclave." Previously, local, state, and federal authorities had provided for relief of varying kinds including poor relief, but allocations of disaster relief were made on a case-by-case basis and after extensive debate (Landis 1998).

63. Moreover, Landis has concluded that contestation over the benchmarks of suffering and relief allocation created the ideological scaffolding for the U.S. social welfare

state. As this suggests, Landis has countered Theda Skocpol's thesis that the American welfare state originated with enactment of Civil War veterans' benefits (1998). On the Civil War veteran's benefits program, see Skocpol (1992). On state formation in the United States, see Skowronek (1982).

64. *First Report of the Treasurer of the Committee of Relief for the Sufferers by the Fall of the Pemberton Mill* (Lawrence: June, 1860), pp. 6-7, 11. *First & Second Reports of the Treasurer of the Committee of Relief, Lawrence, MA 1861;* 77.08.32; Immigrant City Archives, Lawrence, MA.

65. *First & Second Reports of the Treasurer of the Committee of Relief, Lawrence, MA 1861;* 77.08.32; Immigrant City Archives, Lawrence, MA.

66. Storrow and Oliver served together on Lawrence's elected school committee. Oliver eventually became Superintendent of Lawrence schools (Dorgan 1918, pp. 98-99).

67. American Textile History Museum, Lowell, Massachusetts, MSS 117, Box 1 Papers, Reports, and Correspondence, re: Victims, etc. Folder 1.1. Relief Committee—Notes, Minutes (Jan.-Feb.) 1860.

68. J.Q.A. Batchelder, William D. Joplin, Edward P. Poor, Sylvester A. Furbush, Henry Withington, and Elbridge Weston filled out the ranks of the inspectors (Dorgan 1918, p. 57).

69. *First Report of the Treasurer of the Committee of Relief for the Sufferers by the Fall of the Pemberton Mill* (Lawrence: June, 1860), pp. 6-7, 11. *First & Second Reports of the Treasurer of the Committee of Relief, Lawrence,* MA 1861; 77.08.32; Immigrant City Archives, Lawrence, MA.

70. Untitled, January 28, 1860, American Textile History Museum, Lowell, Massachusetts, Box 1, MSS 117, Folder 1.1 Relief Committee—Notes, Minutes (Jan-Feb 1860).

71. American Textile History Museum, Lowell, Massachusetts, Pemberton Relief Committee, MSS 117.2 F4, R18/7: Expense Analysis, From Ledger of Assistance Series: Financial, item 13 in series.

72. Untitled, January 16, 1860, American Textile History Museum, Lowell, Massachusetts, Box 1, MSS 117, Folder 1.1 Relief Committee—Notes, Minutes (Jan-Feb 1860).

73. In practice, however, the relief committee authorized a sub-committee (or the distribution committee) to use its "judgment in distributing clothing to all parties wanting in immediate necessity of the same and when by so doing the Committee may be relieved of further care." Untitled, January 16, 1860, Box 1, MSS 117, Folder 1.1 Relief Committee—Notes, Minutes (Jan-Feb 1860).

74. In the following months, the committee reversed itself and granted "temporary relief" to operatives made destitute by unemployment. Furthermore, the committee approved payments for funerals, medical care and medicine, including "the board and wages of nurses; " as well as for the "board of all injured persons until their recovery; and outlay necessarily incurred. . ." Untitled, January 16 and February 12, 1860, American Textile History Museum, Lowell, Massachusetts, Box 1, MSS 117, Folder 1.1 Relief Committee—Notes, Minutes (Jan-Feb 1860); and *First & Second Reports of the Treasurer of the Committee of Relief, Lawrence, MA 1861,* p. 14; 77.08.32; Immigrant City Archives, Lawrence, MA.

75. *First & Second Reports of the Treasurer of the Committee of Relief, Lawrence, MA 1861,* 14; 77.08.32; Immigrant City Archives, Lawrence, MA.

76. Charles S. Storrow to Edward O'Neil on April 7, 1860. American Textile History Museum, Lowell, Massachusetts, Pemberton Relief Committee, MSS 117, Box 1 Papers, Reports & Correspondence, re: Victims, etc. Folder 1.49 Sampson, Augusta L.

77. *First & Second Reports of the Treasurer of the Committee of Relief, Lawrence, MA 1861, 15;* 77.08.32; Immigrant City Archives, Lawrence, MA.

78. See, for example, the Committee's disposition of claims by Celia Connelly. American Textile History Museum, Lowell, Massachusetts, Pemberton Mill Relief Committee, MSS 117, Box 1: Papers, Reports, & Correspondence, re: Victims, Etc. Folder 1.13 Connelly, Celia Clarke (?).

79. Charles S. Storrow to John Whitty, Esq., President of the Lowell Irish Benevolent Society, December 7, 1860. American Textile History Museum, Lowell, Massachusetts, MSS 117: Papers, Reports, and Correspondence, re: Victims, etc. Folder 1.57 From Relief Committee.

80. Storrow stated that "in the Report of May last, the contributions of the Irish Benevolent Society was entered as $58. The whole amount sent by the Society to the Mayor was $100, of which he personally distributed $42, and the balance only was paid to the Treasurer and came into his accounts." *Final Report of the Treasurer of the Committee of Relief for the Sufferers of the Fall of the Pemberton Mill in Lawrence, Mass. on the 10th of January, 1860* (Lawrence, February 1861), 23. State House Library, Commonwealth of Massachusetts.

81. To Amos A. Lawrence, January 21, 1860, American Textile History Museum, Lowell, Massachusetts, MSS 117, Folder 1.57 From Relief Committee.

82. Ibid.

83. *Final Report of the Treasurer of the Committee of Relief for the Sufferers of the Fall of the Pemberton Mill in Lawrence, Mass. on the 10th of January, 1860* (Lawrence, February 1861), 5. State House Library, Commonwealth of Massachusetts.

84. Storrow again wrote Lawrence, instructing him to hold $13,000 collected by the New England Society so that "some interest could be obtained" on the sum. Storrow explained that the Pemberton relief committee had sufficient monies "for immediate purposes" and would request the fund when it was wanted "at Lawrence." Abbott Lawrence recommended much the same procedure two months later, arguing that "A little interest will not hurt anybody." Abbott Lawrence to Charles Storrow on March 16, 1860 and Charles Storrow to Amos A. Lawrence on January 25, 1860. American Textile History Museum, Lowell, Massachusetts, MSS 117, File 1.57 From Relief Committee and Folder 1.7 Subscriptions for the Victims.

85. Grinnell attributed citywide unemployment to a decline in shipping. Joseph Grinnell of New Bedford, MA to Mayor D. Saunders, Jr., January 24, 1860. American Textile History Museum, Lowell, Massachusetts: Pemberton Mill Relief Committee, MSS 117, Box 1 Papers, Reports, and Correspondence, re: Victims, etc., Folder 1.7 Subscriptions for the Victims.

86. Charles S. Storrow to the Honorable Joseph Grinnell, January 26, 1860. American Textile History Museum, Lowell, Massachusetts, MSS 117, File 1.57 From Relief Committee.

87. Notice, American Textile History Museum, Lowell, Massachusetts, MSS 117, File 1.57 From Relief Committee.

88. Poirier has concluded that disaster narratives ignited a robust, cross-class critique of industrial capitalism on the eve of the Civil War (Poirier 1990, pp. 78, 82-86).

89. Based on these rumors, fearful textile operatives in Lawrence and elsewhere boycotted their places of employment, while city clerics urged congregants to return to work in the mills (Poirier 1990, pp. 79, 90-91; Haskell and Mason 1860, pp. 45-46).

90. According to Clarisse Poirier (1978, pp. 243-244) (and Ardis Cameron, who has reported Poirier's conjecture as fact (1993, p. 18), neither was the Pemberton Mill Relief Committee prepared to impugn Lawrence industrialists. According to a biographer of David Nevins, the Mill's owner when it collapsed, city fathers did not pressure the manufacturer to indemnify disaster victims. Allegedly, they feared that Nevins would disinvest in or close Pemberton Mill. My own research does not support this contention. That said, common sense dictates that the Relief Committee's dependence on industrialists for aid would certainly have had quelled public condemnation of Nevins.

91. According to Storrow, in less than sixty seconds "the [mill] floors . . . five stories in height, suddenly gave way, the walls were overthrown, and stone, bricks, timber, machinery, and this vast crowd lay in one confused mass of ruins." Later that evening, he continued, "a fire broke out . . ." *First Report of the Treasurer of the Committee of Relief for the Sufferers by the Fall of the Pemberton Mill, in Lawrence, Mass., on the 10th of January, 1860* (Lawrence: June, 1860), 5-6. Pemberton Relief Committee, Immigrant City Archives, Lawrence, Massachusetts.

92. Letter to Francis Cogswell, President of the B&M RR, January 18, 1860 American Textile History Museum, Lowell, Massachusetts, MSS 117, File 1.57 From Relief Committee.

93. My argument builds on Susan L. Stoop's cogent interrogation of portraiture as cultural representation. Stoops curated an exhibit on portraiture at the Worcester Art Museum, Massachusetts, during winter 2002-2003. She has argued "that even the most traditional portraits are not always made with the singular goal of likeness but frequently involve elements of performance or role-playing, and degrees of anonymity and abstraction" (2002, Introduction, p. 7).

94. One journalist reported that he accompanied physicians as they visited afflicted operatives in their homes and then wrote up their observations. Borrowing from Michael Denning, I contend that these and other narratives tell us more about the writer and his or her age and milieu than about the subject. Denning has discussed the "ruses" of representation and the importance of the narrator's stance for literary representations of working-class people (1987, pp. 3, 104; Haskell and Mason 1860, p. 30).

95. My reading of Victor Turner and Michael Denning informs my analysis of the disaster narratives as rhetoric (Turner 1982; Denning 1987, p. 7).

96. For a compendium of these materials, see Haskell and Mason (1860).

97. Michael Denning has used the terms genre and conventions interchangeably, arguing that genre mediates between "individual texts and the social and historical situation." He has defined rhetoric as "the stock of commonplaces that are used to persuade and entertain." Frederic Jameson has asserted that genres are "social contracts between a writer and a specific public . . ." I take this to mean that reading publics are both

socialized to enjoy a particular convention, but they also perpetuate and alter it according to their powers of consumption. Based on this I conclude that antebellum readers expected that disaster narratives would mimic popular literary genres (Denning 1987, pp. 74-75, citing Jameson, 223 n7).

98. According to Reynolds, "the shift from doctrine to narrative was not so rapid or pronounced among sermonizers as it was among American tract writers, who by 1850" were responding to Americans' preference for "religious entertainment." Moreover, "conservatives in both fundamental and intellectual camps" eschewed fictionalized theology (1980, pp. 480-482).

99. *Sermon by Reverend E. M. Tappan, at the Freewill Baptist Church* (Haskell and Mason 1860, pp. 41-43).

100. Parker had already established himself as a critic of the excesses of industrial capitalism and its disassembling of workers' bodies (Phelps 1869, p. 80; Frothingham 1874, p. 470; Siracusa 1979, pp. 142-143).

101. Theodore Parker was aligned with freethinking Boston Transcendentalists rather than with the decidedly more conservative Vermont Transcendentalists. See Menand (2001, pp. 68, 247-250), and Sermon by Reverend E. M. Tappan, at the Freewill Baptist Church (Haskell and Mason 1860, p. 42).

102. *First Report of the Treasurer of the Committee of Relief* (Lawrence, MA 1860), 12. Pemberton Mill Relief Committee, First and Second Reports of the Treasurer of the Committee of Relief, Lawrence, MA 1861, 77.08.32, Immigrant City Archives.

103. Storrow concluded by thanking the benefactor for her offer of women's clothing and asked that she send the garments to George P. Wilson, City Missionary. Charles S. Storrow to "Madam," February 4, 1860. American Textile History Museum, Lowell, Massachusetts, MSS 117 Pemberton Mill Relief Committee Series. Box 1: Papers, Reports, and Correspondence, re: Victims, etc. Folder 1.57. From Relief Committee.

104. Byrnes had organized a campaign to raise $1,000 and succeeded in soliciting $950 in subscriptions, a quarter of which was donated by parishioners of a local Catholic church. According to Byrnes, a local organizing committee—"the laboring one"—had overseen the Worcester campaign. Byrnes informed Hoadley that the Committee could easily have "raised more, but for the letter" of Lawrence's Mayor Saunders, Jr., "announcing that more than enough was already subscribed . . ." Edwin Byrnes of Worcester to John C. Hoadley, Esq., January 25, 1860. American Textile History Museum, Lowell, Massachusetts, MSS 117 Pemberton Mill Relief Committee Series. Box 1: Papers, Reports, and Correspondence, re: Victims, etc. Folder 1.7 Subscriptions for the Victims.

105. Edwin Byrnes of Worcester to John C. Hoadley, Esq., January 25, 1860. American Textile History Museum, Lowell, Massachusetts, MSS 117 Pemberton Mill Relief Committee Series. Box 1: Papers, Reports, and Correspondence, re: Victims, etc. Folder 1.7 Subscriptions for the Victims.

106. *Farwell v. Boston & Worcester Railroad*, 4 Met. (45 Mass.) 49 (1842), 59. Alan Hyde has characterized "embodied experience" as bodily phenomena such as pain or sexual pleasure. Alan Hyde, *Bodies of Law* (Princeton: Princeton University Press, 1997, p. 6).

107. O. K. Vates—Air Major's Only Son, "Lines on the Great Calamity at Lawrence, and Fall of the Pemberton Mills, Jan. 10, 1860," Library of Congress, Rare Books and Special Collections Division.

108. Rural women came to Lawrence in search of "sons and daughters in the fated Mill" but, according to the narrator, these women were frequently unable to locate the remains of their children (Haskell and Mason 1860, p. 14).

109. Wood interviewed Dr. Graves, presumably Connelly's doctor, and "several" of her neighbors. He wrote his report on January 30, 1860 while in Lowell, Massachusetts. American Textile History Museum, Lowell, Massachusetts, Pemberton Mill Relief Committee, MSS 117, Box 1: Papers, Reports, & Correspondence, re: Victims, Etc. Folder 1.13 Connelly, Celia Clarke (?).

110. Antebellum Americans of all classes conceived of men as providers of a family wage and women as homemakers and the inculcator of values in children. (On this see Jeanne Boydston 1990).

111. American Textile History Museum, Lowell, Massachusetts, Pemberton Mill Relief Committee, MSS 117, Box 1: Papers, Reports, & Correspondence, re: Victims, Etc. Folder 1.13 Connelly, Celia Clarke (?).

112. Ibid.

113. Ibid.

114. Ibid.

115. Ibid.

116. John Fallon to Charles S. Storrow on October 8, 1860. American Textile History Museum, Lowell, Massachusetts, Pemberton Mill Relief Committee, MS 117, Box 1: Papers, Reports, & Correspondence, re: Victims, Folder 1.34 McCarthy, Ellen F.

117. Ibid.

118. In journalistic accounts, Palmer's first name was spelled as Maurice whereas agents of the Pemberton relief committee spelled it as Morris in their correspondence. I use Maurice in deference to usage by residents of Rochester, N. H., where his family resided (Haskell and Mason 1860, pp. 15, 24); American Textile History Museum, Lowell, Massachusetts, Pemberton Mill Relief Committee, MSS 117, Box 1 Papers, Reports, Correspondence, re: Victims, etc., Folder 1.43: Palmer, Morris H.

119. Clarisse Poirier (1990, p. 7) and Donald Cole (1960, p. 52) have narrated Palmer's death in their accounts of the disaster.

120. Those responsible for republishing Fuller's letter editorialized but little about its contents. Instead, they signaled their interpretation of it by entitling the segment "A Touching Narrative." Rather than resort to melodrama, they observed in a single sentence that the letter "was published a few days after the calamity" and "disclosed the sad circumstances attending the death of one who perished." John H. Fuller, "To the Public," January 18, 1860 (Haskell and Mason 1860, p. 24).

121. A cursory review of the committee's settlements with victims and their dependents confirms the accuracy of this description. *Final Report of the Treasurer of the Committee of Relief for the Sufferers of the Fall of the Pemberton Mill in Lawrence, Mass., on the 10th of January, 1860* (Lawrence, February 1861), 9-23, and especially 20. State House Library, Commonwealth of Massachusetts.

122. On January 28 the relief committee voted that "Mr. Joplin be authorized to proceed to Rochester, N. H. for the purpose of visiting the Palmier [sic] family & to ascertain

its whole condition & report to the Committee what will be best to be done for the effectual relief of said family." Untitled, January 28, 1860, American Textile History Museum, Lowell, Massachusetts, MSS 117, Box 1, Folder 1.1 Relief Committee—Notes, Minutes (Jan-Feb 1860).

123. Her character was suspect, however, as evidenced by Joplin's report that the Palmer family feared that she would return to make a claim on monies settled on the boys. Joplin had recommended that the family appoint a guardian for the boys, in whose name the allocation would be made. The Palmers approached a local judge and requested that he serve in this capacity. American Textile History Museum, Lowell, Massachusetts, Pemberton Mill Relief Committee, MSS 117, Box 1 Papers, Reports, Correspondence, re: Victims, etc., Folder 1.43: Palmer, Morris H.

124. American Textile History Museum, Lowell, Massachusetts, Pemberton Mill Relief Committee, MSS 117, Box 1 Papers, Reports, Correspondence, re: Victims, etc., Folder 1.43: Palmer, Morris H.

125. Duffie's surname is spelled as Duffy in other documents included in the records of the Pemberton Mill Relief Committee.

126. Duffie also instructed Mary to tell their Lawrence creditors that they should not be "uneasy about what I owe them" and "that I will try and do my best to pay them as soon as I posably [sic] can.." Duffie owed two months' rent, or $7, and an additional $39 for other expenses. Thomas Duffie of Fall River to Mary Duffie of Lawrence, February 23, 1860. American Textile History Museum, Lowell, Massachusetts, MSS 117 Pemberton Mill Relief Committee Series. Box 1: Papers, Reports, & Correspondence; re: Victims, etc. Folder 1.18 Duffie, Thomas and Mary.

127. Ann McDonald to Mayor Daniel Saunders, Jr., January, 1860. American Textile History Museum, Lowell, Massachusetts, MSS117 Pemberton Mill Relief Committee Series. Box 1: Papers, Reports, and Correspondence, re: Victims, etc. Folder 1.37 Mulineaux, Hannah.

128. Emphasis added. Ann McDonald to Mayor Daniel Saunders, Jr., January, 1860. American Textile History Museum, Lowell, Massachusetts, MSS117 Pemberton Mill Relief Committee Series. Box 1: Papers, Reports, and Correspondence, re: Victims, etc. Folder 1.37 Mulineaux, Hannah.

129. The letter suggests that the New Hampshire operatives collected $75. Joseph Taylor, H. P. B. Hudson, and B. F. Watson of New Market, NH to Hon. D. Saunders, Jr., January 18, 1860. American Textile History Museum, Lowell, Massachusetts: MSS 117, Pemberton Relief Committee, Box 1 Papers, Reports, and Correspondence, re: Victims, etc. Folder 1.7: Subscriptions for the Victims.

130. I build on David S. Reynolds' argument for this conclusion (1980, pp. 486-487).

131. Michael Denning has established the prevalence and cultural importance of dime novels and story-paper literature (1987). I extrapolate from Susan L. Stoop's analysis of portraiture and especially of the importance of the affordability and reproducibility of media such as photography (2002, p. 7).

132. Not every literary eminence eschewed the popular press. Nathaniel Hawthorne read these stories avidly, much to his son's discomfiture. David C. Reynolds, Beneath the American Renaissance: The Subversive Imagination in the Age of Emerson and Melville (New York: Knopf, 1988), 171, cited in Barton (1998, p. 161).

133. According to Barton, "the media's motto is 'If it bleeds, it leads'" (1998, 156). Barton has grounded his assertions in Singer (1993, ch.3, cited in Barton 1998, p. 170, fn. 2).

134. Petitioning was not the sole preserve of the white and native-born residents of the Commonwealth. On January 16, 1860 the Colored Citizens of the City of Boston gathered at Bethel Church and resolved to dismantle racial barriers to service in the state militia. Thereupon a delegation petitioned the General Court to eliminate the word "white" in statutes governing eligibility for service. Those gathered on the 16th delegated petitioning to Dr. J. S. Rock, Rev. J. Sella Martin, William Wells Brown, and William C. Nell. The legislature approved the requested change in wording and reported out a bill to that effect. Lawmakers were prevented from enacting the bill, however, after being advised that it was unconstitutional. It was alleged that only Congress had jurisdiction over the state militia and eligibility for service. "Petition of Colored Citizens of Boston for removing the word: white from the Statute Book, presented by Mr. Pierce of Dorchester." Rejected Legislation, Packet: "Petition and Reports on Petition" Senate 1860. Drawer 106. Massachusetts State Archives.

135. I am indebted to Debra Osnowitz for her insight about cultures of claims making. Debra Osnowitz to author, August 10, 2001.

136. I draw this conclusion based on my review of the indices for the legislature's handwritten journals and legislative packets for Senate deliberations in 1860. *Journal of the Senate, Volume 81, 1860;* and *Journal of the House of Representatives,* no volume number, 1860; and Senate-1860, Leave to Withdraw/Inexpedient/Next General Court/Indefinitely Postponed/Misc., Drawer 105; and Senate-1860, Rejected, Drawer 106.

137. The thirteenth Amendment prohibited slavery and involuntary servitude, whereas the fifteenth Amendment barred disenfranchisement of males based on "race, color, or previous condition of servitude." *Constitution of the United States of America,* reprinted in Foner (1991, pp. 1199-2000).

138. Likewise, postbellum compilations of U.S. facts, historical figures, and events generally featured an account of the Pemberton tragedy, indicating its historical and cultural significance in even the postbellum period (Barber 1861, p. 264; Phelps 1869; Collins 1871).

139. I contend that "sufferer" also fell out of favor as realism eclipsed sentimentality in U.S. society.

140. Commentary by John Williams-Searle after his presentation of "Bodies Political: Railroaders as Soldiers of Capital, 1870-1908," at the North American Labor History Conference, Wayne State University, 2002, in author's possession.

141. As Charles E. Rosenberg has argued, antebellum physicians and their patients believed that the body and mind were interdependent both functionally and in terms of their well-being. This notion "allowed . . . the multidimensional integration of emotions, family and business circumstances, and individual habits into etiology and therapeutics" (1989, pp. 187-190; Betts 1968).

REFERENCES

Barber, J. W. (1861) *Our Whole Country; or the Past and Present of the United States, Historical and Descriptive.* Cincinnati: Henry Howe.

Barton, M. (1998) Journalistic Gore: Disaster Reporting and Emotional Discourse in the New York Times, 1852-1956. In P. N. Stearns and J. Lewis (eds.), *An Emotional History of the United States* (pp. 155-172). New York: New York University Press.

Betts, J. R. (1968) Mind and Body in Early American Thought. *The Journal of American History, 54:* 787-805.

Blewett, M. (1988) *Men, Women, and Work: Class, Gender, and Protest in the New England Shoe Industry, 1780-1910.* Urbana: University of Illinois Press.

Blewett, M. (2000) *Constant Turmoil: The Politics of Industrial Life in Nineteenth-Century New England.* Amherst: University of Massachusetts Press.

Boydston, J. (1990) *Home & Work: Housework, Wages, and the Ideology of Labor in the Early Republic.* New York and Oxford: Oxford University Press.

Brown, R. D. and Tager, J. (2000) *Massachusetts: A Concise History.* Amherst: University of Massachusetts Press.

Cameron, A. (1993) *Radicals of the Worst Sort, Laboring Women in Lawrence, Massachusetts, 1860-1912.* Urbana and Chicago: University of Illinois Press.

Clark, E. B. (1995) "The Sacred Rights of the Weak": Pain, Sympathy, and the Culture of Individual Rights in Antebellum America. *The Journal of American History, 82:* 463-493.

Cole, D. B. (1960) The Collapse of the Pemberton Mill. *Essex Institute Historical Collections, 96:* 47-55.

Cole, D. B. (1991) *Immigrant City: Lawrence, Massachusetts, 1845-1921.* Chapel Hill: The University of North Carolina Press.

Collins, J. (1871) *Nature's Aristocracy, or, Battles and Wounds in Time of Peace: A Plea for the Oppressed.* New York: Lee, Shepard, and Dillingham.

Dalzell, P. F., Jr. (1987) *Enterprising Elites: The Boston Associates and the World They Made.* New York and London: W. W. Norton & Company.

Denning, M. (1987) *Mechanic Accents, Dime Novels and Working-Class Culture in America.* London and New York: Verso.

Donegan, C. (1984) *For the Good of Us All: Early Attitudes toward Occupational Health with Emphasis on the Northern United States from 1787 to 1870.* Ph.D. Dissertation. University of Maryland.

Dorgan, M. B. (1918) *Lawrence Yesterday and Today (1845-1918).* Lawrence: Dick & Trumpold.

Dublin, T. (1979) *Women at Work: The Transformation of Work and Community in Lowell, Massachusetts, 1826-1860.* New York: Columbia University Press.

Foner, E., Garraty, J. A., and Society of American Historians. (1991) *The Reader's Companion to American History.* Boston: Houghton-Mifflin.

Frothingham, O. B. (1874) *Theodore Parker: A Biography.* Boston: James R. Osgood and Company.

Gordon, D. M., Edwards, R., and Reich, M. (1982) *Segmented Work, Divided Workers: The Historical Transformation of Labor in the United States.* Cambridge, MA and New York: Cambridge University Press.

Hall, P. D. (1997) What the Merchants Did with Their Money: Charitable and Testamentary Trusts in Massachusetts, 1780-1880. In C. E. Wright and K. P. Viens (eds.), *Entrepreneurs: The Boston Business Community, 1700-1850* (pp. 365-421). Boston: Massachusetts Historical Society.

Handlin, O., and Handlin, M. F. (1969) *Commonwealth: A Study of the Role of Government in the American Economy, Massachusetts 1774-1861* (rev. ed.). Cambridge, MA and London: The Belknap Press of Harvard University Press.

Haskell, E. G., and Mason, S. (1860) *An Authentic History of the Lawrence Calamity, Embracing a Description of the Pemberton Mill, a Detailed Account of the Catastrophe, a Chapter of Thrilling Incidents, List of Contributions to the Relief Fund, Names of the Killed and Wounded, Abstracts of the Sermons on the Subject, Report of the Coroner's Inquest, & c.* Boston: J. J. Dyer & Co.

Josephson, H. (1967) *The Golden Threads: New England's Mill Girls and Magnates.* New York: Russell & Russell.

Kann, M. E. (1991) *On the Man Question: Gender and Civic Virtue in America.* Philadelphia: Temple University Press.

Landis, M. (1998) Let Me Next Time Be "Tried by Fire": Disaster Relief and the Origins of the American Welfare State, 1789-1874. *Northwestern University Law Review, 92:* 967-1034.

Levy, L. W. (1957) *The Law of the Commonwealth and Chief Justice Shaw.* New York and Oxford: Oxford University Press.

Linter, S. C. (1948) Mill Architecture in Fall River: 1865-1880. *The New England Quarterly, 21:* 185-203.

Marx, L. (1964) *The Machine in the Garden; Technology and the Pastoral Ideal in America.* New York: Oxford University Press.

Menand, L. (2001) *The Metaphysical Club.* New York: Farrar, Straus, and Giroux.

Mitchell, B. C. (1988) *The Paddy Camps, the Irish of Lowell 1821-6.* Urbana and Chicago: University of Illinois Press.

Murphy, T. A. (1992) *Ten Hours' Labor: Religion, Reform, and Gender in Early New England.* Ithaca and London: Cornell University Press.

Phelps, E. S. (1869) *Men, Women, and Ghosts.* Boston: Fields, Osgood, & Co.

Poirier, C. A. (1978) *Pemberton Mills 1852-1938: A Case Study of the Industrial and Labor History of Lawrence, Massachusetts.* Ph.D. Dissertation. Boston University.

Poirier, C. A. (1990) Aftermath of a Disaster: The Collapse of the Pemberton Mill. In K. Fones-Wolf and M. Kaufman (eds.), *Labor in Massachusetts: Selected Essays* (pp. 77-96). Westfield: Institute for Massachusetts Studies, Westfield State College.

Potter, J. F. (1992) *Factory Inspection and Accident Prevention in Massachusetts, 1879-1912.* M.A. Thesis, University of Massachusetts.

Reeve, P. (1995) *Making Whole That Which Is Lost: The Politics of Class and Citizenship in Labor's Campaign for Employers' Liability Reform, MA, 1881-1912.* Presentation: 17th Annual North American Labor History Conference.

Reeve, P. (1997) *Maximizing Men: Antebellum Commentary on Workers' Bodily Integrity, MA.* Presentation: 19th Annual North American Labor History Conference.

Reynolds, D. S. (1980) From Doctrine to Narrative: The Rise of Pulpit Storytelling in America. *American Quarterly, 32:* 479-498.

Rosenberg, C. E. (1989) Body and Mind in Nineteenth-Century Medicine: Some Clinical Origins of the Neurosis Construct. *Bulletin of the History of Medicine, 63:* 185-197.

Rothenberg, W. B. (2000) The Invention of American Capitalism: The Economy of New England in the Federal Period. In P. Temins (ed.), *Engines of Enterprise:*

An Economic History of New England (pp. 69-108). Cambridge, MA and London: Harvard University Press.

Sellers, C. S. (1991) *The Market Revolution: Jacksonian America, 1815-1846.* New York and Oxford: Oxford University Press.

Singer, E., and Endreny, P. M. (1993) *Reporting on Risk: How the Mass Media Portray Accidents, Diseases, Disaster, and Other Hazards.* New York: Russell Sage Foundation.

Siracusa, C. (1979) *A Mechanical People, Perceptions of the Industrial Order in Massachusetts 1815-1880.* Middletown: Wesleyan University Press.

Skocpol, T. (1992) *Protecting Women and Mothers: The Political Origins of Social Policy in the United States.* Cambridge, MA and London: Harvard University Press.

Skowronek, S. (1982) *Building a New American State: The Expansion of National Administrative Capacities, 1877-1920.* Cambridge: Cambridge University Press.

Stoop, S. L. (2002) *Mask or Mirror? (A Play of Portraits).* Worcester: Worcester Art Museum.

Temins, P. (2000) The Industrialization of New England, 1830-1880. In P. Temins (ed.), *Engines of Enterprise: An Economic History of New England* (pp. 109-152). Cambridge, MA and London: Harvard University Press.

Tomlins, C. L. (1993) *Law, Labor, and Ideology in the Early American Republic.* Cambridge, UK: Cambridge University Press.

Turner, V. W. (1982) Social Dramas and Stories About Them. *From Ritual to Theater: The Human Seriousness of Play* (pp. 61-88). New York City: Performing Arts Journal Publications.

Ware, N. (1990) *The Industrial Worker, 1840-1860.* Chicago: Elephant Paperbacks.

Zonderman, D. A. (1992) *Aspirations and Anxieties: New England Workers and the Mechanized Factory System, 1815-1850.* New York: Oxford University Press.

CHAPTER 7

Regulating Safety, Regulating Profit: Cost-Cutting, Injury and Death in the British North Sea after Piper Alpha

David Whyte*

THE PIPER ALPHA DISASTER

Not long after 9 P.M. on 6th July 1988, a series of explosions tore through the Occidental-owned Piper Alpha oil production platform in the Northern Sector of the British North Sea. With the benefit of hindsight it is now clear that the chances of survival for those onboard had been made slim by a corner-cutting and profit-hungry management regime. Negligent emergency provision and under-maintained critical safety systems were to make a catastrophic situation worse: emergency lighting failed; there were hardly any torches available to the crew; each of the lifeboats was located in the same section of the platform, which also happened to be inaccessible; and no provision had been made for an alternative escape route to the sea. Most people on the platform gathered at the emergency muster point, the accommodation module, which due to its location above the gas compression module also happened to be one of the areas on the platform most exposed to fire and explosion. The accommodation module, constructed from wood and fiberglass, quickly began to burn. The water deluge system—the platform's main defense against fire—failed, but in any case Lord Cullen's report of the official public inquiry was later to conclude that "it is likely that if the deluge had been activated on 6 July 1988 a substantial number of the deluge heads would have been blocked by scale with the result that they would not have been discharged" (Cullen 1990, p. 205). When two life rafts were

*I am grateful to Steve Tombs and Eric Tucker for insightful comments on an earlier draft of this chapter. Any errors and matters of interpretation, are, of course mine alone.

launched, they failed to inflate. The standby safety vessel, a converted fishing boat, had no medical supplies to treat survivors as they were pulled from the sea, and the Tharos, Occidental's state-of-the-art floating fire engine, could not muster sufficient water pressure to reach the flames. In the midst of all of this, those who ignored company emergency procedure and management instructions and sought alternative escape routes actually much improved their chance of survival (Wright 1993).

Occidental's senior management had been warned by their own consultants that the platform would not withstand prolonged exposure to high intensity fire. It was a warning that they chose to ignore after conducting cost-benefit analysis. The company's assessment of the risk of such an incident occurring did not justify the expense of refitting the platform with high-grade fireproofing (Pate-Cornell 1993). The sequence of events that followed the initial explosions illustrate the strictly observed "production first" dictum of offshore management. Managements on platforms connected by the same pipeline chain, the Tartan and the Claymore, declined to shutdown production, and instead continued to feed the blaze with oil as they obediently awaited approval for a costly closure of the pipeline from senior management onshore.

One hundred and sixty-seven were killed in the Piper Alpha explosions and fires; 61 workers survived. Thirty bodies were never recovered from the North Sea due to Occidental's refusal to pay for the excavation of the platform from the sea bed.

There was no prosecution of Occidental, a company that already had a criminal record for killing one of its workers. In September 1987, the company was successfully prosecuted for the death of Frank Sutherland after the company failed to issue a permit to work between shifts. The failure of the Scottish legal system to even consider seriously a prosecution of Occidental for Piper Alpha (the officially recognized technical cause having also involved problems with the permit to work during a shift changeover) is nothing short of a disgrace. This disgrace was greatly compounded by a subsequent civil case, initiated by Occidental in an attempt to recover compensation payments from their contractors and heard in front of the Scottish Court of Session. This law suit, a macabre spectacle of corporate greed which dragged on to become one of the longest in British legal history, forced survivors against their will to recount the events of the 6th July in front of the court. To compound matters, the verdict put an official seal on a version of events that blamed two workers who died on the Piper Alpha for the technical cause of the disaster.

It has emerged since that there was a possible alternative chain of events leading to the technical crisis, evidence that was suppressed by both the public inquiry and the civil court (BBC 1998). Both legal processes established an official version of events that included lengthy criticisms of Occidental, yet still enabled blame to be placed on the dead, and effectively exempted the operating company from legal scrutiny.

This chapter is concerned with the official state response to the Piper Alpha disaster. In particular, it examines the restructuring of the regulatory system, and the industry's counter-strategy. The initial sections of this chapter present an account of the political economy within which the deaths of 167 workers on 6th July 1988 must be understood, before analyzing the impact of the official inquiry into the disaster. The chapter then considers, with reference to data gathered in a series of interviews with offshore safety inspectors, workers, and managers, how a dominant set of assumptions, which can be observed as part of inspectors' "frame" or "worldview," places limits on strategies of regulatory intervention. The chapter concludes by arguing that the translation of this "world view" into regulatory practice can act to undermine the role of workers in guaranteeing their own safety.

For the time being, the chapter returns to the pre-Piper Alpha regulatory context, and traces out some key components of the political economy of the UK's indigenous oil industry.

THE ROOTS OF A SAFETY CRISIS AND THE STATE RESPONSE

Piper Alpha, rather that being understood as a one-off, unpredictable event, is better understood as the culmination of a generalized safety crisis in the industry. The origins of this crisis are in the failure of both the regulatory system and the operating oil companies' management regimes. The elemental origins of the crisis can be found in the political economy that governed the industry during the 1970s and 1980s. W. G. Carson (1982) described the conditions within which British oil policy developed as "the political economy of speed." The speedy development of an industry—central to offsetting Britain's economic decline in the 1970s—came at great cost to the workers, measured in abnormally high rates of injury and death in the sector (eleven times the fatality rate in the construction industry and nearly nine times the rate in mining) (Carson 1982, p. 21).

If the horrific rates of death and injury were one result of the combination of forces which encouraged speedy development, then a second effect was regulatory acceptance, the "institutionalisation of tolerance" (Carson 1982, p. 235), of this appalling toll. Carson measured this in terms of the legal anomalies, jurisdictional gaps, an alarming lack of resources available to the regulatory regime, and a generalized reluctance to enforce legislation. Although his book had little impact on the policy process at the time of its publication, it is telling that many of Carson's core findings (for example on the need for a statutory system of safety representatives, and the recommendation that the Department of Energy's regulatory responsibilities be removed from the sponsoring department) bear a remarkable resemblance to those made by the Cullen Report eight years later.

The offshore drilling and operating companies in the early years of the industry quickly established the use of casualized and sub-contracted labor. The legacy of this structure is that, over the years, the percentage of offshore workers employed as sub-contractors has remained at between 80% and 90%. In the pre-Piper Alpha period, workers were usually employed on short-term contracts that often lasted no longer than a few weeks or months, and contained few contractual rights. Trade union organization was virtually unheard of. Authoritarian, often thuggish, management styles ensured that those who were found to have trade union sympathies, who complained too much about working conditions, or who vocally expressed concerns about safety were run off the platform (in industry parlance, "NRBd"[1]) as a matter of routine. Eighty-three percent of workers on board Piper Alpha on the night of the disaster were sub-contracted (Cullen 1990). They therefore hardly enjoyed a stable vantage point from which to present their concerns to management on questions of safety.

The marginalisation of workers' expertise and knowledge of safety in the offshore management regime was to have catastrophic consequences. In the months preceding the disaster, management ignored a series of reports of gas leaks by workers on the Piper Alpha. On the day of the disaster, two workers complained about a gas smell. Although one received permission by the platform safety officer to down tools, management declined to interfere with work routines and conduct an investigation (*The Guardian* 11 July, 1988).

SAFETY REGULATION AND POLITICAL ECONOMY

The offshore regulatory structure and the labor-market structure, many features of which were unique to U.K. Oil industry in the 1970s and 1980s, were the product of a very specific political economy. This was a period in which productive oil capital enjoyed a structural advantage in relation to policy development in the sector, and in the economy more generally. Prior to the discovery of the United Kingdom Continental Shelf (UKCS) reserves, the oil business had enjoyed a venerable position in British economic history. Long before the discovery of oil in the North Sea, oil had, in the early part of the 20th century, become arguably the single most valuable commodity expropriated from the colonies and the commonwealth. Its value to the British state rose exponentially as oil became the country's main energy source in the latter half of the 20th century.

Since the discovery of substantial reserves in the North Sea, productive oil capital (represented by the operating oil companies, with British and US-owned banks and financial institutions as powerful backers) has held a position as a dominant fraction of capital in the British economic/social system. Productive oil capital helped to re-establish the City of London as a dominant player in the world economy during the Thatcher years (Hutton 1996, pp. 63-64). A commonality of interest between the City of London and the oil business was consolidated in the 1980s with the simultaneous restructuring of the British economy and neo-liberal renewal of capitalist ideology. Becoming a net producer of oil had the effect of strengthening the value of sterling. Monetarist economic policy, most crucially the abolition of exchange controls, allowed the pound to soar to new heights and gave birth to the 1980s credit boom. The restructuring of the British economy had at its heart a reassertion of the dominance of finance capital (as opposed to manufacturing capital), and perhaps the most catastrophic of side-effects of this strategy was the weakening of export markets, a general weakening of British manufacturing, and the concomitant creation of mass unemployment (Alt 1987). A series of attacks on the trade union movement (most visibly the assault on the miners and the print workers in the mid-80s, and the subsequent introduction of a raft of draconian anti-trade union laws) turned the tide in Britain's open class warfare that had been raging with growing intensity for two decades. The consequent sharp rise in the cost of state welfare benefits, coupled with a series of populist income tax reductions, was paid for not only by cuts in other areas of public expenditure but by the oil receipts and the related turnaround in the Britain's balance of payments. There is reason to conclude that the U.K. government's pioneering strategy of neo-liberal economic reform could not have proceeded without oil. Alan Clarke, a veteran member of several Thatcher governments, has since argued that, "without the revenue from oil, there could have been no Thatcherism" (BBC 1997).

The neo-liberal restructuring of the economy of the 1980s augmented considerably the political leverage that had previously been enjoyed by oil capital as a leading fraction of capital during the 1970s. It is in the consolidation of oil capital's hegemonic position that the genesis of the regulatory failure in the pre-Piper Alpha era is to be found.

IMPACT OF THE OIL CRASH

The contractual subordination of workers as a result of the offshore labor market structure had been exacerbated by a chain of events in the market which shook the industry in the mid-1980s. The collapse of the OPEC cartel quota system in 1985 (the average oil price per barrel plummeted from more than $30 in November 1985 to around $10 in April 1986) had a dramatic effect on the industry. In order to defend profit levels, oil companies slashed their operational budgets by between 30 and 40% across the board. The impact on the workforce was devastating. Wage levels fell dramatically and 1986 saw up to 22,000 jobs lost in the industry (Harvie 1994). The operators' response to the oil price crash had far reaching implications for workplace safety in the industry. Funding allocated to ensuring the regular maintenance of plant equipment suffered the same fate. As Lavalette (1991) has noted, offshore safety conditions become particularly volatile during changes in maintenance patterns:

> . . . many of the machines operating on offshore installations are not specif-
> ically designed for the North Sea, rather they are intended for "normal"

> factory working. Yet they are taken into a highly corrosive atmosphere, are squeezed to work as fast as possible and are run for 24 hours a day. The effect of this is to increase the possibility of breakdowns. However, the numerical flexibility that the contract system generates, ensures that manning levels are reduced to their absolute minimum offshore and hence unexpected maintenance demands can cause labor shortage problems. (p. 43)

The intense pressures on safety associated with maintaining production are also partially associated with the operating companies' imperative to avoid periods of shutdown or "downtime." Production shutdown may commonly be the only safe way to maintain plant components integral to the system. Under certain conditions, companies may adopt a "breakdown" or "necessary" maintenance strategy, or delay shutdown in order to alleviate the large costs associated with downtime. It was precisely this type of maintenance strategy that became normalized in the industry during this period.

All available evidence suggests that the post-1985 strategy intensified workforce injuries and fatalities. During the years between 1985 and the end of the decade, the number of workers killed or seriously injured was consistently higher than it had been at any time before in the industry (Woolfson and Beck 1995). The impact of this is graphically illustrated by a Manchester University survey in 1988 which found that "nearly 30% of offshore workers have suffered injuries at work" (*The Guardian* 21 January 1989).

For the consortia of investment, management, and political interests absorbed into productive oil capital, the deaths and injuries suffered by workers may have been an inconvenience, but they did not get in the way of healthy business. The political economy of speedy production and minimal regulatory interference ensured a period of sustained "windfall" profits and, despite a brief dip in profitability following the 1986 price crash, rendered investment risk for the oil companies virtually negligible.

If the chapter so far provides a context for understanding Piper Alpha as a consequence of the oil companies' intense campaign to defend profits, it was also an event that galvanized workers opposition. The only collective bargaining agreements that existed in the industry at the time were the short-term "hook-up" deals made to ensure workforce stability in the early pre-production stage of offshore construction. A series of widely supported and ingenious campaigns of industrial action broke out across the sector in the summers of 1989 and 1990, which sought to establish a serious and ongoing role for trade unions in the safety regime. The campaigns, organized by the then-unofficial shop stewards' committee OILC[2] and based around a series of sit-ins and strikes on offshore platforms, sought to secure as a primary demand collective safety rights. Although it is difficult to estimate the material impact or success of the campaigns of 1989 and 1990 in safety terms, there can be little doubt that in taking this action offshore workers refocused public attention on the Cullen Inquiry and the North Sea oil companies. The campaign conducted by offshore workers confronted management explicitly for their complicity in the toll of deaths and injuries in the industry. In the summer of 1990, Lord Cullen prepared the manuscript of his report with one eye on developments in the North Sea (for detailed accounts of those campaigns and their impact, see OILC 1991 and Woolfson, Foster, and Beck 1996).

THE CULLEN INQUIRY:
RESTRUCTURING THE OFFSHORE SAFETY REGIME

Burton and Carlen have argued that official enquiries into matters of the administration of law and public order "replenish official arguments with both established and novel modes of knowing and forms of reasoning. . . a strategy of discursive incorporation through which legitimacy crises are repaired and the reforms they engender are publicly presented" (1979, p. 8). From this perspective, state public enquiries should be read not as a mechanism for initiating fundamental social change that might prevent a similar chain of events in the future, but as a means of restoring the moral authority of the state and stabilizing the social order in times of crisis. Cullen's role was precisely this: to hone a refined regulatory system which went some way to appeasing public anger and mediating between labor and capital while minimizing any lasting damage to economic or industrial policy.

A key decision made by Cullen was his refusal to reverse Energy Secretary Cecil Parkinson's decision to establish a company-administered system of safety representatives three months after the disaster. Parkinson's knee-jerk response had the effect of stopping in its tracks the long-standing demand for the trade union system that protected all other workers in the United Kingdom. His intervention thus limited the challenge to oil capital at a crucial time. Subsequently, Cullen declined to grant trade unions a central role in Parkinson's system of safety representatives or more generally link safety to trade union rights. Although the Parkinson system was only supposed to be in place for two years before review, Cullen put a permanent seal on the system.

This was not out of line with the general trajectory of reform proposed in the report. Cullen's careful reparation of the legitimacy crisis favored oil capital on most aspects of the new regime. Despite the momentary crisis that placed both oil capital and state regulators under scrutiny, the prevailing balance of social forces in the United Kingdom during the late 1980s meant that the oil companies were in a strong position to resist trade union demands.

Notwithstanding the relatively strong structural position of oil capital, the considerable industrial noise made by the offshore workers' campaign ensured that Cullen could not fail to at least take account of the trade union position. Cullen's report, when it was complete, contained a damning account of the state's regulatory failure and of Occidental's management regime. In perhaps the most vivid example of the Department of Energy safety inspectorate's failure, Cullen recorded how an inspection report following the prosecution of Occidental for the death of Frank Sutherland less than two weeks before the disaster, had accepted that "[l]essons appear to have been learned from the Sutherland fatal incident. A routine inspection in *one year's* time is appropriate" (Cullen 1990, p. 246; my emphasis). For Cullen, inspections on the Piper Alpha ("superficial to the point of being of little use as a test of safety on the platform") were indicative of the wholesale failure of the Department of Energy inspection program to "address the regulatory requirements for dealing with the major hazards" (Cullen 1990, p. 382). The inspectorate, with only seven employees responsible for monitoring and investigation work on all North Sea installations in July 1988 (Cullen 1990, p. 251), was pathetically under-resourced. Trade unions' contributions to the inquiry, echoing Carson, also stressed the irreconcilable conflict of interests or "clientelism" within the Department of Energy, simultaneously the industry's sponsoring department and regulatory authority (Cullen 1990, p. 381). Cullen subsequently ordered the transfer of regulatory responsibility from the Department of Energy to a discrete division of the Health and Safety Executive (HSE). The new regulatory regime would require the state to fund a safety inspectorate of more than 300 staff, around half of whom would be inspectors.

Moreover, Cullen's recommendations would force operators to commit considerable levels of resources to spending on safety technology and risk assessment in the first instance, appeasing the demands for safety.

However, the impetus to re-structure the offshore regime was by no means dominated by "pro-regulatory" forces. As this chapter has already indicated, the prevailing balance of social forces in the United Kingdom in the late 1980s was one in which the labor movement found itself considerably weakened in a relatively short period of time. The institutionalization of neo-liberalism had loosened the influence of organized labor in politics and strengthened the hand of finance capital. For this reason, in some crucial aspects, productive oil capital retained a strong voice in debates on the shape of the regulatory structure. Lacking a political climate in which pro-regulatory forces outside the industry could be harnessed effectively, the offshore industrial action campaigns did not succeed in winning collective bargaining rights on safety. Neither were trade union demands for a new set of clear, minimum legal safety provisions to be successful.

What emerged from Cullen's industrial settlement was a regulatory regime which was to be based around "goal-setting" (Cullen 1990, pp. 390-391). This approach had been enshrined in the British *Health and Safety at Work Act* (1974), the key legislative statute that had never been fully implemented offshore. Goal-setting in the North Sea was slightly different, in that it was to be based upon a monitored self-regulation approach, achieved largely through the preparation of "safety cases."

In contrast to the "prescription" model—the model advocated by the trade unions in their evidence to the Cullen Report—whereby standards of safety are set by detailed minimum standard specifications for plant equipment and safety procedures, "goal-setting" is based upon employers and duty holders (normally the owner of the worksite) setting out a "case" (in the form of a detailed document—"the safety case"—which is based upon numerical risk calculations) which details how risks will be managed and minimized. The regulatory authority HSE must then approve the safety case—often after protracted discussion with the duty holder. The key test that is applied in the consideration of safety cases is ALARP—whether the duty holder has reduced risks to a level "as low as reasonably practicable." Thus, instead of simply complying with a set of predetermined minimum standards, the duty holder is obliged to develop effective and practicable standards suited to the particular requirements of the site. The role of regulator shifts from enforcing legal minima to *assisting* duty holders to comply. Goal-setting and cost/benefit-based standards such as "ALARP" in effect institutionalise consensus (Whyte 2004) or compliance (Pearce and Tombs 1998) models of regulation in which bargaining, persuasion, and negotiation with employers is preferred to law enforcement strategies.

It is significant that Cullen's decision to advocate the goal-setting approach was based largely on the evidence that he heard from prominent individuals in the HSE and the operating companies. The key chapter in the Cullen report, "Future Offshore Safety Regime" (Chapter 21), sets out functional changes in the regime envisaged by Cullen. In this chapter he substantially drew upon the contributions of the HSE, the Department of Energy, and the Norwegian Petroleum Directorate as well as those provided by Conoco, Amoco, Chevron, ICI, and Shell. Although he did consider trade union evidence toward the end of this chapter, detailed contributions submitted to the public inquiry by the trade unions which pointed out the dangers of allowing the oil companies to self-regulate were passed over for the enthusiastic endorsements of goal-setting and self-regulation set out by the oil companies (Cullen 1990, pp. 355-357).

The inquiry undeniably allowed oil capital a leading role in the design of the new regulatory regime, but it was not all plain sailing for the operating oil companies. Cullen was also persuaded to impose some costly obligations upon the companies. The costs of hardware associated with some of Cullen's technical recommendations (notably the provision of fire and blast-proof temporary safe refuges (TSRs) to provide an emergency muster area in the event of major fire and explosion, safety valves on sub-sea and platform production systems, and the costs of quantitative risk assessment and other aspects of the preparation of safety cases) have been estimated variously at £2.3-£2.6 billion (HSE 1995) and £5 billion (Brandie 1994/95). Clearly, whichever estimate one believes, this represented a considerable cost burden for the operating oil companies. This cost also came at a relatively unexpected time, just as the operators were recouping their losses from the 85/86 price crash.

In sum, then, Cullen successfully navigated the industry through its legitimacy crisis, imposing some costs and supporting the least resistible demands of the trade union movement, specifically the establishment of a more adequately funded safety inspectorate, removed from the control of the sponsoring department. However, in so far as the principles underpinning the regime moved further toward a model of "self-regulation" in which the oil companies were to play a role in a negotiated compliance model of regulation, the regulatory settlement also secured the consent of oil capital.

There is some very raw statistical evidence that the Cullen Report had some immediate impact. Between 1991/92 (the year immediately following the publication of Cullen) and 1994/95, the combined fatality and major injury rate fell by 40%. Of course, we must approach those figures with caution, since figures generated by HSE and reported by employers are notoriously vulnerable to under-reporting and manipulation by management, particularly in the context of an offshore contractor/client system which offers high financial rewards for low HSE injury returns (Whyte 1999, pp. 258-261; Woolfson and Beck 1998).

Nonetheless, these data do provide us with a dramatic official picture of offshore safety. It is significant that in the same period, investigations by inspectors rose four-fold (personal communication, HSE Offshore Safety Division (OSD) 8 January, 2000), and the total number of staff in post at the HSE OSD rose at roughly the same rate (see figures cited in Woolfson et al. 1996, p. 378).

CLAWING BACK THE COSTS OF PIPER ALPHA

To the extent that there was a "honeymoon" period following Piper Alpha, it was a short lived one. In the later half of the 1990s, Cullen's goal-setting regime proved to be vulnerable to a new cost-cutting campaign embarked upon by the oil companies. In the aftermath of the oil price crash of 1985/86, individual oil companies had sought to respond in a fragmented and piecemeal fashion to external economic pressures. To recoup the losses following the publication of the Cullen Report however, there emerged a highly organized, collaborative response on the part of offshore operators, which sought to alter the economic conditions that shaped the development of North Sea oil production.

This response involved an immediate counteroffensive against the small number of Cullen's recommendations that could be regarded as "prescriptive." Most notoriously, oil-company lobbying of the HSE achieved swift successes in diluting proposals for a minimum standard of TSRs (Woolfson 1995) and then for the mandatory provision of emergency standby vessels (*Press and Journal* 3 May 1996; and Tombs and Whyte 1998).

This strategy on the part of the oil companies gained momentum under the banner of the collaborative "Cost Reduction Initiative for the New Era" (Crine). The Crine project, organized and initiated by the oil industry trade association, United Kingdom Offshore Operators Association (UKOOA), was first proposed by the industry in 1993 in order to recoup for the oil companies the surplus profit sacrificed to Cullen. Of course, this was not the official rationale for Crine. Rather, it was lauded as a *survival* strategy for an industry reaching maturity and the only basis upon which a "bright future" for operators, contractors, suppliers, workers, and even wellbeing of the nation could be secured (Tuft 1994a, p. 1). "This cost reduction will . . . continue to maximise the remaining recoverable reserves, improve the construction industry's competitiveness in the international arena and thereby help sustain employment at a higher level than would otherwise be possible" (Tuft 1994b). To do so, it targeted a "30% reduction in capital costs" and a "50% cut in operating costs within 2-3 years" (Risley 1995, p. 5).

The implications of Crine for generalized attacks upon conditions, and particular attacks upon safety has been documented in detail elsewhere (Tombs and Whyte 1998; Whyte 1997). The initiative provided an economic rationale for mass redundancies, longer shifts, "multi-skilling,"[3] and cuts in maintenance budgets. At its outset it is hardly surprising that Crine was highly controversial. Public criticism of the cost-cutting initiative by the offshore workers' trade union, OILC, and from some industry analysts, particularly in relation to its safety implications (for example, Mackay 1995; *OILC news release* 17 January, 1996), was a routine feature of media coverage of the industry in the early 1990s.

Perversely, UKOOA and some government ministers promoted the idea that Crine-inspired cost-cutting would actually *improve* safety conditions (for example, see *Lloyds List* 30 November 1994). Jack Criswell in his role as President of UKOOA even went as far as to claim that Crine is "the industry's contribution to safety" (cited in Todd 1996, p. 2). The institutional acceptance of Crine in government circles was a measure of the ability of oil capital to present the initiative both as a survival strategy which would ensure the long term success of the industry, and, by association, a strategy which would also protect the *national* interest. Crine was embraced with considerable enthusiasm in government by both the Department of Energy and the Department of Trade and Industry and by 1995 the latter had proclaimed itself an equal partner in the initiative.[4]

REGULATING PROFIT

Given the concerns about the safety impacts of cost-cutting, Crine provided the new regulatory authority with a very stiff test. And it was a test that the regulator did not appear to relish. Officially, the HSE's position was one of disinterest, broadly reflecting UKOOA's position that Crine would not necessarily impact upon safety. On occasion though it accepted UKOOA's claim that, safety management could become more "efficient" simply by streamlining business (Todd 1996). It was a bizarre position for HSE to take, not least since it contradicted much of HSE's own research that have consistently warned of the dangers inherent in cutting maintenance budgets, over-relying upon contract staff, and employing under-skilled staff (for example, HSE 1985). Indeed, it appears even more ill-judged when placed in the context of the HSE's own evaluation of the safety case regulations which noted, as Crine was beginning to gather pace offshore, "the changes perceived as having a negative effect on safety are in the area of reductions of manning and associated increases in workload" (HSE 1995, p. 32).

In spite of the fact that official figures are treated with extreme caution and even scepticism in many quarters,[5] it continues to be the case that these figures are taken seriously—indeed, accepted as a robust indicator of offshore safety—by the HSE. At a minimum, then, these figures are useful because they provide an official benchmark for measuring broad trends in injuries and incidents and they alert the regulatory authority to safety conditions in the industry. Based on those figures, between 1996/97 and 1997/98 there was a 14% rise in dangerous occurrences, and a 95% increase in major injuries and fatalities.[6]

It is significant for the purposes of our argument here that this dramatic turn in reported injuries and deaths occurred shortly after Crine's lead-in period. The implementation of Crine principles can be traced back to late 1994. It then took around a year for the first cost-cutting measures introduced under the banner of Crine to be implemented. Thus, the years 1996/97 and 1997/98 were significant in that they represent the first two years of operation under Crine-led austerity. It is instructive that during this same period, Crine was highly successful in stabilizing North Sea profit levels. Between 1996 and 1998 the gross trading profits of the North Sea operators were pretty much restored to the pre-price crash windfall levels and annually exceeded £10 billion for the sector (Department of Trade and Industry, *Energy Trends* November 1998).

THE REGULATORY RESPONSE

Clearly, then Crine was having some impact upon the industry. Given that the initiative sought to replicate the dramatic cuts in operational and capital expenditure that the industry witnessed in the pre-Piper Alpha years and given that primary indicators appeared to indicate some deleterious safety effects, it is legitimate to ask how the post-Cullen regulatory regime reacted to Crine.

Prosecutions are not a particularly good indicator of regulatory response, partly because the time lapses between the case being reported to the procurator fiscal (public prosecutor), the case being laid, and finally adjudication, can take many months and often years. A better indicator of the HSE's vigilance is the number of enforcement notices issued.[7] Annual notices issued by HSE OSD fell dramatically from 38 in 1995/96 to 4 in 1996/97 and 12 in 1997/98.[8] This apparent regulatory disengagement is also indicated by the fact that between the calendar years 1995 and 1999 HSE failed to serve a single enforcement notice on any Shell[9]-operated platform, despite evidence of numerous serious safety breaches, not least in the company's Brent field. Some of this evidence was made public in a television documentary and in the testimonies produced by the OILC trade union that had members on the Brent field (for example BBC 1996; *OILC News Release* 28 October, 1999).

It is worth noting that it was also during this period that the inspectorate's burden of monitoring the safety case regime began to ease up. There may still have been some safety case re-submissions to take care of, and this was undoubtedly a major drain on the inspectorate's resources during this period, but the first wave of safety-case work had begun to tail off at the beginning of 1996. The easing of this burden, which enabled the inspectorate to concentrate more fully on inspections and investigations, make it yet more difficult to believe either that HSE were not vigilant about, or acutely aware of, a possible link between Crine and safety.

Evidence from a qualitative survey of HSE OSD inspectors, onshore managers, and offshore workers conducted by the author in the midst of Crine's implementation explored respondents' perspectives on the initiative.[10] Inspectors indicated an acute awareness not only of the issues of safety implicated in Crine, but also about workforce perceptions of those issues. One respondent recalled that at a session he had led at a safety representatives' training course on the role of the HSE, the feedback from the group indicated their most acute concerns focused on aspects of cost-cutting. In particular, safety representatives raised concerns about the downsizing of the workforce, multi-skilling, and the introduction of extended work patterns. Other inspectors reported that workers also raised cost-cutting related issues regularly during inspections. It seems, then, that during a period of comparatively low regulatory activity, inspectors were routinely being made aware of the widely held concerns of workers.

According to Hawkins, an HSE inspector's decision to take enforcement action is conducted within a particular "frame." The frame constitutes a range of forces that bear upon the decision that are external to an individual case under investigation. Those include their personal values and training, and the influence of colleagues. The frame is also determined by "the current political setting, the state of the economy, government ideology about regulation, or the attitudes, values, and policy of the agency . . ." (Hawkins 2002: p. 434). It is those latter features that, due to the particular structural advantage enjoyed by oil capital, outlined above, have assumed a heightened significance in the North Sea safety regime. And it is with Hawkins' insights in mind that the chapter proceeds to explore some features of the regulatory frame in order to uncover a possible explanation for regulatory disengagement during the implementation of Crine.

EXPLAINING REGULATORY DECISION MAKING ON THE FRONT LINE

If we want to understand the "frame" within which regulatory decisions take place, then we are, to some extent, exploring the connection between ideas and the conduct of offshore front-line inspectors. There is a link here to Gramsci's account of the hegemonic process by which ideas become dispersed through the state and civil society which stresses the relation between "common sense" beliefs and "norms of conduct" (Gramsci 1996, p. 424).

We have to take a little care here, since regulatory policy in organizations such as the HSE is rarely coherent or consistent enough to enable us to explain precisely each individual decision by inspectors. Pearce and Tombs have warned against a conceptualization of the regulatory inspector in "caricature, as something akin to an automaton, compelled towards the prosecution of each and every violation detected" (1998, p. 237). The regulation of safety law is, just as the enforcement of other bodies of law, subject to the discretion of law enforcers. Whilst inspectors work within an institutional framework and are bound by policy and by decisions their managers make, particular enforcement decisions made by inspectors and their team leaders respond to particular circumstances and so are always going to differ in some respects from the general position adopted by the institution. Having said this, in order to understand how particular regulatory *norms* of conduct develop we have to explore the degree to which the institution and the individuals who carry out its work share common perspectives and assumptions.

The following analysis seeks not to identify a coherent ideology or unitary worldview that is commonly held by all HSE inspectors—it is hardly likely that such ideological cohesion could exist in any profession. Nor is the purpose to reconstruct a typical worldview which is in any sense "complete." Rather, the analysis presented here identifies some common characteristics of a worldview or "frame" that can be discerned from inspectors' responses during interviews.

Our discussion here is concerned with three sets of assumptions/ideas that appear to connect the worldview of HSE offshore inspectors to HSE policy in relation to the Crine/safety debate.

THREE STRANDS OF A REGULATORY WORLDVIEW

1. Crine, Survival, and the National Interest

The perception of cost-cutting as essential to the survival of the industry was unanimously held among inspectors interviewed. For example, one inspector characterized Crine as "at best an efficiency driver and at worst a necessary evil." Inspectors' uncritical acceptance of the central tenet of Crine's survival philosophy, by default, enables UKOOA and the oil companies to shape some key domain assumptions about what is and is not *economically* possible in terms of safety performance. This is a dangerous road to take, since one effect of the claim to assert the "national interest" may be to render the question of safety as a secondary one (i.e., if Crine is essential for the survival of the industry, then it follows that it is in the national interest that costs must be driven down). It matters less whether Crine is the principal source of an intensifying pressure upon safety conditions in the industry or not. One onshore production manager in a subsequent interview summed up this effect with brevity: "If Britain wants the oil, then we have to get on with extracting the oil and meet the new challenges head on. We have to tighten our belts, and I think the HSE realise this as much as anybody."

At the time of those interviews, however, it was quite possible to find alternative perspectives of the impact of Crine in safety terms, particularly in the accounts of workers and their organizations. It was also possible to find alternative assessments of the economic conditions around which Crine emerged. Some of those accounts demonstrate on one hand scepticism of the necessity of Crine as a survival strategy from within the industry (for example, Mackay 1995), and on the other, the view that rather than an inevitable result of market conditions, Crine is better understood as a highly orchestrated attempt to claw back the costs of the post-Piper Alpha regime from the contractors and supply firms (for example, Foster, Maguiness, and Munro 1994). Moreover, there was an emerging body of evidence in the mid-90s which showed that the North Sea was probably the least likely oil producing zone in the world to suffer the disinvestment or capital flight threatened in Crine statements (Tombs and Whyte 1998). Indeed, despite its maturity, the North Sea is among the most stable oil provinces in the world. Evidence from oil analysts WoodMackenzie in 1998 concluded that most North Sea fields were viable at prices as low as $10 per barrel (*The Scotsman* 23 December, 1998). This equates to around 50% of the bottom-line price required for viability in Crine's doom-laden projections.

This disengagement from debates around viability and survival, rather than representing a *neutral* position, in effect demonstrates HSE's willingness to accept oil capital's version of the economic conditions which structure the industry as harsh "reality," no matter how conflated or fictional this reality might be. HSE's regulatory disengagement from intervention in Crine-led cost-cutting is perhaps reinforced and certainly not discouraged by the government's continued institutional support for Crine under Labor. The Labor government's Oil and Gas Task Force, established in November 1998, just over a year after Labor took power, was dominated by oil industry CEOs and aimed explicitly to escalate and provide political support for Crine. The Task Force was subsequently relaunched in January 2000 under the name PILOT. Crine's successor LOGIC[11] initiative was launched around the same time as the Task Force by Secretary of State for Trade and Industry Peter Mandelson with a £1.6 million government grant (*Oil and Gas Supply Chain News* 17 November 1998, http://www.dti.gov.uk/ogsc/news/news-1.htm). LOGIC and PILOT share the same stated aims: to maintain oil production at 3 million barrels per day, to increase oil and oil supply industry exports by 50%, and to generate new business worth £1 billion every year.

The political urgency with which those institutional imperatives are to be pursued is something which inspectors were acutely aware of. Interviews with inspectors revealed a strongly-held perception that their decisions are likely to have a political impact which extends way beyond the immediate vicinity of the workplace. One interviewee betrayed an alarming degree of obedience to political elites which verged on the paranoid: "You have to be careful, because some of these decisions we can make, if we made them, could land up on the desk of Bill Clinton. These guys have contacts at that level." Other inspectors reported that the political impact of the regulatory process was a feature of balancing enforcement decisions. As one noted:

> You need to bear in mind that you can't go around shutting installations down, these people have injected a lot of money into the economy and potentially will inject a lot more, and we have to bear that in mind—put it into the equation—when we're dealing with them [operating oil companies].

Responses from inspectors indicated that rather than being removed from the regulatory process, wider structural-political questions are intrinsic to the worldview or common sense of inspectors, and have some bearing upon how they conduct their responsibilities.[12]

2. Better Safety is Better Business

A second assumption related more directly to the management of safety under the Crine project is that better safety equals better business. Regardless of the strength of workforce opinion expressed to inspectors in a wide range of fora and contexts (see previously) the consensus among inspectors was that a large-scale cost-cutting project of the magnitude of Crine will not *necessarily* generate safety-related problems. The words of one inspector sum up a widely held view among inspectors: "Crine says, 'we can reduce costs without prejudicing safety.' Well if they can, fine. . . . We are not management consultants, so it's out of our control. To be blunt, it's nothing to do with us."

The claim here is that production-related decisions of management that are not safety-critical can be ring-fenced from those that are. Quite apart from the fact that this approach to safety management is one which has long-since been discredited both by academic and industry experts (Kletz 1988), virtually all of the outcomes of Crine—"multi-tasking," downsizing, cutting back maintenance, withdrawal of emergency cover—fall within the definition of safety-critical. Again, this is a point articulated in HSE's own statements and literature (for example, HSE 1985; see also Slapper and Tombs 1999, p. 142).

The idea that safety can be somehow formally separated from other aspects of the offshore labor process falsely assumes that safety is not integral to the labor process, and that safety conditions are not necessarily related to changes in production regimes. Safety therefore should not be on the same agenda as disputes over shift length, overtime and so on. Indeed, this is another grass-roots HSE position also found in its official discourse. It has already been noted above, but is worth re-iterating that OSD's Head of Policy proclaimed at a Crine conference in 1996 that Crine-related cost-cutting and better business could equate with to better safety (Todd 1996). It is a position which may be interpreted as an attempt to distance HSE from the Crine/safety debate. Inspectors' views on the degree to which Crine would impact upon safety varied, but there was a broadly held consensus that interference in managerial decisions related to cost-cutting was beyond the remit of the OSD.[13]

3. Promoting the "Common Interest"

A third set of assumptions asserts forcefully that workers and managers have a common interest in the management of health and safety. Thus, according one inspector: "The duty holder and the workforce should be working together for the same purpose. We shouldn't have to intervene at this level and it is this relationship that is really out of our hands."

The "common interest" principle is not unique to the offshore sector, nor does it reflect a new ideological formation. It is an idea which can be traced back to early forms of social regulation in the 19th century (Carson 1985; Tucker 1995, p. 103). It is an idea embedded in the western liberal tradition of social regulation. Lord Robens, a latter day architect of British health and safety law, argued successfully for an enduring application of this principle:

> . . . there is greater natural identity of interest between "the two sides" in relation to health and safety problems than in most other matters. There is no legitimate scope for "bargaining" on safety and health issues. . . . (Robens 1972, para 66, cited in Nichols and Armstrong 1973)

It is this idea that provided the foundation for formally enshrining the tripartite regulator/trade-union/employer system of consultation in U.K. workplaces.[14] But the offshore interpretation of the "common interest" principle, evident both in official policy and in interviews with inspectors, has devalued the regulatory role of trade unions. Moreover, the claims made by the "common interest" principle are contradicted directly by the experience of workers. The persistent use of management bullying and the NRB as a means of disciplining and disposing of offshore workers who raise safety concerns is testimony to the fragility of this principle. The widespread use of the NRB against "troublesome" safety representatives in the decade following Piper Alpha has been noted elsewhere (Whyte 1998, 1999). Such incidents are regularly brought to the attention of HSE inspectors, yet the regulator has consistently refused to involve itself, preferring to maintain an artificial partition between "industrial relations" and "safety matters." As one inspector argued: "It's not our job to sort out individual problems. They have to be done through normal routes." One safety representative described his experience of recording his discontent with HSE inspectors after management had refused to discuss safety-critical issues that he had raised: "When the boys from the HSE come out, they'll meet with you and discuss things. If you raise a problem with them, they'll tell you to go through the channels, to go and see your supervisor, and if he doesn't do anything, to go and see the OIM[15]. . . ." This is a common experience shared by offshore safety representatives. One noted of inspections: "I have stopped dealing with HSE because they don't seem interested in the safety rep system."

Inspectors' responses confirmed that they would refer workers with safety problems back to management as far as possible since, in the words of one inspector, it is "management who have the most influence over safety in the workplace." This reflected a strong consensus among inspectors that developing a close working relationship with management was a key aspect of ensuring effective compliance. As one inspector pointed out: "You have to deal with management because the only place that you are going to get action is in the corporate line of command." This approach was rationalized by inspectors with reference to the need to work pragmatically, within the limits of the possible. This position is well illustrated by the operation of an HSE safety telephone "hotline" advertised on official notices posted by the inspectorate on every platform. The hotline encourages workers to report confidentially issues of concern but carefully stresses that complaints should not be logged until platform management are consulted fully about the matter:

> Individuals who have concerns relating to any aspect of offshore safety should immediately raise the matter with their supervisor or the responsible person for the area concerned. It may also be appropriate that the matter is referred to the individual's safety representative. Any individual who remains dissatisfied as to the actions taken following the above should report the matter directly to the Offshore Installation Manager. (OSD, safety notice 5/91 dated 3 May 1991)

HSE practice, then, is underpinned by the assumption that on matters of safety managers, acting rationally, would act in concert with the interests of their workforce. Since it is managers who are the key guarantors of safety, while trade union involvement may be desirable it is not essential to the regime. It is an assumption that locates the causes of death and injury at work not in the capitalist political economy (Moore 1991; Pearce and Tombs 1998, pp. 127-152; Tucker 1990, pp. 179-187), but in organizational pathology, whereby safety problems are interpreted as an unexpected flaw in the organization. Thus, the regulatory process is purged of class conflict and reconstructed as a consensual process—a process which seeks only to persuade and cajole management to do what is assumed to be their best interests anyway. It follows from this logic that regulatory strategies need not fall back upon the adversarial tactics of strict legal enforcement (Dalton 2000).

CONCLUSION

What we have unraveled from the interview data is the existence of a set of assumptions that frame the decision-making processes of offshore inspectors. This set of assumptions places limits upon the feasibility and, indeed, the desirability of a particular course of regulatory action. Regardless of some obvious contradictions inherent in the ideological baggage carried by front-line inspectors (for example, that the "common interest" might somewhere along the line contradict the "national interest" as constructed by UKOOA and the protagonists of Crine), together the ideological claims evident in the regulatory agency at a corporate and a front-line level connect to influence the discretionary decisions that are made during regulatory visits.

Hegemonic rule, it should be stressed, is not achieved in a linear fashion by way of the ascendancy of particular fractions of capital—in this case, productive oil capital. After all, similar versions of the regulatory worldview discussed in the preceding section can be found in other industries at different stages of development. What counts above all for the shape of the safety regime, in terms of the particular form that ideology takes, is the general form that British capitalism takes in any given period. The development of the regulatory system in the oil sector—crudely connected to the emergence of neo-liberal hegemony that had managed to institutionalize self-regulation—is the historical foundation upon which oil capital's autocratic domination of the labor process has been built. When it came to Lord Cullen's public inquiry, it seems that neither the public exposure generated by the post-Piper Alpha crisis nor the trade union strategy could force a break from self-regulation (for a detailed account of the failure of the trade union challenge to oil capital, see Woolfson et al. 1996).

The Crine years (1995-1999) constituted a period in the history of the U.K. offshore oil sector during which the particular claims around the future of the industry were disseminated with some celerity and force. Crine was promoted with an almost evangelical fervor by oil industry and government representatives alike, and in this context, it is perhaps unremarkable that some of the organic "truths" established by Crine—that a cost-cutting program on this scale would not impact upon safety conditions, and that in any case, the industry would not survive without Crine—were accepted at face value by HSE in policy and in practice. In other words, those truths were accepted as "common sense" at various organizational levels of HSE if not by the workforce. The collapse in enforcement activity in the midst of Crine's implementation must be, if not wholly, then at least partially attributed to the success with which oil capital as a leading hegemonic fraction has been able to disseminate and promote its ideas. While it is important to reiterate the warning that those fragments of a regulatory worldview are not shared entirely by all inspectors all of the time, it appears to be the case from the sample here that they do present a dominant group of ideas which connect HSE policy with regulatory practice.

Health and Safety Executive (HSE)

HSE's *de facto* compliance with oil capital on questions of cost-cutting, survival, and the national interest has profound implications. Insofar as Crine defined the commercial realities of the North Sea in the post-Piper Alpha period *and* insofar as this was a definition which appears to have been left unchallenged by the regulator (see also, *Blowout*, Issue 67 May 2002), the result has been that under a negotiated goal-setting regime Crine has effectively shifted the parameters both for safety standards and for regulatory intervention (for a similar discussion of goal-setting, see Dawson, Willman, Bamford, and Clinton 1988, p. 15). In an industry where workers (the large majority of whom remain sub-contracted and casualized) have few bargaining rights and are in no position to present an alternative view of the economic conditions of the industry, goal-setting has effectively allowed the oil companies to dictate the terms of their own compliance to the regulator and to claw back the costs of the Cullen Report.

In the offshore industry, the systematic exclusion of workers from the regulatory process has had calamitous consequences both prior to and in the period following the Piper Alpha disaster. Those conditions are unlikely to change in the wake of the Labor government's flagship industrial relations legislation, the *Employment Relations Act* (1999). One effect of the new law in the context of the offshore trade union vacuum has been to allow employers rather than workers to select the union that will represent the workforce. Ultimately the Act has established a system of selective competition that has enabled employers to set one union off another until the terms of the recognition agreement have been gradually eroded. Some agreements have already excluded safety as a legitimate subject for negotiation. One union, the OILC, has been deliberately excluded from the process by companies that fear its militancy (Woolfson and Beck 2004). Workers will continue to struggle for safety rights in safety committees as atomized individuals and within their trade unions, but with the impending drift toward "sweetheart" deals this may, outside the regular public interventions in debates on offshore safety by OILC and other trade unionists, continue to be a largely hidden struggle.

The enduring legacy of Crine is that new cuts in operational costs in the post-Piper Alpha industry are rarely constructed as anything other than a rational response to market forces. Thus, early in 2002, BP announced the disposal of 500 workers (300 of them working in offshore operations), with an additional 500 contractor redundancies likely, citing the imperative of remaining streamlined in a competitive environment (see *Press and Journal* 22 March, 2002). It was the very same competitive environment which, in 2002, guided BP to award CEO Lord Browne a 66% rise in his annual remuneration to £3,037,000 (*Labor Research* August, 2002). A year later, Shell announced the redundancy of 350 offshore staff—around a fifth of the workforce—to enable the industry to remain "internationally competitive." One trade union leader was unequivocal about the potentially catastrophic effects of the latest campaign of downsizing: "The need to cut costs is the only driver here. Shell will be cutting down on vital maintenance work at a time when their platforms are ageing and . . . that has obvious safety implications. Platforms are beginning now to fall apart. It's a recipe for disaster."[16] In an industry in which long-term profits accumulate to offset short-term losses, a "market-forces" defense for such intense downsizing is indefensible, especially as the widely predicted resumption of high oil prices have brought us to the cusp of another era of windfall profits for the industry. The legacy of Crine is that workers will increasingly pay for the accumulation of those profits—measured by the loss of their lives and their jobs—in spite of the fact that this sector is virtually guaranteed long-term profitability. HSE recorded fatalities and major injuries are at a four-year high; the latest confirmed figures from 2002/03 record 310.4 combined fatalities and major injuries per 100,000 workers. This recorded rate has not dropped below 200 since 1995/96 (HSE 2004).

The public exposure and workers' campaign for recognition following Piper Alpha disaster offered a brief chance to interrupt the structural advantage enjoyed by productive oil capital in Britain to strengthen regulatory protection of workers' health and safety. However, the legacy of a British state-encouraged political economy of speed, the catastrophic disengagement on the part of the regulatory authority, and most important of all, the near-Victorian system of industrial relations has dominated the long-term response to the Piper Alpha disaster, leaving few controls in the workplace. Crine has broadly achieved what it set out to do, and its legacy lives on, formally through the government's PILOT initiative, and informally in the supine, collusive ideology that dominates the regulatory landscape. If this ideology, which seeps into the worldview of the offshore safety inspector and narrows the boundaries of legitimate regulatory intervention, remains dominant and if a rigid system of authoritarian managerial control remains intact, there can be little chance that the upwards trend in injury rates will be reversed, or little guarantee that another major disaster will not occur in the North Sea once again.

ENDNOTES

1. Not Required Back. This expression can be traced back to the early days of the industry when workers had their official working record stamped "NRB," effectively signaling that they would not be employed again by any offshore company. The expression is still used in the industry to describe on-the-spot sacking of workers.
2. Offshore Industry Liaison Committee, which in 1995 formed as an independent trade union in its own right.
3. Observers of industrial relations and the labor process will be familiar with multi-tasking/multi-skilling demands associated with the neo-liberal drive for a "flexible" labor market. What this has meant for offshore workers is the requirement to be available to cover a multitude of jobs, often with negligible training/experience. For example, some workers have reported being sent on four-day scaffolders courses and on return to the platform being expected to carry out the same tasks that previously would have been done by experienced scaffolders. In this context,

as offshore trade unionist and safety expert Ronnie MacDonald has observed, multi-skilling is much more appropriately described as de-skilling.

4. Initially, CRINE annual conferences were jointly organized by UKOOA and the DTI. In 1995, the Department donated £100,000 for the work of the CRINE Office to match the operating companies' funding (*European Offshore Petroleum Newsletter* 30 November 1995).

5. It is difficult to draw any conclusion from those official injury rates, partly for the reasons noted earlier, but also because of changes in the way injury and incident data is collected and recorded. First, RIDDOR (Reporting of Injuries, Diseases and Dangerous Occurrences Regulations) changed the rules for reporting in 1996, thus rendering HSE figures from 1995/96 onwards incomparable with previous years' data. Second, under-reporting and falsification of reportable data is notorious in the industry. According to some close observers of offshore employers, industry-generated quantitative indicators are vulnerable to manipulation and non-reporting to such an extent that it may be no exaggeration to say "they are not worth the paper they are written on" (Woolfson and Beck 1998, p. 15). This is not to say the figures cannot be usefully reconstructed, but it is instructive in this respect that it remains possible for industry interpretations of the figures to suggest that the industry is one of the safest in the country, while other interpretations of the same data regard it as one of the most dangerous (Woolfson et al. 1996).

6. Figures extracted from data in HSE (2001a).

7. Given the high number of incidents and illegalities brought to the attention of the inspectorate, enforcement notices issued by HSE are perhaps as likely to indicate *enforcement activity*—or the degree to which the regulatory strategy is following a punitive course *in response to illegalities*—as they are to indicate rising or falling rates of illegalities *per se*.

8. Figures supplied by HSE OSD (personal contact 21 August, 2001). Notices included in those figures are those which have been served on duty holders in the British offshore oil industry. Notices issued by HSE OSD in other sectors (for example, inshore diving) have not been included.

9. Shell UK Exploration and Production is the second largest operator in the North Sea, with 14 installations currently producing oil.

10. A total of eight interviews with frontline HSE OSD inspectors were conducted in December 1996/March 1996. Data reproduced in this section also draws upon a larger survey of 32 offshore and onshore managers in North Sea operating and contractor companies, and with 100 offshore workers. Interviews with workers and managers took place between spring 1995 and summer 1998. See Whyte 1999 for a detailed description of survey methods.

11. Both PILOT and LOGIC are acronyms, but are never referred to by their full titles, even in source documentation.

12. While the oil industry may appear unique as an industry which enjoys such a degree of structural influence, there are other sectors (for example, chemical production, energy supply, defense) and indeed individual companies (for example, ICI, British Nuclear, BAE Systems) who may be—and have every reason to be—perceived as enjoying similar strategic importance to the domestic economy.

13. Although this is not a clear-cut position to adopt by any means. For one, there is the question of the safety case. In the safety case documents, most of them completed before the introduction of Crine, platform manning levels, safety management systems, and risk calculations had to be approved by HSE inspectors. On the question of manning, Cullen himself was most unequivocal on safety criticality: "UKOOA submitted that it was for the operator to decide the appropriate manning levels for an installation and the appropriate qualifications of personnel . . . while agreeing that this has to be for the decision of the operator, it should be set out for review by the regulator as part of the operator's SMS (safety management system)" (Cullen 1990, p. 371).

14. In the offshore system, the distinctly bipartite character of the industry has sought to maintain some degree of a tripartite facade at a corporate level. For example, some trade unions have always been incorporated into HSE advisory committee structures while remaining frozen out of offshore agreements.

15. Offshore Installation Manager. The senior manager in command of an offshore platform, a position often described as similar to that of a ship's captain.

16. Jake Malloy, General Secretary of the OILC trade union, *The Scotsman*, Tuesday March 18.

REFERENCES

Alt, J. (1987) Crude Politics: Oil and the Political Economy of Unemployment in Britain and Norway, 1970-85. *British Journal of Political Science, 17:* 149-199.

BBC. (1996) *Frontline Scotland.* BBC Scotland documentary, 16 May, broadcast on Scottish network channel.

BBC. (1997) *Newsnight,* 5 October, news daily, broadcast on UK network channel BBC 2.

BBC. (1998) *Ghosts of Piper Alpha: Frontline Scotland,* BBC Scotland documentary, 17 November, broadcast on Scottish network channel.

Brandie, E. (1994/95, Winter) Achieving the Balance Between Safety and Cost Reduction. *Offshore International.*

Burton, F., and Carlen, P. (1979) *Official Discourse: On Discourse Analysis. Government Publications, Ideology and the State.* London: Routledge and Kegan Paul.

Carson, W. (1982) *The Other Price of Britain's Oil.* New Brunswick, NJ: Rutgers University Press.

Carson, W. (1985) Hostages to History: Some Aspects of the Occupational Health and Safety Debate in Historical Perspective. In B. Creighton and N. Gunningham (eds.), *The Industrial Relations of Health and Safety* (pp. 60-78). London: Croom Helm.

Cullen, Lord (1990) *The Public Inquiry into the Piper Alpha Disaster (2 volumes).* Cmnd 1310, London: HMSO.

Dalton, A. (2000) *Consensus Kills. Health and Safety Tripatism: A Hazard to Workers Health?* London: AJP Dalton.

Dawson, S., Willman, P., Bamford, M., and Clinton, A. (1988) *Safety at Work: The Limits of Self Regulation.* Cambridge: Cambridge University Press.

Foster, J., Maguiness, H., and Munro, A. (1994) *Restructuring in the UK Offshore Oil Industry: Partnership or Corporate Powerbroking?*, unpublished paper, University of Paisley.

Gramsci, A. (1996) *Selections from the Prison Notebooks*. London: Lawrence and Wishart.

Harvie, C. (1994) *Fools Gold. The Story of North Sea Oil*. London: Hamish Hamilton.

HSE. (2004) *Offshore Safety Statistics Bulletin 2003/2004: Fatal and Major Injuries to Offshore Workers*. Online at www.hse.gov.uk. Accessed 1 July 2004.

HSE. (2001a) *Health and Safety Offence and Penalties: A Report by the Health and Safety Executive*. London: HSE.

HSE. (2001b) Unpublished, *Restricted Management* internal memo circulated by Taf Powell, Head of the Hazardous Industries Directorate Offshore Division, 16 October, 2001.

HSE. (1995) *An Interim Evaluation of the Offshore Installations (Safety Case) Regulations, 1992*. London: HSE Books.

HSE. (1985) *Deadly Maintenance. Plant and Machinery. A Study of Fatal Accidents at Work*. London: HMSO.

Hawkins, K. (2002) *Law as Last Resort: Prosecution Decision Making in a Regulatory Agency*. Oxford: Oxford University Press.

Hutton, W. (1996) *The State We're In*. London: Vintage.

Kletz, T. (1988) *Learning from Accidents in Industry*. London: Butterworths.

Lavelette, M. (1991) *Some Very Peculiar Practices—Work Organisation and Safety in the North Sea Oil and Gas Industry*. Unpublished paper, University of Aberdeen.

Mackay, T. (1995) Crine Hype Hides Actual Impact. *Press and Journal*, 24 April.

Moore, R. (1991) *The Price of Safety: The Market, Workers' Rights and the Law*. London: Institute of Employment Rights.

Nichols, T., and Armstrong, P. (1973) *Safety or Profit?* Bristol: Falling Wall Press.

OILC. (1991) *Striking Out: New Directions for Offshore Workers*. Aberdeen: Offshore Information Centre.

Pate-Cornell, E. (1993) Learning from the Piper Alpha Incident: a Post-Mortem Analysis of Technical and Organisational Factors. *Risk Analysis, 13*: 215-232.

Pearce, F., and Tombs, S. (1998) *Toxic Capitalism: Corporate Crime and the Chemical Industry*. Aldershot: Ashgate.

Risley, A. (1995, Spring) The Challenges of the Nineties. *Offshore International*, pp. 4-6.

Slapper, G., and Tombs, S. (1999) *Corporate Crime*. Harlow, Essex: Longman.

Todd, I. (1996) Better Business is Better Safety. Paper presented to conference, *Crine: Learning to Survive*, London, 31 January-1 February, 1996.

Tombs, S., and Whyte, D. (1998) Capital Fights Back: Risk, Regulation and Profit in the UK Offshore Oil Industry. *Studies in Political Economy, 57*: 73-101.

Tucker, E. (1990) *Administering Danger in the Workplace: The Law and Politics of Occupational Health and Safety Legislation in Ontario, 1850-1914*. Toronto: University of Toronto Press.

Tucker, E. (1995) The Westray Mining Disaster and Its Aftermath: The Politics of Causation. *Canadian Journal of Law and Society, 10*: 91-123.

Tuft, V. (1994a) *President's Day Address: CRINE—Cost Reduction Initiative for the New Era*. London: Marine Management Holdings Ltd.

Tuft, V. (1994b) Partners in Crine. *Crinewatch*, August.

Whyte, D. (1997) Moving the Goalposts: The Deregulation of Safety in the Post-Piper Alpha Offshore Industry. In J. Stanyer and G. Stoker (eds.), *Contemporary Political Studies* (pp. 1148-1168). Nottingham: Political Studies Association of the United Kingdom.

Whyte, D. (1998) Overcoming the Fear Factor: Workforce Involvement and Health and Safety Offshore. *Public Money and Management,* October-December, pp. 33-40.

Whyte, D. (1999) *Power, Ideology and the Regulation of Safety in the Post-Piper Alpha Offshore Oil Industry.* Unpublished Ph.D. thesis, Liverpool John Moores University.

Whyte, D. (2004) Corporate Crime and Regulation. In J. Muncie and D. Wilson (eds.), *The Student Handbook of Criminology and Criminal Justice* (pp. 133-152). London: Cavendish.

Woolfson, C. (1995) The Deregulation of the British Continental Shelf: The Hidden Agenda. In proceedings of *Offshore Safety in a Cost Conscious Environment from British and Norwegian Perspectives* conference, KNA Hotel, Stavanger, Norway, November 15-16, 1994, Aberdeen: Offshore Information Centre.

Woolfson, C., and Beck, M. (1995) *Seven Years After Piper Alpha: Safety Claims and the New Safety Case Regime.* Glasgow: University of Glasgow.

Woolfson, C., and Beck, M. (1998) *The Lessons of Piper Alpha: Onshore and Offshore Safety in Scotland Today.* Workers Memorial Day Lecture delivered at Edinburgh Trades Council, 28th April.

Woolfson, C., and Beck, M. (2004) Union Recognition in Britain's Offshore Oil and Gas Industry: Implications of the Employment Relations Act 1999. *Industrial Relations Journal, 35*: 344-358.

Woolfson, C., Foster, J., and Beck, M. (1996) *Paying for the Piper: Capital and Labor in Britain's Offshore Oil Industry.* London: Mansell.

Wright, C. (1993) The Effect of Work Group Organisation on Responses to a Total Emergency in the Offshore Oil Industry. In *Workforce Involvement and Health and Safety Offshore: Power, Language, and Information Technology* (pp. 59-62). Proceedings of the international conference, March, Glasgow: Scottish Trades Union Congress.

CHAPTER 8

Courts, Crime, and Workplace Disaster

*Richard Johnstone**

In Australia 23 million working days are lost annually as a result of work-related injury and disease (Industry Commission 1995, p. 17) far exceeding time lost through strikes and other forms of industrial action (Bohle and Quinlan 2000, pp. 6-7). The vast majority of these lost working days are incurred when workers are *individually* injured, killed or made ill at work. Despite the huge costs to employers, workers and the community of workplace illness and injury, estimated at more than A$31 billion each year (Productivity Commission 2003, p. xxii), these individual workplace injuries, diseases, and deaths receive little media attention. Even though the occupational health and safety (OHS) statutes of the Australian States and Territories require serious workplace incidents, injury, disease, and death to be reported to OHS inspectorates (Clayton, Johnstone, and Sceats 2002, pp. 138-144), the response of governments to these individualized workplace disasters is surprisingly muted.

This chapter analyzes one key aspect of the state's response to workplace death, injury, and disease, namely prosecution for OHS offenses in the courts. I argue that court-based prosecution, particularly the sentencing process, operates in such a way as to maintain the "membrane of normalcy" in the face of the potentially egregious affront posed by work-related illness, injury, and death, not only to social normalcy, but also to social legitimacy. Recognizing that these processes stem historically from the social ambiguities of the nineteenth century, the chapter draws on recent empirical work in Australia (principally in the state

*This chapter draws on a large study of occupational health and safety prosecutions in Victoria, Australia: see Johnstone 2003a and 2003b.

of Victoria) on the approach taken by OHS regulators to criminal prosecution of duty holders under OHS statutes after workplace injury or fatality has occurred (Johnstone 2003a, 2003b; see also Perrone 2000). The focus of the chapter is on the magistrates' courts, where the majority of OHS prosecutions in Australia are conducted. The principal questions addressed in this chapter are: what part does prosecution under the OHS statutes play in the state's reaction to workplace illness, injury, and death? How do investigators, prosecutors, and courts (particularly magistrates' courts) "construct" OHS issues? What do these constructions, and overall approach taken to OHS prosecutions, tell us about the role of the criminal law in responding to injury and death at work.

The chapter begins with an overview of the traditional OHS enforcement paradigm, the legal framework for OHS prosecutions, and the contemporary enforcement profile of the Victorian OHS inspectorate. It then shows how most OHS prosecutions are initiated in response to injuries and fatalities, so that from the outset the prosecution is focused on an event and its details, and away from broader issues. It then argues that the sentencing processes in OHS prosecutions systematically "normalize" the traumatic events that motivated those prosecutions. Not only are these individual fatalities and serious injuries not portrayed as "disasters," but lawyers representing defendant business organizations are able to adopt routine mitigation strategies (such as "blameshifting," highlighting the uniqueness of events leading to the injury, and/or showing how the egregious event is a thing of the past and no longer relevant) to reconstruct the facts before the court to argue that their clients exhibit a relatively minor degree of culpability for individual workplace injuries and fatalities. Those work-related injuries and fatalities that result in prosecutions appear to be isolated cases, at worst "bad apples," rather than symptoms of poor OHS management or, at a deeper level, a result of the competitive pressures that modern capitalism places on business organizations to subordinate OHS to production and profit imperatives. This response of the courts to death and injuries at work provides yet another example of the way in which work-related injury and death "are not treated as seriously and as culpably caused as deaths [and injuries] in other circumstances" (Slapper 2000, p. 155) and of the way we "culturally absorb" death and injury at work "as if they are part of life itself" (Slapper 2000, p. 155).[1]

THE LEGAL FRAMEWORK AND HISTORICAL APPROACH TO ENFORCEMENT

The Traditional Approach to OHS Regulation

Since the Victorian *Factory and Shops Act* 1885, and in common with most of Europe and North America, Australian state parliaments have responded to the workplace death and injury toll by enacting statutory standards regulating certain workplace hazards. Until the 1970s and 80s these standards were extremely detailed and technical, focusing mainly on specific measures to be adopted to prevent injury to workers operating dangerous machinery. State inspectorates enforced these standards using a variety of strategies, including formal invocation of the criminal law through prosecution. Building upon the British model, these statutes relied on magistrates' courts as the primary venue for OHS prosecutions. Accordingly these courts, at the lowest level of the Anglo-Australian court hierarchy, have played a major part in the process of examining, constructing, and adjudicating all aspects of the OHS offenses,[2] particularly the determination of whether an offence has been committed, and the appropriate level of punishment.

A notable feature of the early history of Anglo-Australian OHS regulation was the manner in which OHS statutes tacked offenses on to the existing criminal justice system, without any consideration of whether the criminal justice system and its procedures—developed in pre-capitalist Britain to regulate the behavior of individuals (Slapper 2000, Ch. 2)—should be reconstructed to suit the requirements of a regulatory system aimed at controlling business organizations. A further tension developed because the *British Factories Acts* from 1844 (Carson 1979, pp. 53-54; 1985, p. 69) onwards created strict liability obligations. This signaled to a magistracy steeped in traditional criminal law notions of intention (*mens rea*) that OHS offenses were not "real crime." This mindset also mirrored the inspectorate's historically developed views on the "ambiguity" of OHS crime, discussed below.

Elsewhere I have argued that the early Victorian OHS regulators were the heirs of a particular form of OHS regulation that stretched back to mid-nineteenth century Britain (Johnstone 2000). Prosecution was infrequently used by an inspectorate which followed strongly an approach of negotiated compliance through the use of education, advice, and persuasion. Carson (1979) has vividly described this preference for informal action in response to detected contraventions as "the conventionalisation" of OHS crime, where offenses "are accepted as customary, are rarely subject to criminal prosecution and, indeed, are often not regarded as really constituting crimes at all." Further, he used the expression "ambiguity" of factory crime to describe the discontinuity between factory crime and "real crime" (Carson 1980). This distinction between *crimes* and *quasi crimes* or *regulatory crimes* relies upon and reinforces popularly held assumptions about the centrality of the market as a private, autonomous arena in which social relations are governed by voluntary agreements between formally equal individuals, rather than by formal legal rules. Writers like Glasbeek (1986) and Tucker (1990, 1996) have argued that regulatory legislation actually reinforces rather than challenges this conception of the market as an autonomous, self-regulating sphere. The enforcement of OHS standards ultimately rests on the threshold of voluntary compliance within the marketplace, rather than on the threat of externally imposed legal sanctions, which are used as a last resort.

When prosecution was the favored approach in Victoria, the statutory focus on requiring dangerous machines to be guarded meant that machinery guarding offenses resulting in serious injuries were the most likely to go before the courts.

The prosecution statistics in Victoria for the period 1885 to 1979 suggested that the ambiguity and conventionalisation of factory crime permeated not only the inspectorate's decision-making processes, but also proceedings before magistrates. Even though the maximum fines available for offenses under the OHS provisions were very low during the period 1885 to 1979 (in 1979 the maximum fine was A$2,000), the fines imposed by the courts averaged 25% of the maximum fine in the period 1900-1919, and between 10 and 15% of the maxima in the following six decades (see Johnstone 2000).

The Late Twentieth Century Reforms

Reflecting the wave of OHS regulatory reform that swept through Australia from the mid-1970s, in 1985 the Victorian *Occupational Health and Safety Act* (OHSA) was enacted, and replaced the traditional-style *Industrial Safety, Health and Welfare Act* 1981 (ISHWA). The OHSA enacted broad general duties on employers to employees and persons other than employees, namely, self-employed persons, occupiers of workplaces, designers, erectors, and installers of plant, and manufacturers, suppliers, and importers of plant.

These general duties were "fleshed out" by regulations and codes of practice, which at first simply reproduced the detailed technical machinery guarding and other standards in the old *Factories and Shops* and *Labor and Industry Acts* and regulations. Beginning in 1988, however, regulations and codes generally abandoned specification standards, and instead used a mix of general duties of care, performance standards (where a goal or target was set, and the duty holder could decide how most effectively to meet the target) and process standards. The latter prescribe a process or series of steps to be followed by a duty holder in managing specific hazards, or OHS generally. They generally set out hazard identification and risk identification, assessment, and control procedures.

The OHSA also made provision for the election of OHS representatives and the introduction of OHS committees (Part IV).

The OHSA gave OHS inspectors additional enforcement powers, in the form of improvement and prohibition notices, and made provision for the prosecution of directors and senior managers where a corporate offense against the OHSA was committed with their consent or connivance, or was attributable to their willful neglect. The maximum penalties for offences were significantly increased to A$25,000 for a corporation, and A$5,000 for an individual. These maxima were increased to A$40,000 and A$10,000 respectively in 1990. In 1997 the maximum fine for corporations was increased to A$250,000 if prosecuted in the County Court, and A$100,000 if prosecuted summarily in the magistrates' court. In addition, under the general sentencing legislation, courts were empowered to adjourn matters once the charges were proved and, without convicting the defendant, require the defendant to post a recognizance to be of good behavior, and to fulfill other specified conditions, for a specified period. From 1991 courts were also able to impose fines without convicting the defendant.[3]

It is notable that the general duties, particularly the employer's duties, appear to be capable of broad interpretation, and in particular, could be interpreted to require courts to examine all aspects of the work process in determining whether an employer has complied with the duty (Johnstone 1999; 2004, chs. 4 and 5). Further, the OHS offenses differ from the *typical* crime in that they are *inchoate* offenses, requiring no specific harm to be proven, but rather contemplating the possibility or risk of harm. In other words, whether a system of work is safe and without risks to health is an objective question of fact, and does not require proof of an injury.[4] These duties are also examples of the way in which contemporary regulatory law relies on a mix of constitutive and constraining regulation to achieve its ends (Hutter 2001, ch.1). Constitutive regulation is a form of regulatory law which attempts to use legal norms to constitute structures, procedures, and routines which are required to be adopted and internalized by regulated organizations, so that they become part of its normal operations. The aim is for legal norms to infiltrate deep into the organization, requiring it and the individuals within it to act responsibly. Where this fails, the law has the option of intervening more overtly through external regulation and sanctions (restraining regulation).

In principle, then, the OHSA had the potential to mandate that employers and other duty holders adopt and implement the key principles of effective OHS management, which are generally agreed to be:

- demonstrated senior management commitment to OHS;
- the integration of OHS management into core management and work activities;
- the adoption of a systematic approach to OHS management, involving risk assessment processes and an audit system to identify all risks and to determine which require urgent attention;
- the ability of the OHS management system to accommodate to change, particularly changes to work methods, systems and processes, substances, plant and equipment, and changes to the workforce; and
- valuing worker input to the OHS management system (Frick, Jensen, Quinlan, and Wilthagen 2000).

How did the state use this legislative armoury to respond to workplace illness, injury, and death? How did the inspectorate use its enforcement powers to enforce these potentially broad provisions?

THE ENFORCEMENT OF THE OHSA

An empirical study of OHS enforcement in Victoria from 1983 to 1999 (Johnstone 2003a) indicates that the contemporary Victorian OHS inspectorate, consistent with all of the other Australian OHS inspectorates, has continued the British tradition of enforcement through persuasion, advice, and education. Table 1 provides data from the Victorian inspectorate's annual reports in relation to the OHSA. Only in a small proportion of visits were improvement and prohibition notices issued. Even then, improvement and prohibition notices far outnumbered prosecutions.

This enforcement profile reflected the Victorian OHS inspectorate's 1985 *Prosecution Guidelines,* which were operative until the end of 1997.[5] The guidelines specified that the *principal instruments* to ensure compliance with the OHSA were to be improvement and prohibition notices. If alleged offenses could be remedied by the use of notices, "further legal proceedings will not be instituted in the Courts." A failure to comply with a notice "[would] be viewed as a serious matter" and would generally lead to prosecution. The guidelines set out six other circumstances in which prosecutions would generally be taken:

Table 1. Enforcement of the OHSA

Year	Inspection visits	Written observations	Improvement notices	Prohibition notices	Cases prosecuted[a]
1987/88	20307	N/A	1358	350	45
1988/89	11597	2878	1421	337	42
1989/90	16331	3177	2375	1034	45
1990/91	36868	N/A	3343	1647	76
1991/92	45363	N/A	3012	1655	119
1992/93	58746	2777	2851	1004	68
1993/94	70208	1586	1798	870	64
1994/95	48374	N/A	1481	822	64
1995/96	44661	N/A	2001	975	76
1996/97	44703	2281	3219	1040	57
1997/98	N/A	2569	3410	1242	84
1998/99	N/A	N/A	1735	1059	78

[a]These figures only include the number of cases brought, not the total number of informations issued.

Sources: Annual Reports and Industry Commission, 1994, Tables J8, J11, J12, and J20, and Industry Commission, 1995, Tables M17, M19, M22, and M23. Where there were differences in the data, the figure in the Annual Report was preferred. The statistics from 1994/95 onwards were very difficult to ascertain from the Annual Reports, and the figures for workplace visits and notices issued may be inflated. This table was first published in Johnstone, 2003a, p. 90.

(i)   Where the alleged breach has resulted in a fatality or "serious accident";
(ii) The willful repetition of the same offense;
(iii) Non-compliance with a Provisional Improvement Notice;
(iv) Offenses in relation to inspectors under section 42;
(v)   Discrimination against an employee under section 54; and
(vi) "Where the issue of notices is not considered appropriate for ensuring compliance. . . ."

Not only did these guidelines institutionalize the inspectorate's longstanding practice of prosecuting as a last resort, but the focus of the guidelines on prosecution for breaches resulting in fatalities and *serious accidents* institutionalized the event-focused nature of prosecution. The inspector's attention was immediately drawn away from an examination of the broader context of the event, generally the system of work, to focus on the details of the event itself. From 1983 to 1999, 87% of OHS prosecutions conducted in Victoria were the result of an injury or fatality. This suggests that prosecution was used principally as a response to a workplace *disaster*. In the vast majority of these cases, the inspectorate was responding to a single injury or fatality. Interestingly, in the period 1983-1991 only 21 of the 594 cases (under 4%) prosecuted involved a fatality. The vast majority of cases prosecuted (67%) involved incidents where fingers or hands were amputated, lacerated, or otherwise injured. In the period 1992-1999 just over 20% of cases prosecuted involved fatalities. About 30% of cases involved hand injuries and there were far more prosecutions for burns (6%) and harm from chemical exposure (2%). In short, most prosecutions resulted from traumatic injury or fatalities.

Turning to the types of matters prosecuted, in the 1980s about 90% of cases prosecuted involved injuries or fatalities which took place on machines. Not surprisingly, in about 75% of cases prosecutions were taken under the machinery-guarding provisions. In addition, the majority of general duty prosecutions were also machinery-guarding cases. The majority of the remainder of cases consisted of prosecutions for failure to report accidents to the inspectorate. What would explain this prosecution profile? Until the 1980s the inspectorate was traditionally recruited from male engineering sector apprentices, whose work revolved around machinery. The traditional regulatory focus, as noted earlier, had also been on dangerous machinery, and the result was that a significant focus of the enforcement culture was on dangerous machinery.

In the 1990s, the vast majority of prosecutions (about 90%) have been taken under the employers' general duty clause. Nevertheless, even after the recruitment of new inspectors, including women, from a wider range of occupations, and a concerted attempt to broaden the range of prosecutions to include non-machinery issues, still about 40% of cases up until the end of 1999 involved machinery guarding. The two types of prosecution that increased the most during the

1990s were falls (mainly in the construction industry) (15%), workers being hit by flying objects (8%), electrical hazards (5%), explosions (4%), and exposure to chemicals (4%).[6]

Further, 85% of defendants were corporations, the remainder comprising individual proprietors, partners, workers, and corporate officers. Despite the possibility of pursuing general duty prosecutions in the County Court, in the vast majority of cases the parties chose to have prosecutions heard before a magistrate. Until 1991 there were only two cases where prosecutions were conducted before the County Court. Since then the number has increased marginally, so that in recent years nearly half a dozen cases are conducted each year before the County Court. A couple of cases, including the prosecution of ESSO Pty Ltd in 2001 as a result of a major gas explosion at the ESSO Longford plant, have occurred in the Supreme Court. In addition, it should be noted that the vast majority of defendants plead guilty to OHS offenses in the magistrates' courts. The matter then usually proceeds by the prosecutor giving an event-focused summary of the facts from the bar table.

This prosecution profile suggests that the typical OHS prosecution in Victoria is the result of a serious injury to a male worker, involving inadequately guarded machinery, or a fall from height in construction work. It involves a plea of guilty in proceedings before a magistrate, where evidence of the contraventions is provided through the prosecutor's summary from the bar table of the circumstances surrounding the incident. In the vast majority of cases, the court found the charges proved. The central issue, then, was the penalties imposed by the courts.

THE SENTENCING PROCESS

The Victorian OHS statutes left the courts with a broad discretion to determine the appropriate penalty for an OHS prosecution. The only significant limit was the maximum penalty, and the usual sentencing principles developed by the courts (Fox and Freiberg 1999). Given the Anglo-Australian tradition of limiting the role of the prosecutor in the sentencing process to raising the appropriate sentencing principles, and testing sentencing facts raised by defendants, defense counsel tended to control sentencing proceedings. The research showed that the most commonly raised factors were the defendant's safety record, attitude to safety, and cooperation; the role in the accident of the worker or other workers; the suggestion that the inspectorate had overlooked the hazard in a previous visit; the fact that the accident occurred in unusual or unforeseeable circumstances; and the fact that after the accident the defendant looked after the injured person and/or remedied the hazard. What De Prez observes in relation to environmental prosecutions in Britain, is also true of OHS prosecutions in Victoria, namely that the choice of terminology and style of mitigation surely demonstrates . . . what the legal profession and its clients have assumed to be most likely to influence the bench. . . . Such arguments are therefore clearly important in analysis of the social construction of these offences, for they are designed to refute and neutralize the criminalisation of the defendant's activities. . . . The defence, therefore, have the upper hand in being able to reinforce their favored view of environmental offences. (2000, p. 66)

How successful were these strategies? Table 2 outlines the range of sentencing outcomes imposed by magistrates from 1983 to 1999 on defendants once charges under the *ISHWA* and *OHSA* had been proved. Table 2 shows the number of informations adjourned without conviction with the defendant placed upon a recognizance to be of good behavior (and occasionally required to make a payment into the court box or to a charity of the magistrate's choice), the number of fines without conviction (only available to the court after 1992), the number of recorded convictions, and the average fine for offenses under each of the *ISHWA* and *OHSA* during the period of this study. Table 2 also expresses the annual average fine in terms of a percentage of the maximum available fines.

Table 2 shows that where the charges were proved in prosecutions under the *ISHWA* and *OHSA* a conviction and fine was imposed in just over 85% of charges. The average fine over the period of the study was just over 21% of the maximum available fine. The percentage of cases resulting in good behavior bonds from 1983 to 1992 was just over 17%, and over the whole study it was 10%. Given that prosecutions were only launched for what the inspectorate considered to be the most serious cases, and that sentencing law stated that good behavior bonds were not an appropriate form of disposition for offenses under the OHS legislation involving serious injury,[7] the number of charges resulting in good behavior bonds would seem to be remarkably high. If fines without conviction are included in the analysis, the percentage of cases over the entire study where charges were proved but the defendant was given a disposition that did not involve a conviction was just under 15%. Table 2 suggests that fines without conviction are replacing good behavior bonds as the disposition magistrates prefer to express their ambivalence about the true "criminality" of OHS offenses. In the period 1993 to 1999 fines without conviction were imposed in just over 10% of cases where charges were proved.

Clearly magistrates' ambivalence about the criminality of OHS prosecutions influenced their approach to sentencing. But there was far more to the sentencing process than simply an expression of taken-for-granted ideas or deep-seated ideologies about corporate crime. This is where the analysis of court responses to *micro-disasters* to individual workers in OHS prosecutions echoes and replicates processes displayed in the responses of other state institutions to multivictim disasters.

Table 2. An Overview of Sentencing Outcomes for Informations Where Charges Were Proved: 1983-1999

Year and Act[a]	Good behavior bond (GBB)	GBB and payment into court	Fine without conviction	Total convictions	Total charges proved	Average fine	Percentage of maximum fine
1983 (I)	10	3	—	66	79	$294.32	14.45%
1984 (I)	17	5	—	62	84	$367.58	19.19%
1985 (I)	10	13	—	111	134	$426.04	21.96%
1986 (I)	8	1	—	90	99	$402.56	20.94%
1986 (O)	11	2	—	11	24	$1,368.18	10.27%
1987 (I)	2	—	—	—	2	—	—
1987 (O)	14	11	—	56	81	$956.61	7.29%
1988 (I)	—	—	—	1	1	$500.00	25.00%
1988 (O)	5	1	—	43	49	$2,046.00	9.63%
1989 (O)	15	5	—	53	73	$2,181.13	13.28%
1990 (O)	2	7	—	96	105	$2,835.94	22.92%
1991 (O)	4	3	—	147	154	$3,659.86	31.03%
1992 (O)	3	1	—	109	113	$4,248.17	25.5%
1993 (O)	—	—	6	68	74	$6,037.82	29.0%
1994 (O)	4	1	6	75	86	$7,808.41	22.4%
1995 (O)	2	6	10	84	102	$6,585.07	19.7%
1996 (O)	1	3	8	89	101	$7,793.26	20.9%
1997 (O)	1	4	6	88	99	$7,954.56	21.1%
1998 (O)	—	—	19	73	92	$8,123.29	20.9%
1999 (O)	2	—	17	101	120	$14,673.27	26.7%
Total	111	66	72	1423	1669		21.6%

[a]Prosecutions under the *ISHWA* are denoted by (I), and under the *OHSA* by (O).
Source: This table was first published in Johnstone 2003a, p. 202.

THE DYNAMICS OF SENTENCING, AND "PULVERIZATION"

In his study of OHS in the North Sea, Mathiesen (1980, 1981, 1985) noted that "when lives are lost, fundamental questions concerning the activity . . . are often raised" by "conditions which were earlier seen as isolated being placed in relation to each other," for example the relationship between the profit motive and the lack of safety measures or the pace of oil extraction/coal mining. For example, sociological explanations focusing on the work process and the organization of work raise these issues in relation to most OHS issues. As Mathiesen notes, when many people perceive such a totality or context, the activity itself begins to be threatened. It then "becomes important for the representatives of the activity to pulverize the relationships which people begin to see." An effective method of pulverizing such revealing relationships is to "cut the event out of the fabric in which it exists." Just as Mathiesen demonstrates that politicians and business-people engage in this process in response to macro workplace disasters, so I argue that the sentencing process plays a similar role in OHS prosecutions generally.

"Pulverization" in the Magistrates' Courts

Three samples (1986-1987, 1990-1991, and 1997-98) of 200 cases prose-cuted in Victoria (Johnstone 2003a, pp. 11-17) provide strong evidence that during OHS prosecutions, the offenses and the facts that constitute them are decontextualized or ripped out of the fabric within which they are embedded. Mathiesen describes a number of "isolation techniques" that can be used to fulfill this purpose; I have adapted these to show how pulverization principally takes place in the sentencing process, through arguments raised by defense counsel.

(a) The Splintering of the Event

The most important isolation technique is to split up or splinter the event. It is isolated from its context by "splitting or dividing the event into its more or less free-swimming and unrelated bits and pieces." By splitting the specific event from the context within which it occurred, the context fades and recedes into the background, leaving only the details of the event in focus. As demonstrated earlier in this chapter, the OHS prosecution practices and procedures institutionalize this splintering of the event into minor details, because they invariably focus on a particular incident giving rise to an injury or fatality. In all of the 1980s prosecu-tions involving machinery guarding the court focused in minute detail on the technical aspects of whether or not there was a guard, how it worked, and the actions of the worker. This in turn facilitated scrutiny on factors irrelevant to the offense, such as the injured or deceased worker's behavior during the time leading up to the incident, a particular malfunction, or the problems faced by the employer at a particular time.

A 1988 Victorian Supreme Court case[8] further reinforced the tendency to pulverize events. Section 21(1) sets out the general duty of employers, and section 21(2) purports, in five paragraphs (a) to (e), to provide illustrations of the general duty. The Court held that section 21(1) did not create a continuing offense of allowing to subsist a particular proscribed environment, but rather created a large number of offenses (sections 21(2)(a)-(e)) each consisting of some identifiable act or omission which constituted a failure to comply with the general duty of care. The case was decided in the context of the rule against duplicity—an information setting out charges against a defendant may not include more than one offense. Consequently no one information could include more than one of the matters listed in section 21(2) of the OHSA, which hitherto had been seen as merely providing examples of the operation of the overall general duty. In other words, the ruling effectively prevented a single information specifying an all-encompassing offense of establishing a dangerous work process.

Importantly, the case not only decontextualized each resulting offense by limiting the elements that need to be proved to found the offense, but also splintered the different aspects of the work process so that they are seen as discrete items. This might appear to enable the prosecution to seek greater penalties for such contraventions, because the defendant could potentially be found guilty under a number of charges, for each of which the court could impose a fine. But in practice, as noted above, most defendants entered guilty pleas to one or perhaps two charges, and the remainder were withdrawn. Even where multiple charges were successfully pursued, the defendant usually argued that the charges effectively arose out of one incident, and that the level of fine should reflect that. Whether or not the penalty was applied concurrently as if the breach entailed only one incident, or cumulatively on the basis that multiple contraventions were involved, depended on the application of the principle of totality in sentencing. This principle seeks to ensure that a separate penalty is not imposed upon a defendant for each offense with which they are charged if the offenses are similar and arise out of a single incident or episode, or are based upon events which are connected.[9] Consequently, issuing multiple informations did not always increase the total fine imposed, and often significantly reduced the scope of the offenses before the court. In these latter cases, the only benefit to the prosecution appeared to be that at the end of the day the defendant had a greater number of prior convictions.

(b) Blameshifting

A major consequence of splintering was the close scrutiny of the details of the event, which in turn almost inevitably led to an analysis of culpability based on individualistic notions of causation and the allocation of blame. A number of blameshifting techniques were used.

The most common was to blame the worker. When I interviewed magistrates about OHS prosecutions in 1988, each indicated that the moral culpability of an employer for an offense would be reduced if there was evidence that the worker had contributed to the accident. This factor was often used in mitigation by defense counsel, despite the fact that the alleged carelessness of the employee has very little to do with the offense of failing to provide a safe workplace.

Another frequently used technique was to shift the blame onto the state, in the guise of the inspectorate. In mitigation a common factor raised was that the inspectorate had previously inspected the plant without commenting on the hazard under scrutiny. This argument is deeply rooted in dominant ideologies about the role of the state in the prevention of workplace illness and injury. A third blameshifting technique argued in mitigation is that the supplier of plant and equipment had, for example, supplied the employer with unsafe equipment and was therefore responsible for the hazard rather than the employer.

(c) The Good Corporate Citizen

The most basic and widespread plea in mitigation was that the defendant had an excellent safety record and an exemplary attitude to safety, so that the defendant was portrayed as a *responsible* company or person. The plea turned the court's attention away from the event itself, and away from the organization of work, to concentrate on the reputation and attitude of the defendant. Clearly, magistrates accepted that the employer's *good record* (usually meaning that they had no, or very few, previous work-related illnesses or injuries) was an important factor in reducing the defendant's culpability. Most defense counsel in the sampled cases had no difficulty in painting their clients as responsible organizations. Virtually every plea in mitigation involved the defendant claiming a good safety record, and a good attitude to safety.

(d) Individualizing the Event

Fourth, as Mathiesen points out, the event may be individualized by making it into "something unique, something incomparable, something quite special, individual, a-typical." Such a presentation ensures that far-reaching conclusions or generalizations cannot be drawn from the event, because it is far too excep-tional, unique, or abnormal. For example, workplace injuries can be typified as *freak accidents, catastrophes,* or *tragedies,* signifying that each event is something unusual and unexpected, because, in the words of Mathiesen, "if one all the time had to expect tragedies, the activity as a whole . . . would . . . not be initiated in the first place" (Mathieson 1981, p. 58). Further, if an event is unusual, both the severity of the contravention itself and the culpability of the defendant must be reduced, and hence there is less need for the sentencing court to be concerned with punishment, rehabilitation, or deterrence. This plea was usually built into a *good corporate citizen* plea, to emphasize the unusual nature of the incident giving rise to prosecution. In other words, the defendant tried to show that it had a generally unblemished approach to OHS to which the particular event was an exception. An important aspect of the technique was that there was highly detailed scrutiny of the event, without any reference to a systematic management approach to OHS. By focusing on the event, and not the underlying system, defense counsel was able to argue that the exact circumstances of the event were unforeseeable, rather than allowing focus to be on the system, in which case resulting injuries or illnesses would be foreseeable.

In Victoria a classic example of this isolation technique was the *Simsmetal* prosecution in the Victorian County Court.[10] The charges arose out of an incident in which one of the company's furnaces exploded, killing four workers, and severely injuring another seven. The explosion occurred because the company's chemical handling procedures were so defective that sodium nitrate was stored in unlabeled bags in a shed in which potassium chloride was usually stored. A forklift driver transported the sodium nitrate to the smelter believing it be potassium chloride, an accepted and safe fluxing agent. The court, in sentencing, referred to the storage of sodium nitrate in the shed as *evil chance* and the mix up as the *intervention of malevolent chance*. The explosion was portrayed as being the result of bad luck, rather than the inevitable consequence of bad work procedures and practices.

(e) Isolating the Present from the Past and Future

Fifth, Mathiesen argues that to form a total understanding of an event, it is important to perceive the past, present, and future of the event. A total perspective is avoided by isolating the past, the present, and the future of the event from each other. The previous isolation techniques illustrate how this is done: if the event is split up, the contextual past and present are removed from the analysis. If the event is individualized, the event's past is replaced by the mythical past contained in the "good record" and "good attitude."

In sentencing pleas, defense counsel often isolated the event in a favorably reconstructed present. For example, maximum emphasis was often placed on the human or humanitarian response of the employer in looking after the injured worker by, for instance, taking the worker to hospital, visiting the worker in hospital, re-employing the worker afterward, assisting with the worker's rehabilitation, and so on. In virtually every case a key mitigating factor was that after the incident and before the prosecution proceedings the employer had rectified the situation—for example, the employer had guarded the machine as required by the inspectorate. As one magistrate commented to me in an interview, "the courts have to give credit to people who have done the right thing."[11]

Another technique involved isolating the event from its context by relegating it to an outmoded past. This is an extremely common mitigating technique, nearly always accepted by the court. Examples included assertions that since the "accident" the company had replaced the offending machine, engaged a new management team, employed an OHS consultant, or introduced a new OHS program. The suggestion was that the situation that led to the violation has been relegated to the past and will not be repeated.

(f) Anthropomorphizing the Defendant

Even though some defendants relied heavily on the corporate veil to reduce the impact of prior convictions on the assessment of penalty, in many other cases defendants fused the characteristics of the personnel running the corporation with the corporation itself, so that the corporate defendant could gain the exculpating benefit of the admirable human characteristics of its management or directorship. On other occasions, defense counsel gave the corporation human characteristics and qualities, to ensure that the fictional corporate entity received the benefits of a sentencing system that took into account as assessment of the character of the human defendant.

For example, defense counsel were sometimes careful to ensure that the court was aware of the defendant corporation's role in the community—its charitable works and so on. On other occasions, the awards received by personnel within the corporation were attributed to the corporation. Sometimes the fact that the managing director was hard-working and concerned for the welfare of workers was raised as a factor. On one extraordinary occasion in 1986, defense counsel referred to the fact that the managing director's daughter was a member of the Victorian bar, and obviously respectable and law abiding.

These, then, are the isolation techniques, used by defense counsel to transform and individualize the already decontextualized event in the sentencing process. Victorian OHS prosecutors gradually developed strategies to counter these arguments (Johnstone 2003a, ch. 8), but were never able to fully prevent the transformation of the issues.

Countering Isolation Techniques

One strategy adopted by prosecutors was to appeal against sentencing decisions of magistrates that imposed inadequate penalties, although defendants seeking to reduce penalties launched appeals far more often. Prosecutors mostly appealed in cases where magistrates had imposed fines without conviction (Johnstone 2003a, pp. 240-246). In addition to imposing higher penalties in individual cases, prosecutors also hoped that County Court would develop OHS sentencing principles to guide the magistrates' discretion. This was done in a series of cases beginning in 1989, but few, if any, of these principles inhibited the use of the isolation techniques (Johnstone 2003a, pp. 246-258).

Another strategy was for the prosecutor to play a greater role in sentencing, primarily by ensuring that their summaries from the bar table outlined defects in work systems and provided as much context as possible. They also made greater use of their right to challenge submissions put to the court by the defendant, and to emphasize sentencing principles that had been developed by the courts. To support this strategy, efforts were made ensure that inspectors collected relevant sentencing material (such as evidence of contraventions discovered and action taken during previous visits, and the defendant's accident record) during their investigations. There was also much evidence that as the OHS inspectorate's competence in investigation improved during the 1990s, sentencing outcomes improved.

It was also clear that, over time, magistrates became hardened to the mitigating factors raised by defendants, particularly the blameshifting arguments, and unsubstantiated assertions of good corporate citizenship.

Despite these important developments, it was clear that the isolation techniques were difficult to counter. Consequently, OHS prosecution proceedings inevitably failed to connect the event under scrutiny to the totality of which it was part, with the result that OHS prosecutions inadvertently played an ideologically significant part in the political process of shoring up hegemonic social structures. This is not to deny that prosecution plays a crucially important part in the enforcement of OHS statutes (Gunningham and Johnstone 1999, chs. 4, 6, 7), or that, over time, OHS fines increased dramatically in Victoria (see Table 2). Indeed, as new post-1997 maximum penalties took effect, in 2000 and 2001 the maximum penalties imposed by the courts continued to rise significantly (WorkCover 2001, 2002), and there was much anecdotal evidence that increased fines were having a deterrent affect and motivating at least some employers to rethink their attitudes and approaches to OHS. Rather the point here is that the individualistic form of the criminal law not only reduced the level of actual fines imposed when compared to the maxima available, but also played an important role in maintaining the *membrane of normalcy* attaching to OHS injury and disease.

Not only are OHS prosecutions conducted in the lowest level of the court hierarchy, and disposed of quickly and expeditiously, but the process at the heart of the adjudication of these cases—the determination of penalty—routinely "normalizes" the circumstances of offenses through the use of the isolation techniques. Defense counsel in this process focus on the way OHS offences display characteristics not typical of most offenses in the mainstream criminal justice system. The remainder of this chapter develops this argument.

THE FORM OF THE CRIMINAL LAW

The *ISHWA* and *OHSA* were criminal statutes and thus had to operate according to existing rules pertaining to criminal procedure and sentencing. They were principally concerned with the mechanics and details of standard setting, the establishment of the inspectorate, and in the case of the *OHSA*, the functions and powers of OHS committees and representatives. Apart from the penalty structures in the Acts, all other provisions governing the procedural and sentencing aspects of prosecutions were contained in the statutory and common law provisions in the mainstream criminal law. There are a number of consequences arising from an unchallenged adoption by OHS regimes of the processes and procedures of the mainstream criminal justice system.

The Event Focused Nature of the Criminal Justice System

The large majority of prosecutions within the criminal justice system are event-focused, whether they be traffic offenses, theft, burglary, possession of illegal drugs, domestic violence, assault, sexual assault, murder, or any other of the many statutory or common law offences. The rules of criminal procedure have evolved around, and consequently institutionalized, this event-focused nature of criminal procedure. As I argued earlier in this chapter, OHS offenses differ from most criminal law offences in that they are both constitutive and inchoate. In OHS crime the actual injury is a consequence of a work process that has not been organized, structured, and monitored so as to ensure that that is safe and without risks to health. At a deeper level, the issue is the control of the work process by the employer to the detriment of the employee, the prevalence of other organizational objectives (such as short-term or long-term profitability, increased market share, productivity, increased utilization of capital, longer production runs and so on) over OHS objectives, and the failure to practice systematic OHS management.

Despite the inchoate and constitutive nature of OHS standards, OHS prosecutions invariably focused on events. It is far easier for the prosecution to prove that the facts constituting an event are in breach of the statutory provisions than it is to prove that management has failed to organize work so that it is safe and without health risks for workers, or even that a system of work is inherently hazardous, regardless of whether or not ill-health has resulted. The evidence from interviews with magistrates suggested that penalties would be greater if the event resulted in a serious injury. The important points are that this bias toward events and incidents is a direct result of the form of the criminal law, in particular the rules of evidence and procedure, and the fact that most criminal prosecutions are event-focused. The legal form, deeply rooted in individualistic notions of responsibility, is preoccupied with events and details, and with scrutinizing individual actions.

There is, therefore, an institutionalized drift toward constructing OHS issues by focusing on the detailed actions of the actors during the event, rather than focusing on the overall system of work surrounding the event or the underlying organization of work in the workplace. Hale argues that the purpose of legal investigation and prosecution in relation to workplace injuries is to unearth points in the chain of events leading to the damage at which the duty of care was breached. . . . Th[e] punitive orientation to the investigation gives it both its direction and the rules for how far it goes. It is directed at uncovering the truth; something which is seen as objective and of which there is only one version, though what that version is may be disputed. It stops when the culpable actions are found and does not bother to dig deeper to find out why they were carried out. (1997, pp. 6-7)

The Nature of the Trial

In the criminal trial in an adversarial legal system, the competing subjects are the state and the defendant, the latter conceptualized formally as an individual. This form of the trial has the "effect of abstracting the legally relevant 'facts' from their complex social reality, thereby depoliticising the issue before the court" (Sargent 1989, p. 50). McBarnet (1981) notes that "[t]he facts of a case—a case of any sort—are not *all* the elements of the event, but the information allowed in by the rules, presented by the witnesses, and surviving the credibility test of cross examination" (p. 148). Not only is the law event-focused, but its view of the event is partial. This partial focus is endemic to law. The adversarial nature of the trial emphasizes a legally constructed contest between the prosecutor's and defense counsel's version of reality, with little room for the experience of the victim (or indeed the collective issues facing workers) whose interests, different to those of the prosecutor, are marginalized (Sargent 1990, pp. 105-106). Even with the introduction of provisions for Victim Impact Statements in 1994, the victim's interests are simply represented in terms of pain and suffering, rather than more broadly as a participant in workplace processes. As a result the case is depoliticized so that the parties are unable to show the social, economic, or political issues underlying the act in question (Grau 1989, pp. 205-206).[12] This characteristic of abstracting the "facts of the case" from their social, economic, and political context is basic to the form of the criminal law used in contemporary Australia. Law, as Hunt observes, plays an important ideological role in individualizing and decontextualizing the experience of social relations under capitalism (Hunt 1985). Not only are issues decontextualized, but they are then recontextualized

in terms recognizable to the legal gaze, . . . into the form of an individual moral actor for the purpose of fitting the corporate persona into the discourse of criminal law conceptions of responsibility and sanctioning. (Sargent 1990, p. 106)

I demonstrated earlier how the investigation and prosecution of OHS offenses have transformed OHS issues into "terms recognizable to the legal gaze." Not only is the prosecution process event-focused and abstracted or decontextualized, but the sentencing process is extremely open-textured, with very little constraint on the discretion exercised by the magistrate. There is a significant tension in the legal form between the open texture of the rules of sentencing and the magistracy's need to particularize the sentence to the facts of the case at hand. This enables defense counsel and the court both to enunciate the rhetoric of the importance of OHS and deterrence, but at the same time chip away at the defendant's liability by transforming the nature of the issue until it is more in line with individualistic notions of culpability implied in the criminal law. In the Anglo-Australian adversarial system, the parties are largely in control of the process. I have already argued that, at the sentencing stage, control of the process passes to defense counsel, so that in an adversarial system dealing with OHS offenses, defense counsel can further decontextualize and individualize OHS issues and then recontextualize matters within taken-for-granted ideas about the workplace. The result is a divergence or gap (McBarnet 1981, pp. 155-162) between the rhetoric of the seriousness of OHS and the importance of deterrence, and the individual case-based reality of the process, without undermining the value of the rhetoric as ideology.

The Individualistic Criminal Law and the Ideological Role of Mens Rea

A further characteristic of the form of the criminal law is that it has developed over the centuries in the context of traditional street crime committed by individuals. The vast majority of defendants in the criminal justice system are natural persons. But most defendants in OHS prosecutions are corporations. The criminal justice system, however, has assimilated business organizations by regarding them as individual moral actors, in the same way as it deals with natural persons. The criminal law applies to corporations individualistic models of liability, rather than attempting to adapt the legal system to accommodate the collective nature of organizational behavior. It has applied the normal sanctions to corporations where appropriate (for example fines), has discarded others considered to be inappropriate for corporations (imprisonment) but has failed to explore new forms of sanctioning.

The abstracted, event-focused and individualistic nature of the criminal law contributes to another characteristic of the criminal law: its emphasis on traditional notions of *mens rea* as the central component of criminal liability. It certainly makes sense for a criminal justice system focusing on events perpetrated by individuals to adopt an individualistic notion of culpability having at its core the intention, in a broad sense, to perpetrate the event in contravention of the law. But it does not make sense to transfer these notions to OHS crime, where strict liability can be justified because illness and injury are inevitable consequences of work systems organized in a manner that do not take into account OHS considerations.

Sargent (1989, p. 53)[13] has argued that the notion of mens rea is important on the level of rhetoric in that it legitimizes and reinforces the individualistic distinction between "real crimes" based on the violation of accepted social values and mere regulatory, or public welfare, offences which are seen as less morally opprobrious. This perpetuates the relative immunity of corporate offenders, as I argued, with reference to Carson's work earlier in this chapter.

The OHS general duty provisions do require the prosecutor to discuss fault by showing that practicable measures were not taken. The strict or absolute provisions coupled with the notion of practicability, however, limit the prosecutor to having to prove fault as negligence without, in traditional criminal law thinking, having to demonstrate full criminal intention or recklessness. The relative brevity of the prosecution's summary in uncontested cases further limits the prosecutor's ability to highlight the defendant's culpability. At the same time, the broad sentencing discretion given to the court invites defense counsel to mitigate strongly by suggesting that fault is absent, or at least minimal. As I have already demonstrated, sentencing procedure and practice strongly support defense counsel's efforts to reconstruct the offence so as to minimize culpability. In her study of environmental prosecutions, De Prez observes that the strict liability provisions in environmental regulation

> act as a cloak for many defendants, for as the prosecutor is not required to prove "fault," this leaves defense counsel plenty of room to deny culpability in order to attract the sympathy of the bench. (2000, pp. 67-68)

This neutralizing of the culpability of OHS offenders must be seen in the context of the discretion to prosecute. In most cases, prosecutions are taken because the matters represent more serious contraventions, where the defendant has demonstrated clear moral culpability (Carson 1970a, 1970b; Johnstone 2000). The prosecution process itself systematically denies that seriousness (Croall 1988, pp. 312-313). Yet it is difficult for the prosecution to reproduce before the court the factors that may have led the inspector to construct moral blameworthiness.

The form of the criminal law enables defense counsel to reproduce individualist arguments about criminal liability, and to transform issues of culpability from the systematic focus so important in the nature of OHS, to an event-focused "every case is decided on it its facts" approach, with factors to be weighed up against each other. These factors, together with the open texture of sentencing procedure, facilitates—indeed institutionalizes—an approach in which culpability can be decontextualized, transformed and individualized.

Trivializing Occupational Health and Safety

The problems raised for the regulation of OHS offences by the individualistic, event-focused form of the criminal law are exacerbated by the venue of the vast majority of OHS prosecutions, the magistrates' courts. McBarnet (1981, pp. 138-140) observes that there is an ideology of the "triviality" of the matters coming before the magistrates' courts, which are seen to deal with everyday matters, with low penalties and little public scrutiny. The magistrates' courts are at the lowest level of the judicial hierarchy, and traditionally adjudicated "petty crime." Cases are decided quickly and routinely, with a minimum of fuss. A magistrate could hear up to 20 cases in a normal day. Within this setting, how can magistrates fail to individualize OHS offenses and regard them as not being at the upper level of egregiousness? Not only are the magistrates' courts geared for fast summary justice, but the emphasis on guilty pleas—and the fact that most cases are indeed guilty pleas—institutionalizes an analysis of culpability that is primarily based on magistrates' common sense opinions of OHS and on the briefly constructed facts put to the court by the prosecutor and reinterpreted by defense counsel. Most important of all, magistrates are simply not used to imposing large penalties on corporations. Most offences prosecuted have maxima below those in the *OHSA*, and most of their penalties are imposed on individuals with low capacity to pay. The defense strategy of transforming, decontextualizing, and individualizing the issue, indeed, of "pulverising" the facts, was aimed at trivializing the charges. The setting of the prosecutions in the magistrates' courts ensured that the triviality of the offenses was always an issue, and a continual matter for contest.

THE IMPLICATIONS OF DECONTEXTUALIZATION
AND INDIVIDUALIZATION

The matters discussed in this chapter have a number of important implications for the regulation of OHS. This section discusses those implications.

Explaining Low Penalties

All these factors explain why fines for OHS offenses tend to be low, and thus not a serious punishment or deterrent to employers. Magistrates tailor the sentence to the culpability of the defendant. They have difficulty conceiving these offenses to be truly criminal, they are susceptible to careless worker and other blame-shifting arguments, and the key isolation techniques operate to reduce their perception of the defendant's blameworthiness. Once the facts are decontextualized and individualized, and the defendant's good record, cooperation, remorse, and subsequent improvement of OHS performance are put to the court, it is not surprising that penalties are moderate when compared to the available maxima.

Reproducing a Narrow Vision of OHS and
Obscuring the Origins of Occupational Illness

On another level, this study suggests that even though the OHS legislation has the potential to enforce a broad construction of OHS issues, the models of injury causation and OHS management reproduced by the prosecution process are very narrow. This has important implications for the use of the criminal law in stigmatizing dangerous workplace structures. If prosecution is to have the desired impact of improving working conditions, it must be clear to employers that they need to organize the work process differently to avoid legal liability. There needs to be an emphasis on developing an organizational culture and ongoing organizational processes that envisage OHS as an interdisciplinary and broad, systems-based management activity (Bohle and Quinlan 2000; Frick 2000). It is not sufficient to merely change the rhetoric of the law and the content of the substantive legal rules in order to optimize the law's role in preventing workplace illness and injury through criminal regulation. The form of criminal law used needs to be examined and transformed to ensure that the desired approach is constructed at all stages of the process (Gunningham and Johnstone 1999, ch. 7).

Defusing Occupational Health and Safety as an Issue

I argued earlier in this chapter that this study supports the observation that law plays an important role in individualizing and decontextualizing the experience of social relations under capitalism (Hunt 1985). The conflictual nature of work relations is obscured by the decontextualized and individualized nature of the trial, which provides no scope to link particular hazards with the nature of capitalist work relations. The individualistic criminal law form effectively decriminalizes OHS and prevents the criminal justice system from treating equally all forms of socially deviant behavior. The criminal law and concepts of sentencing are not empty vessels that can be filled with whatever content society chooses. In OHS offenses not only do the elements of the offense decontextualize issues of OHS, to the benefit of the defendant, but the sentencing process further transforms and individualizes the offense, and enables the culpability of the defendant to be further sanitized.

At the deepest level, then, the courts' reconstructions of OHS issues play an important role in defusing OHS as a social, political, and industrial issue. The state is heavily dependent on the process of private accumulation of capital, and must create and sustain the conditions of accumulation (Offe 1975). The state must not just be seen as an instrument of the dominant capitalist classes. Its legitimacy depends on it at least giving the appearance of transcending the interests of particular capitalists. It also has to respond to pressures *from below* to maintain the social conditions necessary for capitalist accumulation. Recent critical legal theory has attempted to explain the consensual nature of law, in particular the manner in which it functions to reproduce ideologies supporting capitalist and patriarchal relations of production (Sargent 1990; Simpson and Charlesworth 1995). This in turn has led to a greater examination of the role of law as an institutional site for the production and dissemination of ideologies that reproduce consent for unequal relations within capitalism. Ideologies play a role in defining the way in which social relations are lived and experienced, and in the manner in which political and social conflicts are identified and resolved (Hunt 1985; Sargent 1990, pp. 99-100).

Workplace fatalities, injuries, and disease are potentially disruptive of the social order and to the ongoing process of capital accumulation. Carson and Henenberg argue that

> [t]he relative centrality of work to human experience and the potentially egregious demonstration of stark domination or exploitation represented by occupational health and safety issues cannot but have rendered them one of the most likely locations in which fatigue fractures or pressure cracks could have appeared in the fragile edifice of consent. (1988, p. 1)

They also argue that the fact that such breaks in the hegemonic processes have not occurred is due in some measure to the ideological role played by the early factory legislation, and reproduced in OHS legislation in Britain and Australia in the following 150 years (pp. 2-4). Central to these ideologies is the ambiguity and conventionalization of OHS crime and the fundamental acceptance that OHS is the responsibility of the state, and not part of the industrial relations process. These ideologies are reinforced by dominant workplace ideologies based on the acceptance of the overriding importance of private property, the belief that workplace illness and injury are inevitable by-products of industrial progress and the technological imperative and therefore beyond human control, and by workplace ideologies stemming from a unitary view of workplace relations.

The evidence in this study suggests that the courts themselves play an important role in reproducing consent for key conceptions of OHS, and a narrow model of injury causation. This chapter has shown how key ideologies have permeated proceedings before the courts, and have severely restricted the courts' examination of OHS issues. The ideologies work in two closely related dimensions. At one level the key legal actors, the inspectors, prosecutors and especially the defense counsel and the magistracy, are informed by ideologies which have their origins outside the law, but become an integral part of legal proceedings, legislation, and legal doctrine so that they become virtually unquestioned. The ideologies of the careless worker, of the inevitability of accidents, and of the managerial prerogative are intrinsic to the law, as well as consistent with the way workers and managers experience work. They are taken for granted by defense counsel, magistrates, and by some inspectors and prosecutors. Court proceedings then become the medium through which these are reproduced and disseminated.

On a second level, I have already argued that the form of law itself plays a crucial role in decontextualizing and individualizing the experience of social relations under capitalism. Once the OHS issue is isolated as a disembodied event, and recontextualized within the notion of the defendant's good corporate citizenship, and the dominant ideologies of the careless worker, the inevitability of accidents, and the central responsibility of the inspectorate to discover hazards, the court's understanding of the incident is transformed and individualized, and the courts' perception of the defendant's liability severely reduced. The process of decontextualization and the infiltration of dominant ideologies is not a passive process, where magistrates simply use their taken-for-granted notions of OHS. Rather they are actively encouraged by defense counsel to isolate the event, abstract it from its context, and recontextualize it within the dominant ideological framework. It is not only in the interests of defense counsel to pulverize the event in question, but their training, steeped in legal individualism, reinforces their perceptions of the justness of their case. The court, as I have shown, became the venue of an ideological contest once the prosecutors took up the challenge. The court, therefore, becomes an important site in which meanings of the social world are constructed, contested, and disseminated (Sargent 1990, p. 101).

The isolation techniques discussed earlier enable the courts to play a role in repairing threats to the fragile edifice of consent. The focus of the prosecution on a particular employer and a particular event suggests that what the court is dealing with are isolated instances of unsafe work practices in an otherwise safe industrial world (Sparrow 2000, pp. 182-185), rather than as an example of a more deep-seated problem concerning the priorities given to the provision and maintenance of working environments that are safe and without risks to health. Once again this is a characteristic of the capitalist legal form. The focus is always on individual legal subjects—in this case individual defendants—not on the nature of work organization in general. The events themselves are explicable through a series of blameshifting and isolation techniques, and the defendant is usually represented as having dealt with the problem. In fact the process of pulverization of the defendant's liability often goes further to suggest to the court that if these are the worst instances, then things cannot be too bad. The event-focused nature of prosecutions (and their location in the magistrates' courts) also suggests that even if the prosecution, or indeed the magistrate, challenges the defendant's construction of its own liability, the challenge itself is isolated to this particular defendant and the particular circumstances.

The court is seen to be dealing with the issue, and convicting offenders, while at the same time sanitizing the issues so that the underlying activity, the production of goods and services, is not threatened. In other words, the court plays a major legitimating role in OHS, but the underlying issues are largely untouched. Of course, to maintain legitimacy, the law must appear to be just and effective.

This explains why, from the late 1980s in Victoria, harsh criticisms of magistrate's penalties for OHS offenses were met by the government increasing penalties, discussing the possibility of creating an industrial magistracy,[14] and considering the use of the "criminal law proper" to prosecute offenders.[15]

It has also ensured that there have been occasional significant and highly publicized prosecutions in the intermediate and superior courts. In each of 1989 to 1992 there was a single County Court prosecution, and two in 1994. From 1995 there have been four to six such prosecutions annually. Only one of these cases has been well publicized and attracted a large fine. In 1989, after an explosion which killed four workers and injured seven others, the highly publicized prosecution of *Simsmetal*[16] in the Victorian County Court resulted in a total fine of $48,000 for three charges, by far the largest penalty of the 1980s. But as the discussion of *Simsmetal* earlier in this chapter showed, the County Court, in its determination of penalty in that case, did nothing to counter the major isolation techniques.

Prosecutions at the level of the Supreme Court have been even more exceptional. In 2001, again as a result of a highly publicized gas explosion which killed two workers and seriously injured eight others and brought the State of Victoria to a standstill, the Victorian Supreme Court in *DPP v ESSO Australia Pty Ltd*[17] imposed a total of A$2 million for 11 contraventions of the OHSA, including a number of maximum penalties to some of the charges. The ESSO prosecution was altogether exceptional (Hopkins 2002). It was the first contested OHS prosecution at Supreme Court level. Exxon owned the defendant. The incident itself cut gas supplies to the city of Melbourne for two weeks, and the explosion aroused national and international interest (Kletz 2001). The prosecution followed a Royal Commission (Dawson and Brooks 1999; Hopkins 2002) in which the presiding Commissioner, a respected former High Court judge, found that ESSO had "manifestly" violated the law. At the Supreme Court trial ESSO made no attempt to explain what had caused the explosion, leaving it to the prosecution to prove this, and showed no corporate remorse in response to the explosion. Both of these factors weighed heavily against ESSO in the sentencing verdict of the Supreme Court. ESSO has since been subject to extensive civil litigation by victims of the explosion, and from customers suffering economic loss from the loss of gas supply. It was almost as if the incident had unanimously been labeled a disaster, and the defendant's conduct egregious.

Both of these prosecutions were extremely important, and showed the potential of highly publicized proceedings in higher level courts. Both to some extent appeased critics of the OHS regulatory authorities' benign approaches to OHS enforcement. But both cases were unusual multi-victim, highly publicized explosions—traditional disasters—and both had environmental impacts upon the public. While such cases undoubtedly have an important deterrent role, their rarity suggests one of the dangers of these highly publicized "show trials." During the period 1983 to 1999 there were 1100 prosecution cases in Victoria, and in each the processes described in this chapter were operative, resulting in inadequate fines and a decontextualized understanding of OHS. The *Simsmetal* and *ESSO* cases, while providing valuable publicity and something of a general deterrent effect, did little to establish sentencing principles which challenged the isolation techniques outlined earlier in this chapter. They were so unusual as to be in danger of providing unwitting legitimacy for an OHS enforcement system in which OHS court prosecution does not focus sufficiently on a systemic approach to OHS management, and falls far short of a minimal role for OHS prosecution as the "benign big gun" beneath which OHS regulators encourage voluntary compliance from duty holders (Ayres and Braithwaite, 1992, ch. 2; Gunningham and Johnstone 1999, chs. 4, 6, and 7).

ENDNOTES

1. Quoting Kinney, Weiss, Sufalko, Gleason, and Maakestad (1990, p. 27).
2. Since the 1980s higher-level courts, the intermediate level County Court of Victoria, and the Industrial Relations Commission of New South Wales, have heard more serious OHS prosecutions in Victoria and New South Wales respectively. Nevertheless, the vast majority of OHS prosecutions in Australia are conducted before magistrates.
3. *Sentencing Act* 1991 (Vic) ss 7(f) and 8.
4. *R v Australian Char Pty Ltd* (1996) 64 IR 387 at 400; and *Haynes v C I and D Manufacturing Pty Ltd* (1995) 60 IR 149 at 158.
5. New guidelines were introduced from 1998, but had little impact upon this study.
6. For the gender implications of this approach to prosecution, see S. Jamieson (2000) and Johnstone (2003a, p. 96).
7. See *Curtis v Email Limited* (1970) 12 AILR 194; *Tucker v Mappin* Unreported, Industrial Relations Commission of Victoria in Court Session (Marshall P), Case No 91/1983, 21 November 1983; and *DPP v Pacific Dunlop Tyres Pty Ltd and Goodyear Tyres Pty Ltd, trading as South Pacific Tyres*, unreported, County Court of Victoria (Fricke J), 22 November 1991.; *Schultz v Tamworth City Council*(1995) 58 IR 221 at 229. For relevant sentencing principles developed in New South Wales, see Thompson (2001, pp. 88-89).
8. *Chugg v Pacific Dunlop Limited* [1988] VR 411, affirmed in *R v Australian Char Pty Ltd* (1996) 64 IR 387.
9. See *WorkCover Authority (NSW) (Inspector Mulder) v Yass Shire Council* (2000) 99 IR 284 at 295 (Wright J); Thompson (2001, p. 62-4).
10. *R v Simsmetal Limited,* unreported, County Court of Victoria (Villeneuve-Smith J), Melbourne, 9 March 1989.
11. Interview with author.
12. Referred to in Sargent, 1989, p. 51.
13. See also Norrie (1993, pp. 88-89) and Slapper (2000, ch. 2).
14. See Industrial Relations (General Amendment) Bill 1988 (Vic), ss 22 and 23; Industrial Relations Bill 1990 (Vic), Part 11.
15. See Department of Labor, Occupational Health and Safety Division, Central Investigation Unit, *Prosecution Policy*, 25 June 1990; and the Bill brought before the Victorian Parliament in 2001 to introduce the crime of corporate manslaughter.
16. *R v Simsmetal Limited,* unreported, County Court of Victoria (Villeneuve-Smith J), Melbourne, 9 March 1989.
17. (2001) 107 IR 285 (Cummins J).

REFERENCES

Ayres, I., and Braithwaite, J. (1992) *Responsive Regulation: Transcending the Deregulation Debate.* New York: Oxford University Press.

Bohle, P., and Quinlan, M. (2000) *Managing Occupational Health and Safety in Australia* (2nd ed.). Melbourne: Macmillan.

Carson, W. G. (1970a) Some Sociological Aspects of Strict Liability and the Enforcement of Factory Legislation. *Modern Law Review, 33*: 396-412.

Carson, W. G. (1970b) White Collar Crime and the Enforcement of Factory Legislation. *British Journal of Criminology, 10*: 383-398.

Carson, W. G. (1979) The Conventionalisation of Early Factory Crime. *International Journal of the Sociology of Law, 7*: 37-60.

Carson, W. G. (1980) The Institutionalization of Ambiguity: Early British Factory Acts. In G. Geis and E. Stotland (eds.), *White Collar Crime: Theory and Research* (pp. 142-173). London: Sage.

Carson, W. G. (1985) Hostages to History: Some Aspects of the Occupational Health and Safety Debate in Historical Perspective. In W. B. Creighton and N. Gunningham (eds.), *The Industrial Relations of Occupational Health and Safety*. Sydney: Croom Helm.

Carson, W. G., and Henenberg, C. (1988) The Political Economy of Legislative Change: Making Sense of Victoria's New Occupational Health and Safety Legislation. *Law in Context, 6*: 1-19.

Chugg v Pacific Dunlop Limited [1988] VR 411.

Clayton, A., Johnstone, R., and Sceats, S. (2002) The Legal Concept of Work-Relatedness in Australian OHS and Workers' Compensation Systems. *Australian Journal of Labor Law, 15*: 105-153.

Croall, H. (1988) Mistakes, Accidents, and Someone Else's Fault: The Trading Offender in Court. *Journal of Law and Society, 15*: 293-315.

Curtis v Email Limited (1970) 12 AILR 194.

Dawson, D., and Brooks, B. (1999) *The ESSO Longford Gas Plant Accident: Report of the Longford Royal Commission*. Melbourne: Government Printer for the State of Victoria.

De Prez, P. (2000) Excuses, Excuses: The Ritual Trivialisation of Environmental Prosecutions. *Journal of Environmental Law, 12*: 65-77.

Department of Labor Occupational Health and Safety Division, Central Investigation Unit. (1990) *Prosecution Policy*, 25 June.

DPP v Pacific Dunlop Tyres Pty Ltd and Goodyear Tyres Pty Ltd, trading as South Pacific Tyres, unreported, County Court of Victoria (Fricke J), 22 November 1991.

Fox, R. G., and Freiberg, A. (1999) *Sentencing: State and Federal Law in Victoria* (2nd ed.). Melbourne: Oxford University Press.

Frick, K., Jensen, P., Quinlan, M., and Wilthagen, T. (eds.). (2000) *Systematic Occupational Health and Safety Management: Perspectives on an International Development*. Amsterdam: Elsevier.

Glasbeek, H. (1986) *The Maiming and Killing of Workers: The One Sided Nature of Risk Taking in Capitalism*. Jurisprudence Centre Working Papers, Department of Law, Carleton University, Ottawa.

Grau, C. W. (1989) Whatever Happened to Politics? A Critique of Structuralist and Marxists Accounts of State and Law. In P. Bierne and R. Quinney (eds.), *Marxism and Law* (pp. 196-209). New York: John Wiley and Sons.

Gunningham, N., and Johnstone, R. (1999) *Systems and Sanctions: Regulating Workplace Safety*. Oxford: Oxford University Press.

Hale, A. (1997) Introduction: The Goals of Event Analysis. In A. Hale, B. Wilpert, and M. Freitag (eds.), *After the Event: From Accident to Organisational Learning* (pp. 1-10). Oxford: Pergamon, Elsevier.

Haynes v C I and D Manufacturing Pty Ltd (1995) 60 IR 149.

Hopkins, A. (2002) The ESSO Longford Trial. *Journal of Occupational Health and Safety— Australia and New Zealand, 18*: 3-67.

Hopkins, A. (2000) *Lessons from Longford.* Sydney: CCH.

Hunt, A. (1985) The Ideology of Law: Advances and Problems in Recent Applications of the Concept of Ideology to the Analysis of Law. *Law and Society Review, 19*: 11-37.

Hutter, B. M. (2001) *Regulation and Risk: Occupational Health and Safety on the Railways.* Oxford: Oxford University Press.

Industrial Relations Bill 1990 (Vic).

Industrial Relations (General Amendment) Bill 1988 (Vic).

Industry Commission. (1995) *Work, Health and Safety.* Industry Commission, Melbourne. Vol I.

Jamieson, S. (2000) *The Future of Our People: Women and Prosecution for Work Injury in NSW.* Unpublished SJD thesis. University of Sydney, Sydney.

Johnstone, R. (1999) Paradigm Crossed? The Statutory Occupational Health and Safety Obligations of the Business Undertaking. *Australian Journal of Labor Law, 12*: 73-112.

Johnstone, R. (2000) Occupational Health and Safety Prosecutions in Victoria: An Historical Study. *Australian Journal of Labor Law, 13*: 113-142.

Johnstone, R. (2003a) *Safety, Courts and Crime.* Sydney: Federation Press.

Johnstone, R. (2003b) Safety, Courts and Crime: Occupational Health and Safety Prosecutions in the Magistrates' Courts. *Policy and Practice in Health and Safety, 1*: 105-127.

Johnstone, R. (2004) *Occupational Health and Safety Law and Policy* (2nd ed.). Sydney: Law Book.

Kinney, J. A., Weiss, K., Sufalko, Gleason, A., and Maakestad, W. (1990) *Criminal Job Safety Prosecutions.* National Safe Workplace Institute: Kansas City.

Kletz, T. (2001) *Learning from Accidents.* Oxford: Gulf.

Mathiesen, T. (1980) Kunsten å isolere en ulykke (translated as The Art of Isolating an Accident). In B. Eggen and H. Gundersen (eds.), *Nordsjøtragedien* (translated as *The North Sea Tragedy*) Oslo: Pax Publishers.

Mathiesen, T. (1981) Disciplining through Pulverization. In *The Hidden Disciplining: Essays on Political Control.* Oslo: T. Mathiesen.

Mathiesen, T. (1985) *Die Lautlose Disziplinierung* (The Hidden Disciplining). Bielefeld: AJZ Verlag. (I have benefitted from an English translation by the author of this work.)

McBarnet, D. (1981) *Conviction: Law, the State and the Construction of Justice.* London: Macmillan.

Norrie, A. (1993) *Crime, Reason and History: A Critical Introduction to Criminal Law.* London: Weidenfeld and Nicolson.

Offe, C. (1975) The Theory of the Capitalist State and the Problem of Policy Formation. In L. N. Lindberg, et al. (eds.), *Stress and Contradictions in Modern Capitalism. Public Policy and the theory of the State.* Lexington, MA: Lexington Books.

Perrone, S. (2000) *When Life is Cheap: Governmental Responses to Work-Related Fatalities in Victoria 1987-1990.* Unpublished Ph.D. thesis. Department of Criminology, The University of Melbourne, Melbourne.

Productivity Commission. (2003) *National Workers' Compensation and Occupational Health and Safety Frameworks Interim Report,* Melbourne: Productivity Commission.

R v Australian Char Pty Ltd (1996) 64 IR 387.

R v Simsmetal Limited, unreported, County Court of Victoria (Villeneuve-Smith J), Melbourne, 9 March 1989.

Sargent, N. (1989) Law, Ideology and Corporate Crime: A Critique of Instrumentalism. *Canadian Journal of Law and Society, 4*: 39-75.

Sargent, N. (1990) Law, Ideology Social Change: An Analysis of The Role of Law in the Construction of Corporate Crime. *The Journal of Social Justice, 1*: 97-116.

Schultz v Tamworth City Council(1995) 58 IR 221.

Sentencing Act 1991 (Vic).

Simpson, G., and Charlesworth, H. (1995) Objecting to Objectivity. In R. Hunter, R. Ingleby, and R. Johnstone (eds.), *Thinking About Law: Perspectives on the History, Philosophy and Sociology of Law.* Sydney: Allen & Unwin.

Slapper, G. (2000) *Blood in the Bank: Social and Legal Aspects of Death at Work.* Aldershot: Ashgate/Dartmouth.

Sparrow, M. K. (2000) *The Regulatory Craft: Controlling Risks, Solving Problems and Managing Compliance.* Washington, DC: The Brookings Institution.

Thompson, W. (2001) *Understanding New South Wales Occupational Health and Safety Legislation* (3rd ed.). Sydney: CCH.

Tucker, E. (1990) *Administering Danger in the Workplace: The Law and Politics of Occupational Health and Safety Regulation in Ontario, 1850-1914.* Toronto: University of Toronto Press.

Tucker, E. (1996) Worker Health and Safety Struggles: Democratic Possibilities and Constraints. *New Solutions,* Winter: 61-69.

Tucker v Mappin Unreported, Industrial Relations Commission of Victoria in Court Session (Marshall P), Case No 91/1983, 21 November 1983.

Victorian WorkCover Authority. (2002) *Recent Prosecutions 2001.* Melbourne: VWA.

Victorian WorkCover Authority. (2001) *Recent Prosecutions 2000.* Melbourne: VWA.

WorkCover Authority (NSW) (Inspector Mulder) v Yass Shire Council (2000) 99 IR 284.

CHAPTER 9

Blame and Causation in the Aftermath of Industrial Disasters: Nova Scotia's Coal Mines from 1858 to Westray

"when the slaughter is wholesale"

Susan Dodd

The Westray coal mine exploded in May 1992 in Plymouth, Nova Scotia, killing 26 men. When I interviewed relatives of men who died at Westray, as part of a study on the aftermath of industrial disasters in 1997, I was shocked by the freshness of their grief. Most family members feared the impending report of the inquiry: they believed it would blame the dead men for their own misfortune (Dodd 1999, 2001). This anxiety was remarkable because it was not supported by the inquiry testimony. In fact, witness after witness had testified to the incompetence and recklessness of the mine operators and the dereliction of duty by regulators. Why then, were relatives so anxious about the impending report? Of course, incomplete mourning, prolonged exposure to public scrutiny, and shaken confidence in Canadian law all contributed to relatives' pre-report anxiety.

I argue here that an even more fundamental source of this anxiety lay in culturally grounded practices evident in bureaucratic reports on workplace fatalities and injuries. Westray family members were bracing themselves against a longstanding practice of blaming miners for their own injuries and deaths. This is not to say that relatives necessarily knew the contents of previous reports, but rather that their five-year struggle to protect their men's good names gave them intimate knowledge of the strategies of bureaucratic capitalism. Perhaps they sensed that a space for critique that had been opened by the disaster would be closed by the release of the report.

Reviewing reports from Nova Scotia's coal mines contributes to our understanding of the culture of disaster aftermaths and the ideological work of inquiries in particular. I begin with an analysis of reports on coal mine disasters from the first report of the Nova Scotia Mines Inspectorate in 1858 to the report on the 1979 explosion in Devco Colliery Number 26 in Cape Breton. I turn then to a close reading of the Executive Summary of *The Westray Story*. Mapping practices of reporting on coal mine disasters in Nova Scotia allow me to analyze the ideological work aimed at containing public reflection on the class violence exposed by mine disasters. Disasters such as Westray and those that preceded it in Nova Scotia's coal mines call into question three fundamental socio-economic presuppositions:

> . . . first, that risk is a natural and unavoidable consequence of productive activity in general, and staple extraction in particular; second, that private economic activity is preferable to public activity; and third, that occupational health and safety is an area in which workers and employers share a common set of interests and objectives, a consensus. (Glasbeek and Tucker 1999, p. 72)

Inquiry reports attempt to reinstate these presuppositions—to help them regain transparency within "legitimate" public discourse.

READING INQUIRY REPORTS

In this chapter, I read inquiry reports as literary works. Inquiry reports manage the social disruption caused by disaster by drawing on a stock of available stories and character types. Routine bureaucratic reporting—the day-to-day housekeeping of administrative memos and databases—operates unproblematically until disaster strikes. Inquiry reports supplement such normal, day-to-day bureaucratic record-keeping. In the aftermath of large-scale deaths and injury, reports on disasters work to limit, substitute, and redirect the public memory of the causes of disaster. That is, reports aim to limit reflection on bureaucratic capitalism as the cause of the disaster, to substitute this explanation with a more individualistic one, and to redirect attention from radical change onto minor legislative reform. This is particularly true where the disaster is evidently caused by the exploitation of workers by owners, with government collusion.

Disasters are typically followed by a proliferation of causal explanations for large-scale loss of life and property, some of which lay blame at the feet of employers and government. Inquiries and their reports work to put these explanations back into bureaucratically manageable order. In any socio-historical situation, numerous causal representations of problematic events are available, though some are more readily available than others. The most plausible of these are what discourse analysts call "prior plausibility structures" (Green 1993). Prior plausibility structures are the familiar tunes of ordinary language: they are the narratives, figures of speech, and character types that we unreflectively expect.

These are not the *only* ways to represent reality, but they are the most likely to give readers a sense of literal meaning. When none of the readily available prior plausibility structures asserts itself, doubt ensues. Doubt about how to account for people, things, or events presents a "cultural coding problem" (Green 1993).

A cultural coding problem occurs when people are unsure about how to interpret something. Usually, this entails a confrontation with someone or thing that will not rest in a culturally legible category but for which numerous interpretations seem equally plausible. Any person or thing that does not fit snuggly into an established character type or role—any boundary crosser—presents a "cultural coding problem." When the exploitative relations of coal mining become manifest in the deaths of workers, "coal miner" presents a cultural coding problem. Are the men who died victims? Are they villains? Were they actively involved in producing the conditions that led to their deaths? Were they passive and if so, does this make them blameworthy? Or are there more complex social and cultural forces at work here? If so, what are they? How can they be changed, and by whom?

Inquiry reports attempt to put people and things back into place. They entertain the most obvious plausible causes, and stabilize public memory by asserting one story as clearly, undeniably the *only* explanation. Accident reports work to limit reflection on the human costs of coal mining by managing the cultural coding problem of worker injury and death. Just as people use impression management in attempts to conceal our sense of vulnerability and to constitute an image in face-to-face interaction, literary conventions of reports work to suppress the anxieties caused by bureaucratic capitalism's failure to prevent predictable accidents (Bloom 1975; Green 1992; Dorothy Smith 1990b, 1999). To give readers a sense that they are looking *through* the report, as through a clear window onto an objective reality, reports play on prior plausibility structures. They do this by using familiar vocabulary and grammar, and by following the rules of inquiry reports as a genre of bureaucratic writing (Green 1992, p. 104).

Each report considered here reflects the literary genre of inquiry reports. Every inquiry report, as such, must present grounds for its own authority, including a definitive account of events consisting of causal chains that identify the source of the disaster (somewhere other than in the structure of bureaucratic capitalism). An inquiry report, as such, must also produce recommendations that, if followed, should prevent another disaster. Much of a report's authority is expressed in the literary conventions by which the historical account of the disaster is given. Each report is a picture of the practices of attributing blame and determining causation that dominated at the time the report was written. By reading reports from inquiries into coal mine injuries and deaths as literary works, we get a snapshot of some of the most potent cultural work of capitalism as it responds to the potential crisis of widespread reflection on exploitation-unto-death of workers by owners.

In reading each report, I have been attentive to the following: a) the ways in which the crisis is depicted; b) the report's claims to have gathered a mass of evidence from which it will discover that future accidents can be avoided by increased administrative control; c) the author-commissioner's self-presentation as having traveled to discover the root causes of the disaster; d) the integration of common sense with the bureaucratic and scientific account; e) and the construction of character types through the transformation of particular people and events into general cases (Fairclough 1995; Green 1992, p. 113).

THREE WAVES OF REPORTS FROM
NOVA SCOTIA'S COAL MINES

Historically, the wretched pay and dangerous work of mining has been in tension with the economic importance of coal. This tension brings the conflict between workers and economic structures to light in unsettling ways. To manage this conflict, sometimes the state uses open force, as in the early 20th century clashes that culminated in the fatal shooting of William Davis in Cape Breton in 1925 (Earle 1989). Sometimes the state compromises, as with gains negotiated through trade unions. And sometimes, along with overt force and compromise, government and owners aim to control knowledge and to shape public debates. This is particularly the case following mining disasters, when the public reconsiders the human costs of coal mining.

Reports passed through three overlapping phases that correspond to three "waves" of occupational health and safety regulation (Tucker 1995, p. 245). The principle goal of the first-wave (1830-1879) was to regulate market activity—in this case, to ensure that the mining companies met their financial commitments to the province. The second wave of occupational health and safety regulation (1880-1969) began when relief societies and other community-based means of managing contingency were standardized and administered by government. This second wave was characterized by weak direct state regulation of workplaces. The third wave of occupational health and safety regulation (1970-present) is characterized by mandated partial self-regulation including the "internal responsibility system" of joint management-worker committees. Now, government agents are characterized as facilitators rather than police or regulators. With the withdrawal of even the pretense of external regulatory enforcement, many occupational health and safety activists wonder whether or not their efforts have backfired. Has placing workers on committees simply implicated them in management decisions, drawing their opinions and language into an elaborate feedback mechanism that reproduces existing workplace conditions? (Doug Smith 2000). Have regulatory bodies become empty shells—window dressing for governments too cowed to interfere with the engines of economic development? The 1992 Westray explosion in Nova Scotia certainly raised such questions for many.

Regardless of the model of occupational health and safety employed in Nova Scotia coal mines, each wave is marked by disasters when, as the 1874 report on the Drummond disaster put it, "the slaughter is wholesale."[1] The 1873 disaster in the Drummond mine killed 60 boys and men, and was the largest major disaster in the first wave of regulation. The second wave of regulation was marked by numerous large-scale disasters: 1880 in the Albion Mine (44 dead); 1891 in Springhill (125 dead); 1917 in Dominion Cape Breton (65 dead); and 1918 in the Allan mine in Pictou county (88 dead). Numerous smaller-scale disasters filled the decades until two Springhill disasters in 1956 and 1958 (39 and 75 dead, respectively) marked the end of coal mining in Springhill. Coal mining petered out during the third wave, due to diminished demand for Nova Scotia coal. Nonetheless, there were two major disasters at Devco in Cape Breton in 1979 (12 dead) and Westray in Pictou County in 1992 (26 dead).[2]

In some ways, there is very little mystery about the material cause of coal mine disasters. The tunnels of a coal mine can collapse in a "fall" or even heave in a "bump." Methane gas can creep out of the mine's porous rock walls, accumulating in nooks and crannies undisturbed by flowing air where the gas then ignites or explodes. Gas explosions produce noxious gasses. Sometimes a gas explosion will shake coal dust into the air then ignite it in a second gunshot-like blast. Fires can start in coal dust and rage in the pit.

As we will see, the forensic project of discovering the "cause" of a coal mine disaster is not a matter of solving a science problem so much as searching for a culprit. A culprit, that is, who draws attention away from the sacrifice of human life in the pursuit of personal profit. The representation of the cause of disaster must, above all re-establish confidence in the ability of bureaucratic capitalism to reflect on itself and reform. The facts of the matter must be prepared so that they can recede from public view.

The First Wave: Miner as Imprudent (1858-1879)
"A recklessness by no means uncommon"

The overall tone of the inaugural Report of the Inspector of Mines in 1858 was exaltation, particularly with the General Mining Association (GMA), which held the rights to Nova Scotia's mineral resources from 1826 to 1858.

> Before turning from the works of the Mining Association, it is proper to observe, that the different collieries seem to be conducted with great skill and ability by the managers at the respective works. They have uniformedly rendered me every necessary assistance in my capacity of superintendent of mines.

> Every department seemed perfect in itself, while the harmonious action of all the parts shews (sic) the perfect triumph of mind over matter, and proves to a demonstration, that "knowledge is power." Mr. Scott, of the Albion Mines, by the aid of his superior scientific and practical attainments as a mining engineer, has, to the astonishment of every person acquainted with the supposed difficulty of the task, effected an achievement in science, which it

> was thought impossible to perform—namely, the re-opening of the crushed mines. Not only has he succeeded in re-opening these works, but he has now brought them to such a state of efficiency, that they promise to yield an unfailing supply of excellent coal. (Nova Scotia 1858, pp. 384-385)

This is the story of heroic, exceptional 19th century men of science winning a struggle against nature. Nature could be harnessed, if only workingmen could be reformed. The report continues:

> Mr. Brown, of the Sydney mines, has I believe, been superintendent of the works there for the last twenty-five years. Under his able, judicious and scientific management, every difficulty seems to vanish, and the collieries under his control appear to be conducted upon the most approved principles of modern skill and economy. The agents also seem to be well qualified for their respective positions. During the past year but one casualty occurred at the Sydney mines, and two at the Albion mines,—all of which I regret to say, proved fatal. That at the former colliery resulted from the carelessness of the deceased, who fell down the shaft while the pit was at work. The accident at the latter place was occasioned by the sudden escape of fire damp from the strata, which, however, was confined to a narrow space, into which unfortunately, the sufferers imprudently ventured with naked light, although it seems they had been warned that indications of inflammable [sic] gas had been discovered in that locality. (Nova Scotia 1858, pp. 384-385)

Two explanations of the cause of injury and death dominated in the early reports: misfortune and worker imprudence. Neither management's nor government's responsibility was ever included among possible contributing factors. However, even the earliest reports anchored management's legitimacy in commonsense judgment. For instance, the mines report for 1859 described two casualties in a Cape Breton mine, and found it "gratifying to know . . . that no blame seems to attach to any of the overmen or others connected with the colliery, as will appear from the verdict of the coroner's jury . . ." (Nova Scotia 1860, p. 290). The deaths were linked with the assertion of the blamelessness of the company's agents, and with the jury's commonsense legitimation of that fact. Any further possible criticism was dwarfed with a "speculative and visionary" account of the "colonial aggrandizement and prosperity" Nova Scotia's mineral deposits held for the future. The report reminded the reader that "this is the age of improvement," and "the great tide of emigration is still setting to the west" (Nova Scotia 1860, p. 290).

By the early 1860s, statistics were already the medium used to represent normal operations: "There have been no particular observations made respecting the conditions [of the mines], beyond what the statistical returns present" (Nova Scotia 1862, p. 35). Statistical tables, including tables on "accidents" (as of 1873) and productivity (tons/workday) began to be used with increased frequency. Tables numbered and dated each accident, named the worker, identified the mine, classified the material cause (e.g., "Fall of coal" or "Explosion of gas"), and categorized the result (i.e., "Recovered" or "Died"). For each, the report provided an explanatory paragraph that named the worker, described his work and his particular act of imprudence or misfortune, and concluded with the consequences to him and others (Nova Scotia 1872, p. 20). The 1862 Report made no mention of attempts to minimize accidents; they were presented as the unavoidable consequence of humanity's fallen nature.

By 1873, an unfavorable comparison of Nova Scotia's statistics with Great Britain's evoked an aspiration to extend administrative control (Nova Scotia 1873, p. 28). Further, the later report displayed concern about the quality of its statistical evidence and taxonomic practices because the distinction between fatal and non-fatal injuries did not capture the full impact of disabling accidents:

> It will be noticed, on referring to the table, that besides fatal accidents, several very serious ones happened, which in their consequences are almost as disastrous as if they had been fatal. Men have been maimed for life, and the burden of their future maintenance thrown on their relatives and friends. This part of the list, full as it is, I have every reason to believe is incomplete, and that the report of several casualties has been withheld! (Nova Scotia 1873, p. 28)

In each of the categories under "Fatal Accidents," moral failure by workers "caused" the casualties: "carelessness or inattention to orders," and "gross negligence" accounted for all five explosions of gas. "A recklessness by no means uncommon in the handling of powder by miners" led to one death and serious injury. "Most of the casualties caused by falls of coal and stone were due to the neglect of the persons injured . . ." (Nova Scotia 1873, p. 30). In a death most difficult to attribute to worker imprudence, the report conceded that the fall of a particular kind of stone "is always sudden and their position in the roof often escapes the eye of the most experienced miner." The flaw remained, of course, situated in the "eye" of the generalized miner. "Accidents in the Shaft" were described also as failings by each particular man: "he missed his foothold"; he "lost his hold"; "[t]he deceased is said to have been subject to fits of giddiness after smoking much. A pipe was in his mouth when he fell"; the deceased "was incautiously leaning" (Nova Scotia 1873, p. 32). The report presented "illustrations of the utter recklessness with which men will expose their lives to dangers, when the dangers, although acknowledged imminent, are familiar, invisible and temporarily doubtful" (Nova Scotia 1873, p. 32). Any sense of the men as collective (as a positive attribute) was undermined by the report's descriptions of individual folly leading others to ruin. The repeated "finding" that the cause of each injury was a moral failure of the injured constructed the "imprudent worker" as an inductively discovered regularity.

The 1874 mines report demonstrates that the Drummond mine disaster that killed 60 men and boys disturbed somewhat the routine practice of blaming the miners. The evidence of this disturbance is noteworthy, but minimal in comparison with the later *Westray Story*. The report emphasizes the importance of extending the bureaucratic power of the inspectorate over both workers and management. Before presenting the disaster, the 1874 report began by explaining the effectiveness of the newly introduced standardization of weighing and recording the amount of extracted coal, to secure the province's income through royalties. "Last year I was not in a position to know that any owner or agent had previously sent either intentionally or through negligence sworn returns which were inaccurate, but I am now prepared to show that the returns on a large output for the year 1872 from one concern were 20 p.c. incorrect . . ." (Nova Scotia 1874, p. 6).

The report then described an English precedent, "relative to the liability of colliery owners for the default of their servants under the *Mines Regulation Act, 1872*" (Nova Scotia 1874, p. 17). Paternalism was eroding slowly, and metaphors of the body convey the shift of the "burden" from managers' shoulders onto "those in subordinate positions." The workers' hands now held "the safety of their own lives and the lives of the working men." The authority did not shift to free individuals, however, but to carefully monitored workers. Finely detailed rules were needed to monitor and discipline workers' movements. The report told a moral tale, where imprudence and death resulted from the absence of such finely detailed regulation. It was clear that when the men's social lives "infiltrated" the mine, conventional craft practices could not save the men from their own imprudence.

Along with increased surveillance of the company's accounting, the 1874 report stressed the need to certify mine managers. Certification was represented as a "watchfulness" whereby future generations' interests would be "protected from waste and lavish consumption." "The employment of certificated managers" could slow the waste of a public good. The precedence for such interference in relations between "masters and mates" was drawn from maritime enterprises, and justified as a means of fitting men who could be "trusted" into appropriate positions.

Given that this was a report on the deaths of 60 men and boys, the report was remarkably mild in stating its uncertainty about the efficacy of granting companies the "trust" of public goods. However, though the report noted the "low" character of miners and mining communities, it entertained the possibility that "many among the working miners, who, possessed of the natural ability and determination to succeed, would strive to improve their position, by strenuous efforts in their spare hours. . . ." Democratic acknowledgment of the "natural energy of character" among some workers demanded mobility within the hierarchical structure, and simultaneous binding of the successful to a bureaucratically administered certification system. This, in turn, would "elevate" the "general standard of education in the mining community" and "improve" the moral tone— in part, by engaging the men's leisure hours. This preamble put into play the prior plausibility structure of worker imprudence in that it implied that a contributing cause of the disaster was the firemen's ignorance. With a controlled extension of "book learning, we might then hope that great improvements would take place in the safety of our mines." As administrative ambitions grew stronger, so did demands for an overarching formality, visible to the bureaucratic eye as certifications and mine plans (Nova Scotia 1874, pp. 8-9).

Finally, the report turned to mine-by-mine reports from the deputies. Under "Pictou County," reporting began with an account of worker radicalism. The 1874 report likened strikes and disasters in their production-curtailing effects: "The bright prospects with which the coal trade of this county opened were early marred by strikes, and later in the spring the lamentable explosion at the Drummond colliery destroyed all hopes of the output exceeding that of the previous year. The falling off amounted to 38,767 tons, and the sales decreased 51,433 tons" (Nova Scotia 1874, p. 11).

Appended transcriptions of the Coroner's Inquest attested to the care of the overman, but the verdict expressed "our regret that [blasting] powder was permitted to be used in the level worked by [miner] Robert McLeod." The manager had to "suppress" his "prudential fears" in order to "run risks which he hoped by care and attention to divert from leading to serious accidents." The manager's excellence was such that it would prepare "to meet all ordinary contingencies arising from the proper use of powder," and yet could not overcome the contingency of worker imprudence; that is to say, McLeod's imprudence in his implied "carelessness or a desire to save labor. . . ." The workmen were presented as imprudent as a group, having "not only not objected to, but required" the use of blasting powder in order to increase their extraction speed and hence income. Further entrenching this sense that the men consciously chose to make money instead of protecting their lives and the mine, the report found "the minds of the colliers were disturbed" by comparing their own situation with the "high rate" of wages in England. Even the manager's empathy for the workers was a source of contagion from the imprudent workers: managers had given the workmen an opportunity to continue to use powder in the mine, but "its gross misuses" in their hands prevailed over management's "exceptional care."

The ambivalence of state-controlled relief measures were evident in the reports' conclusion that "the inevitable law of averages" meant that mining fatalities would increase, and as wages were such that no nuclear family could reabsorb a married, now widowed, daughter, Nova Scotia needed an accident fund. A further benefit of the fund, the report noted, would be its ability to manage expressions of empathy (and shared class interest) following fatalities. Hence, the report concluded with a section titled "Colliery Accident Fund" that endorsed the bureaucratization of gift giving:

> After an occurrence such as that at the Drummond, when the slaughter is wholesale, the sympathies of the people at large are with the families of the sufferers, and contributions of money are freely made for their relief. But when a single fatality occurs—the public attention is not drawn to the trials suddenly imposed on the widow and orphans, and to their need of assistance. Beyond the temporary aid afforded by their local subscription, the care of

her support is left entirely to her relations, who, most probably, are ill able to bear the additional expense. This system of alms-giving is manifestly unfair, and tends to blunt the natural pride of a people accustomed to fairly earn their daily bread.

While still the recollection of the terrible disaster is fresh in the minds of our mining people, I desire to point out to them a system of relief that has been proposed in England, and partly carried out in South Staffordshire; which is, that each district should establish a district permanent insurance fund for the relief of sufferers by colliery accidents. The scheme adopted supplies the required aid, as the payment of a just claim, and not as a gift of charity. Consequently it meets with the approval of all classes interested, and the inevitable law of averages has shown that a proportionate number of fatalities are here, as well as elsewhere, incidental to the growth of the coal trade. (Nova Scotia 1874, p. 37)

The 1874 report contrasted the noble coal mining family, those who "fairly earn their daily bread," with those who received alms. Bureaucratic fear of producing dependents instead of disciplined workers was suggested by conceptual slippage between corpses and those who receive alms. The report lauded the cooperation of managers and yet fretted about the underreporting of accidents, thus legitimizing extended bureaucratic reach. According to "the inevitable law of averages," fatalities would increase, so Nova Scotia needed an accident fund. The fund would help people who were injured in smaller accidents with no wave of sympathy from the general public. A further benefit of the fund would be its ability to manage expressions of sympathy (and so shared class interest) following mass fatalities. As usual, following a disruptive loss of life, this report appended transcripts from the Coroner's inquest testimony, to ground its authority in commonsense experience and judgment.

In the first wave of accident reporting in Nova Scotia coal mines, inspectors gave triumphant first-person accounts of harmonious mines operations. Fatalities were thought to occur whenever miners escaped from the benevolent control of their managers—those 19th century men of science and genius. The physical "cause" of accidents was to be found at the hands of miners. The moral cause was in their souls, in poor judgment, ignorance, or greed. A routine mines report constructed a stereotype of a miner as a person incapable of self-rule and simultaneously attributed those qualities to everyone who dug coal. The reification of routine bureaucratic reality reporting works unproblematically in two directions: embodied individuals are transformed into a category of bureaucratic writing, while that category is read back into day-to-day life. A so-called "healthy" bureaucratic regime is characterized by the smooth functioning of such translation between particular individuals and general categories, and back. Routine mines reports were sufficient to report on typical workplace deaths, while broader reports were needed as the 1874 report put it, "when the slaughter is wholesale."

THE SECOND WAVE: MINER AS ANOMALY (1880-1969)
"what is inevitable cannot be unjust,
though there may still be room for generosity"

In the second wave of workplace regulation, the source of the problem caused by coal mining was identified increasingly with coal mine culture, and less with individual fault. The second wave of accident reporting reflected increasing state regulation of workplaces and workforces. The reports looked to the absence of technology and administration as explanations for disasters and so "found" that disasters could be avoided with more machinery, closer monitoring of workers in all aspects of their lives, and more careful bureaucratic reporting on workplace activity.

The 1880 mines report on the deaths of 44 men and boys in the Albion Mine clearly emphasized a turn to technological means of managing contingency. Once the 1880 report had located the ignition of the explosion (among miners who waited for their picks), it presented a table of provincial governments' contributions to a relief fund to close down the relief question, and then turned to an extended discussion of technological developments. The report looked to technology to overcome the contingencies of human agency and material conditions in mines. For example, electric lights were seen as offering the promise of "the removal of the temptation held out to workmen to tamper with the safety lamp" (Nova Scotia 1880, p. 27). The report cautioned, though, that technical developments only heightened the need for managerial watchfulness.

As the administrative regime developed, it aspired to deepen its control over workers' day-to-day lives. Boys were drawn into schools and out of the coal mines; miners' certification requirements were instituted; contract negotiations between unions and companies became regulated; housing was monitored for sanitation; even the collection and distribution of injury benefits was bureaucratized. In all these developments, people's lives were stabilized even as they were controlled. The substitution of state bureaucracy for conventional practice was evident particularly in reports at the turn of the century when administration replaced and/or supplemented paternalism. As a result, inquiries studied mines, miners, and mining communities from numerous angles.

The 1891 mines report included a "Report on the Springhill Disaster" that killed 125 men and boys. Written by mines expert Edwin Gilpin, this report presupposes its authority to present the facts. Its technical language suggests that this report was not aimed at a general readership. While the machinery and management of the mine were found to have been excellent, Gilpin was disturbed by the "latitude allowed by shot firers to miners in respect to charging holes before they were examined" (Nova Scotia 1891, p. ii). A shot firer produced the spark of the disaster:

> His body was found, with those of the men working in the bord, near the entrance to the place. The shot in the stone had been fired. This, coupled with

the direction of the course of the explosion, showed with reasonable certainty that it had its origin in the bord, and that the shot fired by Wilson was the direct cause of the explosion. (Nova Scotia 1891, p. iii)

While Gilpin attests to Wilson's good reputation, he attributes the explosion to Wilson's mistake coupled with an accumulation of gas in an unusual stone formation that occurred because "the pit was idle the preceding day" (Nova Scotia 1891: p. iv). Though "the general opinion of the witnesses was that the shot firer was a careful man," Gilpin maintains, "the weight of evidence appeared to be that there had been an overcharge of powder." Gilpin concludes:

> That the shot gave evidence of having been a more or less flaming one; that it ignited the gas lodged in the roof stone; that this combination of gas and powder flame acting on an atmosphere charged with a small percentage of gas and fire floating dust derived from the lower bords, caused an intense flame sufficient to propagate itself until it reached an intensely explosive state. (Nova Scotia 1891, p. iv)

Two further observations disturbed Gilpin. Open lights were used not far from areas where safety lamps were required, so "men who are furnished with locked lamps are naturally inclined to be sceptical as to their value if they know that within a short distance open lamps are permitted" (Nova Scotia 1891, p. iv). Worse still, men knew the stone was gassy, but did not report this to management (Nova Scotia 1891, p. v). A jury of "practical coal miners" also concluded that the explosion was accidental, emphasizing the role of the unusual stone. The report appended transcripts from the coroner's inquest and concluded with a table listing the names, ages and "persons dependent on him," i.e., each dead man. As a result, we see that Gilpin presupposes his own authority as a producer of knowledge about mines, though the report grounds itself ultimately in the transcribed interviews with men of practical experience and class identity with the dead. The cause of the disaster was the deed of one man, but also the attitude of workers who are imprudent wherever authority fails.

The Gilpin Commission's 1895 *Report on the Cause, History and Effects of Fires in Pictou County Coal Mines* was the earliest report I encountered that had an identity distinct from the yearly Nova Scotia mines report. Commissioner Gilpin anchored his authority in his personal knowledge of the district (Nova Scotia 1895, p. 12). Appended testimony revealed that the commissioners pieced together the history of fires, the tunnels connecting mines, and quality and quantity of inaccessible mines in the Pictou coal fields from the experiential recollections of miners:

Q. And the only fire you did see was the fire in the Foster pit?
A. I did see it and felt it. I got right home dead. I was unconscious that night and the next day." (Nova Scotia 1895, p. 43)

The questions asked of miners were fact-focused, while those asked of local businessmen were more speculative, e.g., "Is it worth while looking to the opening of the mines to increase the business?" (Nova Scotia 1895, p. 67).

In the 1895 report, management was found to lack "cooperation," and uncertainty about the company's management of Nova Scotia's coal was the problem the report aimed to resolve. Company agent (and former provincial mines inspector) Mr. Poole presented mines manager Mr. Wills as fundamentally imprudent, consistently endangering "the safety of the pit," and misrepresenting the extent of his "expertise" (Nova Scotia 1895, p. 104). The fire in the pit was imbued with devilish agency: "I only have heard of one place where fire and water will live together" (Poole, in Nova Scotia 1895, p. 77). Though Gilpin's 1895 report effaced worker agency, its findings about the layout and condition of the old mine works and the quality and quantity of coal remaining were grounded in experiential knowledge appropriated from older miners. The miners' memories held details about techniques, conditions, and errors that were absent from company records.

1900-1919

From the turn of the century on, the very society produced by mining is presented as a kind of disaster in inquiry reports. Mining produced troublesome people in troublesome communities, and inquiry after inquiry was established to address the problems they posed. In testimony before the 1908 Commission on *An Act Respecting Old Age Pensions and Miners' Relief Societies*, an administrator of an existing relief society responded to the commissioner's concerns that benefits were being paid to men who did not deserve them. The commission was concerned about inconsistencies in doctors' approaches to possible malingerers, and local relief societies' inconsistencies in distinguishing valid from false claims:

> We sometimes turn down the doctor's certificate. We had considerable trouble about that and appointed a committee to interview the doctors. I have interviewed a doctor myself. The doctor said that if a man told him he had a pain in his back and jumped every time he touched him that he had to take the man's word for it. He said there was nothing in his profession in a case of that kind to entitle him to say that the man had no pain. The doctor said our committee would have to be the judges. (Nova Scotia 1908, p. 24)

The commission noted a lack of official statistics about the ages and length of employment of coal miners in Nova Scotia. Miners testified that they could not get life insurance through normal schemes because of the danger of their work, and called for a publicly funded pension scheme.

The 1916 mines report begins with a description of conferences held in Halifax and Sydney on the topic of mine safety: "This conference was unanimous in declaring that the conference held at Halifax had been the means of awakening a feeling in every one that upon him rested a responsibility for the care of his own life and that of his fellow workmen" (Nova Scotia 1916, p. 13). The Sydney conference, entitled "Safety First," adopted a resolution committing provincial and municipal governments, coal companies, and workers to a "movement . . . where all directly interested in coal mining are brought together for the purpose of cooperating to reduce the number of accidents in the coal mines" (Nova Scotia 1916, p. 13).

The Workmen's Compensation Board was established in 1916, in time to report on the deaths of 65 men in Cape Breton in 1917 and 88 men in Pictou County in 1918. The mines report deals with the 1917 deaths of 65 men and boys in Cape Breton with a four-page "Special Report" with no testimony.[3] It concludes with the banal recommendation that the *Coal Mines Regulations Act* should be enforced, especially with regard to the measurement and records of gas conditions, and government inspectors should monitor compliance by company mine examiners more closely (Nova Scotia 1918). These same recommendations would be made in 1980, following the Devco disaster. They would be repeated in 1997, following the Westray disaster.

1920-1949

There were fewer large-scale disasters in the decades between 1920 and 1950, though the fatality rates per million tons of coal remained consistent with earlier times. Inquiry reports of this period concentrate on coal mining as a socio-economic problem that required state intervention of various forms to fix.

In the 1920s, Nova Scotia coal fields became hotbeds of labor radicalism. Burgeoning class-consciousness resulted from unusually strong common cultural ground among workers, a threat to wages and hence to subsistence, an explicit focus on profit maximization by owners, the truck system of credit at company stores, and Marxist political critiques (Frank 1993; Earle and McKay 1989). Inquiries of the period focused on resolving—or at least containing—the struggle for higher wages, and on more democratic control in the workplace. One of the commissioners of the 1925 Duncan Report into Nova Scotia's coal industry linked the threat of popular uprising and even of the separation of Nova Scotia from Confederation with systematic favoring of central Canadian industry. One economist strongly suggested that the government needed to keep Nova Scotia coal miners working or face the possible disintegration of the Dominion (Addendum from Hume Cronyn, in Nova Scotia 1926, p. 153). As central Canada boomed with industrial development, "a wage war was raging in the Nova Scotia coal fields." The threat presented by coal miners and mining threatened the Dominion itself, and thus the radicalism of coal miners provided the Province, as an entity, with bargaining power with the rest of the country (Nova Scotia 1926, p. 146). As the "problem" of coal mining and miners was represented increasingly as broadly social in origin, a more sociological treatment began to replace the more individualistic, sin-based explanations of the first wave of accident reports.

The 1924 report, referring to the rock fall in Inverness that killed four men, found that one problem in the mine was men working the backshift without the Examiner's report being made available to them. In an example of what would become a preoccupation of later reports, the report raised the possibility that the viability of the mine operation itself was put into question by the costs of safe production.

Direct blaming of miners receded somewhat in the 1920s and 1930s with an increased focus on the failure of management to read or interpret signs given by monitoring equipment. Reporting on the deaths of seven men in the Allan mine, Pictou County, the 1930 mines report found that the mine had lacked "a competent man" to respond when the fan stopped clearing methane gas from the rock face (Nova Scotia 1930, 111). The report on the deaths of six men in a 1931 explosion at the Victoria Coal Company in River Hebert, began with a process of elimination. After ruling out an overcharged shot and any permitted open light in the area, it turned to an eyewitness: "Garfield Stevens is the only man who got out alive, who was working in that section on the morning of May 11th at the time the explosion took place." The commissioners interviewed him at his house but discovered that "he was not in condition to question as much as we would like to," so the inquiry was postponed. When Stevens was able to testify, he reported that the shot firer had lit a match absent-mindedly, and ignited accumulated gas. The commissioners found a list of violations of *The Coal Mines Regulations Act*: there was no underground manager or overman; the company had altered the site prior to the investigation; there had been insufficient ventilation to dilute gasses in the mine's air; there had been poor reporting of earlier gas detection; there was poor management in the use of explosives in the mine (Nova Scotia 1931, p. 209). In 1933 when five men were killed in the Joggins mine, the mines report dealt with the matter simply, according to longstanding convention: "I regret to report that five fatal accidents occurred at this mine during the year" (Nova Scotia 1933, p. 69). There was no Special Report in this instance. Again, in 1935 when seven men died in the Allan Mine in Pictou County, the "cause" was found to be a blown out shot. No blame was laid, though the Acadia Coal Company was shown to respond to the disaster by establishing a rescue station in the mine (*Commission on Acadia Coal* 1938, p. 49). The relative disinterest of the mines reports in such fatalities suggests that they did not sufficiently pose a legitimation crisis to require the reinvigoration of dominant cultural codes. The existing prior plausibility structures that saw the men as somehow responsible would ensure ideological continuity.

The 1940s were comparatively disaster-free, unless one counts the overall malaise in the coal industry. Mechanization was essential if Nova Scotia coal mines were to continue operating, and recognizing this fact only reinforced the call for unions to work with management and government (Abbott 1989, p. 42).

The 663 page "Carroll Commission on Coal" (Canada 1946) reported in detail on the coal industry across Canada, with great volumes of statistical support. In recounting Nova Scotia's history, the commission noted, "A series of strikes also tended to keep production down, the most serious being in 1925 when production fell to 3,843,000 tons" (Canada 1946, p. 65). The report rejected the UMW's call for nationalization of the coal industry, as stated in a complementary recommendation by one of the commissioners: "I believe the situation should be considered as a challenge to private enterprise, and that the government assistance should be continued subject to the private interests making a genuine effort to reorganizing these operations" (Canada 1946, p. 591). The commissioners found that dissatisfaction among Dosco workers was rooted in a desire to get rid of a particular group of managers rather than for nationalization (Canada 1946, p. 592).

"Elaborate machinery" had been put in place by which grievances were negotiated (Canada 1946, p. 316), however "[a]dditional steps [were] necessary to end the industrial warfare which [had] been going on in the Nova Scotia coal fields for generations" (Canada 1946, p. 592). The UMW was called upon to "take whatever steps necessary to strengthen its internal discipline" (Canada 1946, p. 317). The mine workforce was aging, as young men enlisted or sought employment elsewhere. While recognizing the decline of the coal industry, the report noted that "youth" was needed in the mines (Canada 1946, p. 314). Just as the unmined coal should be left if contemporary markets did not demand it, there should be a standing reserve of workers available to extract it.

As coal mining in Nova Scotia lacked both economic and social justification, government and unions needed to collaborate to sustain employment in the face of the threat of capital flight. In the passage below, scarcity problems were substituted with attitude problems in men and managers:

> Employee-employer relations are a matter of emotions as much as a matter of fact: they vary from time to time and from place to place, depending upon factors of human personality as much as upon logic and factual circumstances. In one sense the other two main problems [involving the mine workers], living standards and productivity are aspects of the problem of achieving cooperation for there are no more important determinants of the nature of relations between men and management than the trend of earnings of the men and the trend of productivity of the industry. Also important in determining the state of relations at any given time are the history of past relationships and what the men and management each believe to be the present attitude and degree of efficiency of the other in the mutual enterprise. (Canada 1946, p. 315)

The final administrative move for the Carroll's 1946 report with regards to coal mining in Nova Scotia was to tie individual "prosperity more than ever" to "a maximum cooperation between management and labor, progressive leadership by each is essential" (Canada 1946, p. 318). Joint committees were considered, though it was recognized that these could work only in particular circumstances:

"The success of such committees is dependent upon the personalities of the men involved and the good faith of men and management alike. It is too much to expect that joint production committees will function satisfactorily unless the atmosphere is such that collective bargaining functions smoothly" (Canada, 1946, p. 318). Management/government-miner conflict had become "labor relations" and Nova Scotia workers needed to recognize this or be left behind.

Though there was no single, large-scale mine disaster in 1948, the mines report explained, "there was a total of 38 fatal accidents during the year, eight more than in 1942. The fatal accident rate per 1,000,000 tons of coal raised was 6.46. Excluding those lives lost in major colliery disasters, this is the highest rate since and including 1900. No figures are available for comparison with earlier years" (Nova Scotia 1948, p. 14). Besides a simple statement of this fact, a record of the statistics for the year, and the conventional listing of names, occupation, mine, and cause of accident, there is no further treatment of these fatalities in the report.

1950s and 60s

In the mid-1950s, two major mine disasters in Springhill, Cumberland County (1956, 1958) killed over 100 men, and drew international attention to Nova Scotia mines. The 1957 report on the Springhill explosion opened speculation that the men imprudently caused their own deaths, then foreclosed this possibility by declaring that no one was in a state of non-compliance, though managers and inspectors had known of the misplaced electrical cord that was cut, and then sparked the blast. The report described surviving miners' heroic, death-confronting rescue-recovery efforts, and thereby demonstrated the workers' hierarchical harmony with the managers and inspectors who coordinated the emergency efforts. The cause of the 1956 Springhill explosion was described by its royal commission:

> The Commission considers that there was no single or particular defect in the working of the mine or any particular failure to comply with any regulation of the Coal Mines Regulation Act which caused the explosion. The explosion resulted from an unfortunate combination of circumstances for which no blame can be attached to any individual.

> Hereinafter set forth is a statement of the factors and circumstances which the Commission feels contributed to the cause and origins of the explosion or which might contribute to explosions in the future. Recommendations are given with a view to preventing or avoiding the happening of a similar tragic occurrence in Nova Scotia which may provide for greater safety in mines. (Nova Scotia 1957, p. 10)

While the commission found that "there was not complete or strict compliance" with regulations, there was no blame to be laid. The material cause that sparked the explosion was found to be a power cable that was severed, sparked, and ignited available gas and dust. Though both management and inspectors had known about this unsafely placed cable, no blame was laid. In fact, the rescue-recovery efforts were clear evidence of the organic unity of the community:

> The manner in which the whole of the community of Springhill met this disaster is a matter of particular comment. The great courage and fortitude which was made manifest during the time of the disaster won the admiration of all Canadians. The whole community shared in the united effort that was put forward to save the men who were below ground. For a long period of time it was not known what number, if any, were alive. The Commission wishes to refer to the efforts made by the mine rescue teams, the bare-faced miners as well as the great display of leadership and resourcefulness that was shown by so many officials of the Company, the Department of Mines and the Union officials. The courage and bravery shown by so many during the disaster and following days is a matter of great pride to everyone who knows what took place. At no time was there any dissension as to what steps should be taken in the work of rescue and the efforts of all were united.

> We wish to refer to the leadership given by members of the clergy of all faiths, and to the professional skill of physicians, nurses, and to comment on the help of many others who assisted in the rescue and comfort of men employed in the rescue work during the critical days. The fact that so many were saved was wonderful and is itself the greatest tribute that can be paid to all those persons whose skill and bravery will be forever remembered.

> The Commission wishes to express its deepest sympathy to the wives and families of the men who were lost. The Commission considers that every effort was made by all those who took part in the rescue work to make sure that everything was done to save as many men as possible. (Nova Scotia 1957, p. v)

The tragic romance of coal miners' toughness and solidarity was reinforced further by the "Springhill miracle" of 1958 when twelve men were rescued following six and a half days, and six men were rescued following eight and a half days of radio broadcast and televised rescue-recovery efforts (Beech et al. 1960; Brown 1976, p. 53). In the manner of all other commissioners, (when possible), the 1958 commissioners went to "the place of upheaval" (Nova Scotia 1958, p. 6). The bump interfered with the extension of scientific knowledge: "The closing down of the mine after the tragedy which has been the subject of this investigation, has made it impossible to carry out experiments of the nature suggested. It has to be remembered that there are still no adequate instruments for measuring stress in the solid" (Nova Scotia 1958, p. 6). This report separated human agency from the material conditions of the disaster more completely than other accident reports. Certain knowledge of the "cause" was to be found through further penetration of the rocks, new devices for measurement, and re-readings of seismographic charts from Halifax universities. The stress conditions in the roof, walls, floors, and coal face of the mine were already an object of scientific interest, and the report was able to marshal an impressive collection of texts documenting the coal company's collaboration with experts in efforts to minimize bumps in the Springhill operations.

Both Springhill mines, No. 2 that suffered the bump in 1958, and No. 4 that exploded in 1956 killing 39 men, were closed by the time this report was presented. The "whole of the continent" was sympathetic; the survival of many was "a matter of some wonder." "Comfort" was all the report could offer bereaved families, besides the hope of avoiding or anticipating such upheavals in the future:

> The two mines, Nos. 2 and 4, are now closed, and as such mines constituted the main earning power of the community, economic factors have required very serious consideration. The sympathy of the whole of the continent has been made evident. . . . The period of time during which groups of the men were entombed and the subsequent rescue has been a matter of some wonder. There is general rejoicing that a number of the men were rescued after undergoing hardships of an unbelievable nature. To the wives and families and relatives of the men who were lost, very deep sympathy is extended. Little can be said at this time to comfort the dependents. However, it is hoped that investigations of this nature may lead in some measure to understanding the reasons for this tragedy and possibly lead to mining practices and methods which may avoid or anticipate upheavals or bumps. (Nova Scotia 1958, pp. 7-8)

Determinations of cause of death, and lists of men killed (or references thereto) were followed by "commendations" of the men involved in rescue operations. The tragic circumstances of the disaster and deaths provided a dramatic opportunity for the cooperative attitude of workers to be affirmed through their confrontation with death during the rescue attempts (Nova Scotia 1958, pp. 26-27).

The presentation of the rescue-recovery effort was very dramatic, particularly for the reader acquainted with mining terminology. Given the constant media coverage in the nine days' rescue efforts, and international attention including a visit to the mine and selected miners' homes by Prince Phillip, public knowledge of mining terminology was undoubtedly at an all-time high (Brown 1976). The race to re-establish ventilation and communication and to provide equipped men for the search depended on tremendous coordination and knowledge of dangers peculiar to a collapsed coal mine. The mine's behavior was described as "violence." Each discovery of another pocket of live men was described with accounts of heroic efforts and reminders that the mine environment was potentially responsive to any shifts in pressure, especially the digging necessary to search for survivors and bodies. The subjective experience of the workers was utterly insignificant in the report's efforts to establish the causal chain of events: "We have set out in narrative form the history of the area, the geological structure, and statements of the events which occurred immediately before the tragedy and the heroic and splendid efforts that were made by a great many people in the rescue work. The fact that the mine and the place of the disaster was of very great depth is a matter of significance" (Nova Scotia 1958, p. 52). As the report found no non-compliance with any laws, the "facts" were presented unproblematically as a geological puzzle peculiar to Springhill and the depth of the mine. The wisdom of mining at such depth was not questioned: "with the deepening of mines . . . in all parts of the world it is necessary to correlate all available information in the hope that some conclusions can be reached with respect to the causes giving rise to these situations" (Nova Scotia 1958, p. 6). Nonetheless, the two mine disasters marked the end of commercial coal mining in Springhill.

In the 1950s and 1960s, Pictou County coal mines closed, while Cape Breton mines remained open under Devco. Once most mines were closed in Pictou County (by 1972), nostalgia developed that linked the hard, honest, dangerous work of coal mines with a cultural (almost ethnic) destiny (see Ryan 1992, p. 124). Along with such nostalgia grew, it seems, a sense of entitlement to coal mining that contributed to hostility towards Devco-employed Cape Bretoners, and ultimately to the remarkable public funding provided to the developers of the Westray mine.

THE THIRD WAVE:
THE WORKER AND INTERNAL RESPONSIBILITY (1970-Westray)
"the most important thing to come out of a mine is a miner"

The 1980 *Report of the Commission of Inquiry in to the Explosion in the No. 26 Colliery, Glace Bay,* Nova Scotia was the closest to *The Westray Story* in its time and findings. The findings of the material causes of the two explosions were remarkably similar. However, compared to *The Westray Story*, the explanation for the 1979 explosion and deaths of 12 men was relatively unproblematic. Often written in highly technical language, the 1980 report was targeted at readers with technical mining know-how. The report identified a web rather than a point of causation; the physical source of the disaster was a chain of events that began when the continuous miner struck rock at the coalface, sparked, and ignited gas and coal dust. The chain of physical causes was put in motion through poor coal mine housekeeping and so the joint imprudence of miners and managers. That imprudence was supplemented by the ignorance and apathy of regulators. At another level, the explosion was found to be caused by the absence of a blueprint: there was no ventilation plan for drawing the explosive methane gas away from the coal face. The overall cause, though, was found to be community dependency on continued coal production.

Ironically, the 1980 report "found" a lack of knowledge of the laws. It attributed this to ignorance rather than willful non-compliance on the part of Devco. "Almost no one was aware of many of the applicable safety regulations" (Canada 1980, p. 18). Furthermore, "without provision of any evidence to the contrary, silence indicates assent by the chief [Department of Labor] inspector"

(Canada 1980, p. 28). As well, it was found that the Chief Inspector had given a permissive interpretation of safety regulations to the management of Devco:

> This type of interpretation on [sic] a regulation gives substance to the doubts expressed by the labor union representative about the authority of the Regulations and . . . of the Canada Labor Code as well as the ability of Labor Canada to enforce the statutory requirements. The fact that the unions were not even included in the list of those provided a copy of the letter which deals with the safety and lives of the persons whom they represent, can easily be interpreted as a special accommodation to management. (Canada 1980, p. 28)

The 1980 report also found confusion in the hierarchy of managerial responsibility and, as one witness was quoted as saying, an absence of the craft knowledge that had been present "when we were mining by hand" (Canada 1980, p. 79). The mining community was found to be in a state of decay; the culture of safety had not survived mechanization and had become an empty formalism.

At the level of reports, this melancholy recollection of a lost troop of highly self-disciplined miners is entirely mythical and became a venerated norm only with the development of the internal responsibility system of occupational health and safety. It was accompanied by the myth of the lost strong regulatory agency. The organizational pathology in No. 26 had been such that workers had lost confidence in Labor Canada agents, who were closely associated with the company. Also, the report found that workers were afraid they would be fired if they spoke frankly about unsafe work conditions. As usual, the ameliorative imperative was an extension of bureaucratic control in mines.

In a remarkably gentle reproof to errant bureaucrats, the report recommended that Labor Canada agents should "enforce the Act and Regulations in a firm, consistent and objective manner, free from the effects of former loyalties, personal associations and other social pressures brought about by residing in the coal mining community" (Canada 1980, p. xiii).

Incomplete record keeping or workers' manipulation of safety devices interrupted readings from instruments and, therefore, the commission could not depend on technological representations of underground conditions. The transmission of disciplinary work practices was found to lack bureaucratic rationality, and, as the report noted, "'training by association' . . . perpetuates the unsafe as well as the correct habits" (Canada 1980, p. 80). The mine lacked an adequate ventilation plan: "Because the system evolved, there was no approved long-term ventilation plan" (Canada 1980, p. 30). Production bonuses were associated with unsafe practices, including means of blocking the methane detection device. However, the larger ventilation problem was the "cause" of the explosion, and there was no proof that workers rigged the methanometer during the fatal shift. Before the explosion, the UMW had published "a declaration of non-support for anyone caught tampering with the equipment" (Canada 1980, p. 26). Nonetheless, it was found that workers lacked background on how to properly read their working environment through the monitoring devices. Hence, the report recommended further worker training. Community determination to save jobs was implied to have contributed:

> Production of coal was given a priority over almost all other considerations. This was of such importance in the community that frequently the first question asked of the Commission, particularly in the initial stages of the Inquiry before the public hearings commenced and before any information was offered was, "will the mine be closed?" (Canada 1980, p. 32)

A human drama of a narrow escape by some workers who left the coalface early was interwoven with technical details. The "brushers" rushed to leave early, thereby indicating normal slack "housekeeping." Reactions of the dead men were read through traces left on the machines: (the continuous miner was off), and their actions deduced from the corpses' positions relative to their equipment. The bodies were treated as evidence toward establishing the most probable material cause of the explosion, rather than as indices of the men's potential culpability. Though the report stated that the men died within 15 to 20 seconds of the initial spark at the coalface, the cause of death was not stated explicitly (except in the coroner's report, in the Appendices).

1990s: THE WESTRAY STORY

I argue elsewhere that the release of The Report of the Westray Mine Public Inquiry provided great relief for many relatives of the dead men (Dodd 2001). The report marked the beginning of a withdrawal of many key representatives of the families from public life. The narrative structure and characterizations of actors within the report set the stage for the return of family members to private life, and for the focus on legislative reform. The Report channeled a broad-ranging social and political critique into a campaign for legislative reform that demanded government acceptance of the Report's recommendations. As we will see from a careful consideration of the literary practices of *The Westray Story,* this report was called upon to manage a potential crisis. Compared with the first, sketchy reports on mine fatalities in the mines reports, *The Westray Story* is a luxury item. Its elaborate presentation suggests that the aftermath of the disaster was severely disruptive, or at least potentially so.

The Westray Story: A Predictable Path to Disaster is a boxed set of four volumes, in soft cover. On the cover of each volume is a reproduction of a charcoal sketch: a mine, slightly luminescent before a darkening sky. White letters etch the title and author's name in the twilight above the mine. This was a folksy interpretation of the icon of the post-explosion mine: the photo that dominated television, newspaper representations of the disaster. So, before opening the report, the reader was cued to the aspirations of the text to reconfigure public memory of the explosion and its aftermath. She was reminded also of the media event, of hearing about the explosion, then coverage of the search, the end of the search, then the litany of legal processes. She was reassured, further, that above the murky image of the mine lay a crisp, white explanation:

The Westray Story
A Predictable Path to Disaster

The image had come to represent the social breach of the Westray explosion signaling the legitimation problems that accumulated "under" this image in the explosion's aftermath. The title, "*The Westray Story*," stated the report's claim to fix the causal chain leading to the disaster and the associated characters' relative roles and culpabilities. The subtitle "*A Predictable Path to Disaster*" continued this claim. The title promised that stabilizing **The Westray Story** would attach a causal chain leading back to particular, culpable agents. At least, the sub-title qualified, insofar as they failed to "predict" and turn from the "path to disaster." The spatial representation of the causal "path" to the disaster linked an indefinite number of agents together on the path of predictability, and thus raised the question of responsibility for foresight.

The report identified its author, the Westray Mine Public Inquiry, and more particularly, Justice K. Peter Richard, Commissioner. The Province of Nova Scotia was not mentioned on the cover page. (Compare that with the report of the Marshall Inquiry which has the Nova Scotia coat of arms on its cover.) Thus, the commissioner came to stand for the inquiry in a synecdoche reflecting the report's orientation towards systemically embedded individual responsibility.

A demand for collective identities was met on page iii, with a dramatic black bar slashing almost the width of the page. White letters emerging from black read:

"The most important thing to come out of a mine is the miner."

Frédéric Le Play (1806-1882)

French sociologist and inspector general of mines of France

By invoking the memory of a sociologist-inspector, the report claimed scientific objectivity and the right of administration. It also raised the specter of influence against which the report struggled. The expert's quote was the report's claim to membership in an international science of workplace health and safety. It linked the report also with more immediate precursors, notably the Ham Report (Ontario 1976) and the Burkett Report (Ontario-Canada 1981).

While the quote seemed to support the struggle to remember particular men, it cast them in their economically useful roles, implicitly berating the government for not retrieving the bodies (men-cum-miners-cum-*things*). Hence, the report berated the government for permitting the failure of the disciplinary function of the mine as a means of producing docile workers: "the most important **thing** to come out of a mine is the **miner**." Having constructed the individual deceased men as "miners," the report then stabilized them as passive and thus at once innocent *and* complicit in the production and reproduction of a workplace culture of imprudence. More important than the simple economic production of wealth (via energy-producing coal) was the (re)production of a docile workforce. From people, the mine was to produce "miners" as well as mining families committed to reproducing the disciplinary workplace. The Westray mine failed in that its brutality was too transparent: it was too deadly, too quickly. LePlay's "monographs"—studies of workers' domestic lives centered on finely detailed household budgets of exemplary families—were part of a 19th century backlash against the use of statistics to stabilize social life as an object of scientific knowledge and administrative intervention. However, as Hacking argues, resistance to statistical representations of "normal" human life had the unintended effect of extending the statistical reach into human life:

> LePlay's household budgets were descriptions of individual families that were representative of the workers of a region. They say a lot about how the family lived, its needs, its pleasures, its possibilities. LePlay thought that he could deduce from the budget the state of the family and its prospects. Engel's[4] budgets were something entirely different. They were measures of populations, not of "social species" in the style of Balzac or LePlay.

> The taming of chance seems irresistible. Let a man propose an antistatistical idea to reflect individuality and to resist the probabilification of the universe; the next generation effortlessly coopts it so that it becomes part of the standard statistical machinery of information and control. (Hacking 1990, p. 141)

LePlay's tragic replaying of this dialectic of resistance and co-option, individual and statistically enforced norm, set the tragic plot for *The Westray Story*. With this opening reference to LePlay—mineralogist turned sociologist-bureaucrat (as Inspector of Mines)—the report began an ambivalent self-relation evident in a couple of identity problems. First, it was a clear statement that the report needed "scientific" legitimation beyond its evidentiary contents. Also, the report was cursed with the anxiety of its own futility—an anxiety evident in the juxtaposition of LePlay's centuries-old warning about safety, with the "predictability" of the Westray accident. Finally, the LePlay citation set the tone for the report's work of recasting the embodied knowledge of miners and family members in financially manageable terms. Just as LePlay translated the familial lives of workers into detailed domestic budgets, the Inquiry report translated the human loss at Westray into an aberration in governmental accounting.

The next facing page (vol. 1, p. v) continues with the black bars, this time, highlighting a terse statement of fact at the top of the page, and a dedication at the bottom. The factual anchor of the document is this:

At 5:20 am on 9 May 1992
the Westray mine exploded taking the
lives of the following 26 miners.

The normative frame opened by the Le Play quote (vol. 1, p. iii) of a progressing international science of mining health and safety was punctuated by this breach of the norm. The report's reporting began at this moment. Establishing the parameters of the focus of this report, this page cast the "mine" as an agent that exploded and took lives. It took not the lives of men, but of miners. The names of the dead followed, listed in alphabetical order, with their ages at the date of death. This was the first of the Nova Scotia accident reports that I saw that listed the deceased before the findings of the inquiry. In other reports, names were listed by company number in an appendix to the main report. The individuals, brought together by the fact of Westray's breach in the normative practices of safe mining, were the ground on which the monument of *The Westray Story* stood. Again cast in a black bar, the report anchored its legitimacy in commonsense experience.

This Report is dedicated to their memory.

This stated commitment to the "memory" of the men moved to textually "settle" a belief about the Westray explosion that would limit, and re-present, possible narratives of causation along with their associated characters and relations between them. It recognized the family members' fears that their men's reputations—their "memory"—was in jeopardy.

The report's narrative began with three pages, without title. This began by repeating the punctuation of time effected by the explosion. However, the report changed the temporal rhythm to that of an ordinary day, and thus focused on situated life: "In the early morning of 9 May 1992. . . ." Further, the report moved the breach out of the international history of mining health and safety into a precise locale: ". . . a violent explosion rocked the tiny community of Plymouth. . . ." A "tiny community" was acted upon, and violently agitated by an explosion. The shock waves moved outward: ". . . just east of Stellarton, in Pictou County, Nova Scotia." Having begun from the impact on the living, the report looked to the dead: "The explosion occurred in the depths of the Westray coal mine"—thus the cause of this explosion remained hidden from natural vision.

All this was prior knowledge, shared by reader and report. The first "new" point established the report as authoritative interpreter in the continuation of this sentence: "The explosion occurred in the depths of the Westray coal mine, *instantly* killing the 26 miners working there at the time" (vol. 1, p. vii, emphasis added). This was the second, belief-fixing move of the report. It continued the implicit criticism of the government's failure to get "the most important thing" out of the mine, by the imperative of establishing time of death. Without this, there could be no rest for the ghosts that continued to haunt the families (Dodd 2001). The report sealed the mine, and thoughts of the men's last moments authoritatively putting the ghosts to rest: "*instantly killing* the 26." At the same time, with the delivery of this "new" information, the report simultaneously claimed authority to illuminate the obscure causes of the explosion, deaths, and social disruption, and shifted speculation away from the men's suffering and their reflections on death.

In the more detailed account of the "propagation" of the explosion that followed pages later, the *Executive Summary* conceded a more articulated account of the deaths that admits speculation about the dying men's experiences. Hence, "instantly killing" was a substitution for a sequence of possible experiences, as follows:

- The gas would be ignited in much the same way that the spark from the flint of a cigarette lighter will ignite the gas emitted from the lighter reservoir.
- The ignition caused a rolling flame to travel . . . consuming all the oxygen in the roadways and leaving deadly quantities of carbon monoxide in its place.
- The rolling flame did not develop into a methane explosion, although it did increase in intensity.
- . . . three factors combined to cause the flame to propagate into a methane explosion . . .
- The resulting shock wave then created . . . a full-blown coal-dust explosion.
- The resulting coal-dust explosion then moved rapidly through the entire mine, causing death and devastation in a matter of a few seconds. (vol. 4, p. 22)

In the untitled introductory pages, the report suggested that the time of death coincided with the spark. Having dedicated itself to the "memory" of the men, and authoritatively fixed the time of death, the report set the minimal conditions for further "factual" reporting. That is, it evaded potential violence by meeting family members' urgent demand that the men be honored in public following their prolonged subjection to scrutiny and speculation during the aftermath.

Justice Richard assumed the role of reporter, offering himself as an author in the first person: "On 15 May 1992, I was appointed by Order in Council to inquire into and report on this disaster." *Commissioner* Richard was conjured into existence, as such, by a document—an Order-in-Council (vol. 1, p. vii). In assuming sole authorship of this introduction to the report, the commissioner became the synthesizing character holding together and thus limiting the manifold voices represented in the text. At the same time, the commissioner laid an experiential claim to represent all those who delivered testimony before him during the inquiry hearings. The "original fullness of meaning"—all the possible perspectives of witnesses and commentators—was limited by the commissioner's sole authorship. This became *his* story (Green 1992, p. 23). By assuming the authorial position, the Commissioner-character continued in his role of "host" and "moderator" in a truth-telling forum. He was an anthropologist of coal mining culture, and as with all social science reports, his subjects could not talk back (Dorothy Smith 1999).

The description of the commissioner's fieldwork was filled with images of domesticity and the unique collectivism of the coal industry:

> The industry is very close-knit with an interdependence, camaraderie, and fellowship that may be unique in modern-day business. And people in the industry, at all levels, regard what occurred at Westray as a personal matter affecting them as if it had happened in their own backyard. It is for them a family tragedy. I suspect that these attitudes have deep historic roots. (vol. 1, p. vii)

The report contributed to the romance of coal mining, part of the broader genre of romances about primary resource industries. "All levels" shared "deep historic roots" in the industry. Of course, some work and die, others manage and move on, still others profit then reinvest without ever seeing the mine; this separation too has "deep historic roots." As well, "people . . . at all levels" in the industry were identified with the family members of men who were killed. It affected them all as if it happened "in their own backyard," and "as a family tragedy." This metaphor stretched plausibility, particularly given that the explosion occurred quite literally in one family's "own backyard." Their loss was horribly real—the figurative relationship of the real parents and their "miner-son" with the rest of the "coal industry family" was hardly plausible. The metaphor only worked if the metonymy connecting the particular young man with "miner" in general had been established. The report worked on this metonymic relationship, following the tradition of mine accident reports by linking all workers together under the exigencies of "survival." In this, of course, the report affirmed its membership in the genre of coal mine accident reports by substituting the articulation of diverging interests with an integrated model of social relations. The report continued:

> There are few industries in which one's safety, indeed one's very survival, is so inextricably linked to the attitudes, practices, concerns, and behaviour of fellow workers. Truly, in the underground coal mining environment, you are "your brother's keeper." The miner who sneaks a smoke while underground is risking the lives of his fellow miners. On 7 December 1992, the flick of a cigarette lighter underground caused the death of eight miners at the Southmountain Coal Company in Virginia. (vol. 1, p. vii)

Having laid the question of the timing of the deaths to rest in the second sentence, the report brought the question of worker responsibility into play, but deferred explicit judgment of the Westray dead. Compare this with the decisive opening sentence of the Marshall Inquiry's *Digest of Findings and Recommendations*: "The criminal justice system failed Donald Marshall, Jr. at virtually every turn from his arrest and wrongful conviction for murder in 1971 up to, and even beyond, his acquittal by the Court of Appeal in 1983" (Nova Scotia 1989). In detailing the interdependence of coal miners, the report moved from intentional acts (i.e., "attitudes") to psychologically produced acts that were not necessarily self-willed or even conscious (i.e., "behavior"). Anxiety about the responsibility of the Westray dead for their own and others' deaths was brought into play. "Truly, in the underground coal mining environment, you are 'your brother's keeper.'" This resonated in the anxious direction of worker imprudence and families' ethical responsibility; beyond that, in the direction of broader social responsibility for Westray; beyond that, in the even broader direction of questions about inter-personal responsibility in the rest of society; and finally, beyond that to questions about the just "order" of the universe. Appropriating the story of Cain and Abel, the report transformed the imperative of caring for others into a self-care that was dependent on mutual monitoring. The report then recounted a parable of worker imprudence, an act of selfish indulgence that the report presented as leaving a clear causal link to the deaths of his eight coworkers. The report did not let the Westray workers off the hook just yet, but left the possibility of their culpability in play.

However, setting up a contrast with the Virginia case with its (ostensibly) clear, easily established chain of causation, leading unproblematically to worker imprudence, the report began to distinguish Westray from *that kind of* tragedy. The Virginia case was given as an archetypal breach of the normative practices of "the underground coal mining industry" that began with worker imprudence. Having made the association between lifestyle risks and workplace risks noted in the Burkett Report, *The Westray Story* held that the Westray case was something other than the Virginia case.

And so, the report moved to generalities, away from personalities and individual moral failings (or missed chances for heroism). "The Westray tragedy is regarded in the industry as a black mark against coal mining in general rather than as a merely localized event" (vol. 1, p. vii). Since the Westray tragedy was a threat to coal mining "in general," it was essential to the industry itself that this "tragedy" be reconstituted in memory as an aberration.

Having gone native, the commissioner "received a remarkable degree of cooperation from the industry, which, while being most encouraging, underscored the solemn responsibility [he] had assumed" (vol. 1, p. vii). As an initiate into the secrets of this obscure culture, the commissioner assured readers that the coal industry was *not* a conflict-ridden culture. His "solemn responsibility" was to heal disintegration among workers, owners and regulators (or, rather, to quiet any antagonism), the knowledge-making authority of technological expertise, and the impartiality of law. The report's work of reconstituting this code, thereby returning its transparency, began here, once the particular characters were stabilized into a coherent entity, "the coal industry." The breach of the explosion was to be healed by identifying the author-Commissioner-character at once with the coal industry's life-world and its history within social science. Once reified, the mine industry was an "anxious" agent, willing to learn to "prevent" tragedy in the future. "The coal industry—miners, managers, operators, and regulators—is most anxious to determine what can be learned as a result of this tragedy and what can be done to prevent another" (vol. 1, p. vii). Working with, rather than against, the hypostasized "coal industry" (including regulators) was the best way to move beyond "this tragedy" toward "what can be done to prevent another."

These three pages interwove class interests. The report referred to a common "backyard," and described what occurred at Westray as "a personal matter" for "people in the industry." "The coal industry" as a whole "is most anxious to determine what can be learned" and to "determine" "what can be done to prevent another" such "tragedy."

The report turned now to another report for validation: *Towards Safe Production* (Ontario-Canada 1981). With the specter of the imprudent Virginian worker's failure to practice safe production, the report opened outward to other jurisdictions and inward to the prudential responsibilities of workers. However, since "the entire thrust of the [1981 Burkett Report] is to increase and to promote safe practices in mines" (vol. 1, p. vii), the *need* for a Westray report was an indictment of its precursor and the policy effectiveness of inquiry commissions generally. The Westray commissioner stated: "As I read *Towards Safe Production*, I was impressed with the clarity and wisdom" of the definition of government responsibility for mine regulation (vol. 1, p. vii). The multi-jurisdictional character of global capital means that transnational corporations have institutional knowledge of manifold regulatory environments. Governments, as regulators, are more idiotic. That is, policy reports display surprise at the regulatory discoveries of policy reports produced even in jurisdictions of very close proximity. After invoking *Towards Safe Production*, the report clearly delineated the range of action available to regulators around mine safety:

> The only completely safe mine is a closed mine. By the same token, the only completely safe aircraft is on the ground with the engines off. The only truly safe automobile is the one parked in the garage. Once a mine is open, there begins the constant process of trade-off between production and safety. From the chief executive officer to the miner at the working face, the objective must be to operate the mine in a manner that ensures the personal safety of the worker over the economic imperatives of increased production. The two seemingly competing concepts—safety and production—must be so harmonized that they can co-exist without doing harm to each other. (vol. 1, pp. vii-viii)

Without the "trade-off" of worker safety, there could be no "production." This suggested that the riskier the mine, the more the productive potential. At the extreme end of "perfect" safety was stasis. Again, the report noted the need and potential for "harmonizing" the "objectives" of the C.E.O. and the "miner at the working face." Safety and "economic *imperatives*" were in tension. The regulator's role was to effect this (impossible) "harmonization" without "harm." (A "trade-off" implies a zero-sum game—when one interest gains the other loses; a "harmony" implies a full expression of interests working in concert with one another.) The report continued:

It is here that the regulator must assume the role of monitor and aggressively ensure that the balance is understood and maintained. In this sense, the function of the regulator is both instructive and supervisory. As one provincial mine inspector in Ontario told me, "Ideally, if we perform our duties properly we will eventually work ourselves out of a job." As I read *Towards Safe Production* I was impressed with the clarity and wisdom of this regulatory role. (vol. 1, p. viii)

The "trade-off" was now a "balance." Still, the "ideal" presented by the Ontario regulator was one of monitoring and instructing—as if corporate entities needed to be "instructed" in how to maximize safety in the workplace. The Nova Scotia Mines Inspectors' failure to do their jobs at Westray was brought into play here, and thus the report came close to naming some of the prime suspects for direct-line culpability, only to remain in the realm of generality. The mines inspectors' failure to "monitor and aggressively ensure that the balance" was "understood and maintained" came into play in contrast with the Ontario regulator's pious "ideal." Whereas the report brought the possibility of worker culpability into play in contrast with a negative example (the imprudent worker), it brought the possibility of inspector culpability into play in contrast with an ideal (the Ontario inspector who wanted to work himself out of a job).

The Commissioner-character acknowledged the report's legitimate origins, and replied with virtual short-temper: "The Order in Council that established this Inquiry gives me power to 'inquire into . . . whether the occurrence was or was not preventable.' Of course it was" (vol. 1, p. viii). This was the third belief-fixing move of the report. It eliminated the providential possibility from the range of causal explanations of the explosion. And, having admitted the omnipresence of contingency, authoritatively asserted that the "occurrence" was within human control. "For this Report we have chosen the title *The Westray Story: A Predictable Path to Disaster* to convey that message. The message is that the Westray tragedy was predictable and, therefore, preventable" (vol. 1, p. viii). Tragedies, in the Aristotelian sense, must be predictable, but not preventable in the sense that this report means. Classically speaking, tragedies must be the necessary outcomes of the actions *proper* to their characters. "All human happiness or misery takes the form of action; the end for which we live is a certain kind of activity, not a quality. Character gives us qualities, but it is in our actions—what we do—that we are happy or the reverse" (Aristotle, *Poetics*, 1450a20). The real tragedy here may be the administrative optimism of the report itself: "The Report contains recommendations and suggestions aimed at avoiding a similar occurrence in the future" (The Westray Story, vol. 1, p. viii).

Having brought into play and problematized some of the categories of prime suspects for direct-line culpability, (i.e., workers, regulators, C.E.O), the report closes this possibility off: "Anyone who hopes to find in this Report a simple and conclusive answer as to how this tragedy happened will be disappointed (vol. 1, p. vii)." To win the stable redemption of their men's characters, family members would have to relinquish their right to identify other individual culprits.

The report stated as common sense that the "*Westray Story*" (as it called itself) was "a complex mosaic of actions, omissions, mistakes, incompetence, apathy, cynicism, stupidity, and neglect" (vol. 1, p. viii). The report denied any single causal line from individual human action to the explosion and deaths. It lumped together those "serenely uninformed (the willfully blind) or the cynically self-serving" who sought such a simple causal line. Thus, the report suggested commonality between the former premier Donald Cameron and some family members' demands for retribution. Tangled together, the report closed at once the possibility that the men would be blamed, as well as any hope for tracing responsibility back to policymakers and entrepreneurs: "It was clear from the outset that the loss of 26 lives at Plymouth, Pictou County, in the early morning hours of 9 May 1992 was not the result of a single definable event or misstep" (vol. 1, p. viii).

Having closed the way to retribution, and constructed the "harmony" among "all levels" of the ideal "close-knit" "coal industry," the report considered the role of the management at Westray. At the same time, the report reflected on the conditions necessary for its own reportage. This attempt at transparency about the conditions necessary for the report's colloquial "20/20 vision" stated, though in disguise, its very good reasons for anxiety about its own potency as a map for reform:

> This Report has been written with the benefit of hindsight, which, as the saying goes, provides 20/20 vision. Many of the incidents that now appear to fit into the mosaic might at the time, and of themselves, have seemed trivial. Viewed in context, these seemingly isolated incidents constitute a mind-set or operating philosophy that appears to favour expediency over intelligent planning and that trivializes safety concerns. Indeed, management at Westray displayed a certain disdain for safety and appeared to regard safety-conscious workers as the wimps in the organization. To its discredit, the management at Westray, through either incompetence or ignorance, lost sight of the basic tenet of coal mining: that safe mining is good business. As one mining executive remarked to me in June 1996 during a mine visit to Alabama, "We could not afford to operate an unsafe mine, due to the high cost of accidents and downtime." Certainly, the validity of this concept was never more obvious than in the horrible aftermath of Westray. (vol. 1, p. ix)

A cursory glance at the use of the expression "Union Carbide in Bhopal" in business ethics literature gives a sense of this line of thinking (Dodd 1995). One of the stabilizing notions in the aftermath of industrial disasters is that corporations suffer financial setbacks due to the cost of the deaths. At best, this is highly contentious. This paragraph baldly contradicted the report's construction on page viii of a "trade-off" between safety and production. As well, in the excerpt above, the report hedged around blaming Westray management: note the qualified nature of the phrases "a certain disdain" and "appeared to regard." Management at Westray was depicted in passive terms; they "lost sight" "through either incompetence or ignorance." Thus, the report repressed the possibility of a cold-blooded "trade-off" of safety for financial gain. In asserting that safe production is "good business" in a strictly monetary sense, the report turned to an authority beyond the text. A mine owner from Alabama was imported to prop up this assertion. Even then, it lacked plausibility; only a Canadian's conviction that "we" are less exploitative than any Alabama mine owner could lend this statement credence.

The report did not rest easily with its own assertion:

> The tale that unfolds in the ensuing narrative is the *Westray Story*. It is a story of incompetence, of mismanagement, of bureaucratic bungling, of deceit, of ruthlessness, of cover-up, of apathy, of expediency, and of cynical indifference. It is a tragic story, with the inevitable moments of pathos and heroism. The *Westray Story* concerns an event that, in all good common sense, ought not to have occurred. It did occur—and that is our unfortunate legacy. (vol. 1, p. ix)

CONCLUSION

Inquiry reports do not bury facts as much as they prepare facts for burial. Industrial disasters expose the fact that working people die while owners profit, and this creates the potential for political crisis. Inquiry reports play an ambivalent role in the aftermath of disaster: they expose the conditions that led to the deaths and at the same time they work to render the public memory of these conditions safe for capitalism. They manage the fact that a long line of inquiries have "found" similar—even identical—causes of workplace fatalities, and that there would have been no accident if existing laws had been enforced. They divert attention from companies and regulatory structures by shifting focus onto individual managers, inspectors, and workers. They characterize some workers as "obedient" and "cautious," others as "imprudent," and so aim to drive wedges into solidarity by characterizing the individual workers as types of people, or characters that reflect cultural prejudices. The threat that the dead and injured may be blamed places intense pressure on relatives in a contest over the honor and memory of the dead. As well, family members struggle against the transformation of their particular man into a character type and then a statistic (Dodd 1995, 2001).

As we saw repeatedly in the reports, individuals who work in mines are reified into the category of "miner." "The miner" then assumes characteristics of its own, in a hyperbolic ascription of agency to a concept; e.g., "The miner tends to ignore workplace risk." Finally, the report demands that such "miners" need more extensive bureaucratic monitoring. Thus, the report presents an extension on bureaucratic capitalism as the solution to any problem with bureaucratic capitalism. Reports limit reflection of the class antagonism of bureaucratic capitalism, they substitute the systemic crisis with the story of an aberration, and they represent themselves—and increased bureaucratic control—as the resolution to the crisis.

Each report works to engage its readers in the fiction that its recommendations are both sufficient to prevent another disaster and likely to be implemented and enforced. This is an embarrassment because inquiry after inquiry has "discovered" the same problems and recommended the same solutions only for disaster to "strike" again. Each report must convince its readers that it really has "discovered" something new about the cause of the disaster, and that its recommendations are equally new insights into possible preventative measures. The key message must be that the disaster was caused by ignorance rather than a failure of political will, or that where there has been a failure of political will, this, too, is an aberration that has been "discovered" and can be prevented now, and only now that the inquiry has done its work.

The Westray Story brought great relief to many relatives of men who were killed in the mine. Though family members knew that many of their key demands were not met by the report, they experienced an affirmation of their sense that the men were not responsible for their own deaths (Dodd 2001). Media critics praised *The Westray Story: A Predictable Path to Disaster* as a hard-hitting report that traced the ultimate cause of the explosion and deaths deep into organizational malaise in the Nova Scotia Labor Department, and patronage between developers and government. Reports often provide opportunities for trade unions and other interested groups to seize upon particular recommendations to further an agenda for change. My argument here is not that inquiries and their reports are never useful, but rather that their primary function is to legitimize bureaucratic capitalism. This is true especially in light of the probability that the key recommendations will not be enforced even where they are adopted.

The tragedy of *The Westray Story*, as with more than a century of reports that preceded it, lies not only in the deaths and damage. The tragedy of such bureaucratic reports lies also in the vain aspiration of their authors and readers: we seek to settle the crisis of the aftermath *without* losing the impetus for change. Yet to settle on the terms given in inquiry reports means precisely to lose that impetus.

ENDNOTES

1. Deaths per million tons of coal produced varied little from 1900 to the decline of Nova Scotia coal production in the 1950s. Annual death rates ranged between 1.24 to 6.45 in the highest years of coal production, with disasters in 1917 and in 1918 raising the rates for those years. Nova Scotia Mines Reports.
2. See Table 1 *Coal Mine Disasters, Nova Scotia 1873-2003 (4 or more fatalities)* for a more complete list. Also see Table 2 *Some Key Dates in Nova Scotia Coal Mine Regulation* and Table 3 *Selected Commissions of Inquiry Pertaining to Nova Scotia Coal Mines.*
3. MacEwan describes the report of the Provincial Department of Mines as "a lengthy and technical document" that "accused the Dominion Coal Company, as a corporate entity, of responsibility for the deaths; also accused were Alex MacEachern, company superintendent for the New Waterford District, Angus R. MacDonald, manager of

Table 1. Coal Mine Disasters, Nova Scotia 1873-2003
(4 or more fatalities)

Date	Place	Number killed	Cause
1873	Drummond Pictou Co	60	Explosion of gas
1878	Sydney Mines CB	6	Explosion of gas
1880	Albion Pictou Co	6	Flood
1880	Albion Pictou Co	44	Explosion
1883	Vale Pictou Co	7	Explosion
1885	Vale Pictou Co	13	Explosion
1891	Springhill No 1 Colchester	125	Explosion
1899	Caledonia CB	10	Explosion
1905	Reserve Mines CB	5	Explosion
1905	Dominion No 2 CB	4	Explosion
1908	Port Hood CB	10	Explosion
1914	Drummond Pictou Co	7	Boiler explosion
1917	Dominion No 12 CB	65	Explosion
1918	Allan Mine Pictou Co	88	Explosion
1924	Allan Mine Pictou Co	4	Explosion
1924	Inverness No 1 CB	4	Roof fall
1930	Victoria CB	7	Explosion
1931	Victoria CB	6	Explosion
1932	Maple Leaf No 4 Colchester	5	Explosion
1935	Allan Pictou Co	7	Explosion
1938	Princess Glace Bay CB	21	Cable break, rake
1943	Dominion No 2 CB	4	Men fell
1952	McGregor Pictou County	19	Explosion
1952	Dominion No 20 CB	7	Explosion
1954	Springhill No 2 Colchester	5	Bump
1956	Springhill No 4 Colchester	39	Explosion
1958	Springhill No 2 Colchester	75	Bump
1979	Devco No 26 CB	12	Explosion
1992	Estray Pictou County	26	Explosion

Sources: Nova Scotia 1873-1980; Grice, 1980).

Table 2. Some Key Dates in Nova Scotia Coal Mine Regulation

Date	Event
1720	Commercial coal mining begins at Cow Bay
1825	General Mining Association (GMA) monopoly begins
1851	Combination of Workmen no longer illegal
1858	Inspector of Mines Office established
1858	GMA monopoly ends
1864	New *Combination of Workmen Act*
1864	Provincial militia intervene in Cape Breton stroke
1864-1876	At least four strikes at Sydney Mines
1868	Strike at Cow Bay, CB
1873	*Coal Mines Regulation Act* (general engineering requirements)
1879	Provincial Workmen's Association (PWA) in Springhill
1887	PWA wins non-compulsory check-off of union dues in some mines
1888	*Mines Arbitration Act* sets up Arbitration Board
1893	An *Act For Further Encouragement of Coal Mining* creates Dominion Coal Company (Domco) in CB
1900	*Coal Mines Regulations Act:* miners to be paid in legal currency, but check off of store debts, rent, etc. allowed—truck system extended
c1900	Coal cutting machines introduced
1907	*Industrial Disputes Investigation Act,* Canada (IDIA)
1909	United Mine Workers of America (UMW), District 26 formed
1909	Strike by UMW at Domco, PWA & scabs continue work, militia presence
1910	UMW workers return to work; first NS *Workmen's Compensation Act*
1913	UMW District 26 Charter revoked—lack of membership
1914-1918	World War One
1915	*Workmen's Compensation Act* Nova Scotia—no fault coverage, WCB
1917-1919	United Mine Workers of Nova Scotia (UMWNS) formed, amalgamated with PWA to become district 26, UMW
1920	British Empire Steel Corporation (BESCO) formed, controls most steel and coal production in Nova Scotia
1921	"Montreal Agreement" increased wages and "peace obligation," i.e., no strike

Table 2. (Cont'd.)

Date	Event
1922	29% wage cut recommended; UMW calls slowdown, then 100% strike; Cape Breton county a "police zone" with troops and provincial police
1922	17% wage regained, strike ended
1923	Miners on strike in sympathy with steelworkers, militia again in Sydney, District 26 leaders McLachlan and Livingstone arrested for "seditious libel," UMW International revokes District 26 Charter, strike ends
1920-1925	Strikes (at least 58 in the Sydney coalfield) negotiations, UMW District 26 reinstated, militia and police presence
1925	Striker William Davis shot and killed by company police
1926	*Industrial Disputes Investigation Act* (Nova Scotia)
1927-1937	*CMRA* amended for obligatory union dues check-off
1928	BESCO becomes Dominion Steel and Coal Company (DOSCO)
1937	*Trade Union Act* employers required to recognize trade unions etc.
1938-1939	Glace Bay strike against mechanization, machinery removed
1938-1940	Wildcat strikes
1939-1945	World War Two, federal regulation of coal industry
1944	Federal law grants rights to union membership, certification, and a "peace obligation" for the duration of a contract
1947	District-wide strike of miners in Nova Scotia, ends without state force, with slight pay increase, production bonus, and willingness to mechanize
1947-1951	Mechanization, decline in mine employment
1950s	Steep decline in coal mining in Nova Scotia
1967	Devco created (Crown corporation purchased DOSCO's mines)
1989	Westray coal mine begun in Pictou county (opened in 1991)
2001	Last underground coal mine closed in Nova Scotia

Sources: Nova Scotia. *Department of Mines Annual Reports;* Abbott 1989; Robertson 1994; Frank 1993; Stanley 1993; MacEwan 1976).

Table 3. Selected Commissions of Inquiry Pertaining to
Nova Scotia Coal Mines

Date	Commission	To inquire into and report on:
1886	Labor Com	All questions arising out of the conflict of labor and capital
1895	Gilpin Report	The cause, history, and effects of fires in the Pictou Coal Mines
1908	Miners' Pensions	
1910	Hours of Labor	
1917	Workers Compensation	
1925	Duncan Com on Coal	
1926	NS Submission: Maritime Rights	
1932	Duncan Com on Coal	Income, wages, hours, conditions; costs of production, etc.
1934	Jones Economic Com	N.S.'s economic welfare within Confederation
1938	Carroll Com on Acadia Coal	The financial position and affairs of the Acadia Coal Company etc.
1946	Carroll	The coal industry in Canada . . .
1957	Explosion Springhill No. 4	
1958	Springhill Bump	
1966	Donald Com	The Cape Bretin Coal problem
1976	Ham Com (Ont.)	Health and safety of mine workers
1980	Explosion in No. 26	Explosion in the No. 26 Colliery, Glace Bay, Cape Breton
1981	Toward Safe Production or Burkett Report (Ontario-Canada)	Safety in Mines and Mining Plants in Ontario
1997	The Westray Story	Causes of the Westray mine explosion and deaths

No. 12 colliery, and MacLeod MacIntosh, provincial deputy inspector of mines."
He refers to the 1917 Mines Report, though I found no report to match this description.
MacEwan continues, describing charges laid against these officials and against the
company (MacEwan 1976, p. 49). Charges were later dropped.
4. Engel was the director of the Prussian statistical office.

REFERENCES

Secondary Sources

Abbott, K. (1989) The Coal Miners and the Law in Nova Scotia: From the 1864 Combination of Workmen Act to the 1947 Trade Union Act. In M. Earle (ed.), *Workers
and the State in Twentieth Century Nova Scotia* (pp. 24-46). Halifax: Acadiensis.

Aristotle. (1941) *The Basic Works of Aristotle.* R. McKeon (trans.). New York: Random
House.

Beech, H. D., and Lucas, R. A. (eds.). (1960) *Individual and Group Behaviour in a
Coal Mine Disaster.* Washington: National Academy of Sciences—National Research
Council.

Bloom, H. (1975) *A Map of Misreading.* New York: Oxford University Press.

Brown, R. D. (1976) *Blood on the Coal: The Story of the Springhill Mining Disasters.*
Windsor: Lancelot.

Dodd, S. (1995, July) Restitching Reality: How TNCs Evade Accountability For Industrial
Disaster. *Alternate Routes, XII,* 23-63.

Dodd, S. (1999) Unsettled Accounts After Westray. In C. McCormick (ed.), *The Westray
Chronicles* (pp. 218-249). Halifax: Fernwood.

Dodd, S. (2001) *The Writing of 'The Westray Story': A Discourse Analysis of the
Aftermath of the Westray Coal Mine Explosion.* Ph.D. Dissertation. Toronto: York
University.

Earle, M. (1989) "Down with Hitler and Silby Barrett": The Cape Breton Miners'
Slowdown Strike of 1941. In M. Earle (ed.), *Workers and the State in Twentieth
Century Nova Scotia* (pp. 109-144). Halifax: Acadiensis.

Earle, M., and McKay, I. (1989) Introduction: Industrial Legality in Nova Scotia. In
M. Earle (ed.), *Workers and the State in Twentieth Century Nova Scotia* (pp. 9-23).
Halifax: Acadiensis

Fairclough, N. (1995) *Critical Discourse Analysis: The Critical Study of Language.*
London: Longman.

Frank, D. (1993) The 1920s: Class and Region, Resistance and Accommodation.
In E. J. Forbes and D. Muise (eds.), *The Atlantic Provinces in Confederation*
(pp. 233-271). Toronto: University of Toronto.

Glasbeek, H., and Tucker, E. (1999) Death by Consensus: The Westray Story. In
C. McCormick (ed.), *The Westray Chronicles.* Halifax: Fernwood.

Green, B. S. (1992) *Knowing the Poor: A Case-Study in Textual Reality Construction.*
Brookfield: Gregg Revivals.

Green, B. S. (1993) *Gerontology and the Construction of Old Age.* New York: DeGruyter.

Hacking, I. (1990) *The Taming of Chance.* Cambridge: Cambridge University.

MacEwan, P. (1976) *Miners and Steelworkers: Labor in Cape Breton.* Toronto: Samuel
Stevens Hakkert and Company.

Robertson, I. R. (1994) The 1850s: Maturity and Reform. In P. A. Buckner and J. G. Reid (eds.), *The Atlantic Region to Confederation* (pp. 333-359). Toronto: University of Toronto Press.

Ryan, J. H. (1992) *Coal in Our Blood: 200 Years of Coal Mining in Nova Scotia's Pictou County.* Halifax: Fomac.

Smith, Dorothy. E. (1990a) *Texts, Facts and Femininity: Exploring the Relations of Ruling.* New York: Routledge.

Smith, Dorothy. E. (1990b) *The Conceptual Practices of Power: A Feminist Sociology of Knowledge.* Toronto: University of Toronto.

Smith, Dorothy. E. (1999) *Writing the Social: Critique, Theory, and Investigations.* Toronto: University of Toronto.

Smith, Doug. (2000) *Consulted to Death: How Canada's Workplace Health and Safety System Fails Workers.* Winnipeg: Arbeiter Ring.

Stanley, D. (1993) The 1960s: The Illusions and Realities of Progress. In E. J. Forbes and D. Muise (eds.), *The Atlantic Provinces in Confederation* (pp. 421-459). Toronto: University of Toronto Press.

Tucker, E. (1995) The Westray Mine Disaster and Its Aftermath: The Politics of Causation. *Canadian Journal of Law and Society, 10*: 91-123.

Government Documents

Canada. 1886 Royal Commission on Relations between Labor and Capital.

Canada. 1946. Coal Industry in Canada. (Carroll).

Canada. 1966 The Cape Breton Coal Problem. (MacDonald).

Canada. 1980. Explosion in No. 26 Collier Glace Bay, Nova Scotia on February 24, 1979.

Nova Scotia. House of Assembly Journals 1848-1940.

Nova Scotia. Department of Mines, Annual Report (1858-various years)

Nova Scotia. 1895. Report on the Cause, History and Effects of Fires in the Pictou County Coal Mines. (Gilpin).

Nova Scotia. 1908. Report on Miners' Pensions.

Nova Scotia. 1917. Workmen's Compensation.

Nova Scotia. 1925. Commission on Coal. (Duncan).

Nova Scotia. 1926. Submission to the Royal Commission on Maritime Rights.

Nova Scotia. 1932. *Commission on Coal.* (Second Duncan).

Nova Scotia. 1934. *Economic Commission.* (Jones).

Nova Scotia. 1938. Commission on Acadia Coal. (Carroll).

Nova Scotia. 1957. Explosion in Springhill No. 4.

Nova Scotia. 1958. The Bump in Springhill No. 2.

Nova Scotia. 1989. Royal Commission on the Donald Marshall, Jr., Prosecution

Nova Scotia. 1996. Occupational Health and Safety Act. Halifax: S.N.S.

Nova Scotia. 1997. The Westray Story: A Predictable Path to Disaster: Report of the Westray Mine Public Inquiry. (Richard).

Ontario. 1976. Health and Safety of Mine Workers. (Ham).

Ontario-Canada. 1981. Towards Safe Production: Safety in Mines and Mining Plants in Ontario. (Burkett).

CHAPTER 10

Accountability and Reform in the Aftermath of the Westray Mine Explosion

Eric Tucker

DEATH IN THE DOMINION

The Westray mine exploded on May 9, 1992 killing all 26 miners who were working underground at the time. It quickly became apparent that the explosion was not an unforeseeable accident, but rather the predictable result of unsafe and unlawful mining practices, and lax regulatory enforcement. Inadequate ventilation allowed methane concentrations to reach explosive levels and coal dust had been permitted to accumulate. A spark, most probably from an underground mining machine striking a rock, ignited the gas, growing into a rolling methane flame that in turn ignited the coal dust, causing a coal-dust explosion. The mine inspectors knew of these hazardous conditions. During the summer of 1991, without making a formal order, they demanded that the company produce a stone-dusting plan to address the coal-dust hazard. By March 1992 nothing had been done. At that time the inspectors first became aware of dangerous levels of methane, but nothing was done. The next inspection took place on April 29, 1992. Finding that the coal dust problem still had not been addressed, the inspector finally issued a formal order requiring the company to clean up the hazard immediately and to produce a coal-dusting plan by mid-May. Ten days later, the mine exploded (Glasbeek and Tucker 1993; Jobb 1994; Richard 1997).

Within a short time of the explosion, the victims' families, trade unionists, and others began demanding accountability and reform. They wanted to know who was responsible for creating the hazardous conditions in the mine and why they had been allowed to persist. This demand for accountability was not just directed at individuals, but also at organizations and systems. Numerous institutions of redress were mobilized: an inquiry was established; criminal charges were laid against Curragh Inc. (the legal owner of the mine) and two of its on-site managers;

workers' compensation payments were made to the surviving families; damage actions were brought by the families of the dead miners; and campaigns were conducted to change the law. Yet, more than 10 years later, no individual or organization has been held criminally or civilly liable for the deaths of the miners and the occupational health and safety (OHS) regime has changed little. In 2003, however, the criminal law was amended by the so-called "Westray Bill," which purports to make the prosecution of health and safety crimes easier. In short, it seems that while legal accountability was evaded, and the reform-inducing producing potential of this disaster was partially blunted, the specter of egregious criminality going unpunished for apparently technical reasons so threatened the legitimacy of the law that legislators eventually felt compelled to respond. This chapter seeks to explain how this happened.

It begins with a model that identifies some key factors that influence responses to disasters. The model is then applied to the Westray aftermath, examining in greater detail the prosecution of criminal charges, compensation to the victims' families, the inquiry's recommendations in regard to the OHS regime, and regulatory and legislative changes. The final section draws some brief conclusions.

DETERMINANTS OF THE PUBLIC OUTCOMES OF OHS DISASTERS: A WORKING MODEL

While there is now a large body of literature that explores the causes of disasters, much less attention has been paid to the study of their effects on public policy. This chapter proceeds from the assumption that once an event has come to be socially constructed as a work disaster (see earlier chapters) it has a potentially disruptive social effect; it may generate demands that individuals and organizations, typically celebrated for their entrepreneurial finesse and lauded for their contribution to the economic well-being of society, be branded as wrong-doers or criminals for the harm their wealth-producing activities have caused. As well, such events may make visible and call into question, in a dramatic and public way, the acceptability of the existing OHS regime and the criminal laws that apply to corporate misconduct in the workplace. Thus, there is a need to inquire into the factors that influence whether and to what extent work disasters will be crisis producing in the above senses.

It is also necessary, however, to explore the factors that influence the state's ability to manage these crisis tendencies. How and to what extent are state institutions and actors able to contain political harm and reassure the public that the government is not giving employers and corporations special treatment? How and to what extent can those who demand redress effect a de-legitimation of existing institutional arrangements and their underlying assumptions and social relations, and obtain redress? Figure 1 depicts a model for studying both these sets of OHS disaster outcome determinants.

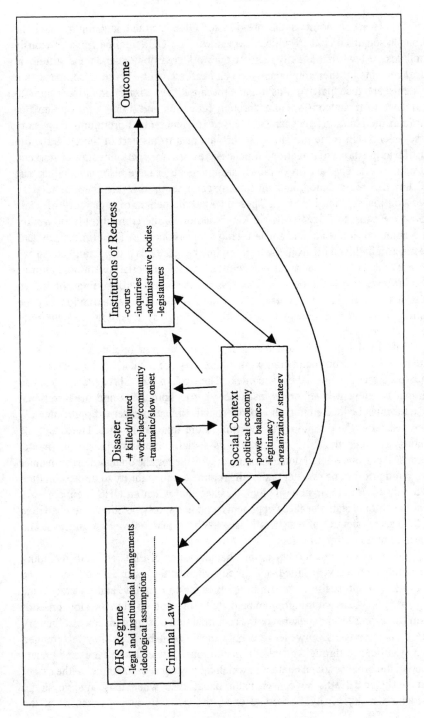

Figure 1. Determinants of the public outcomes of a working disaster.

The starting point is the pre-disaster OHS/criminal law regime and the broader social context in which it operates. The OHS regime most obviously includes the laws that directly regulate the work environment and the institutional arrangements for their implementation and enforcement. Workers' compensation systems are also part of this regime because they almost invariably aim to influence OHS outcomes, either through education and promotion programs or through their funding mechanisms (e.g., experience-rated premiums or penalty assessments). In some jurisdictions, tort law also forms part of the OHS regime insofar as the threat of litigation influences the behavior of employers and workers. In addition to legal and institutional arrangements, I have also included as part of the OHS regime the dominant ideological assumptions that shape regulatory decision-making and behavior. These include the beliefs of regulatory officials about the causes of hazardous working conditions, the compatibility or worker and employer interests, and social relations of production. The criminal law has been partially hived off from the OHS regime because it is not typically construed as part of it. This is because the behavior that results in worker deaths and injuries is not viewed with the same seriousness as analogous wrongdoing committed outside the workplace. Of course, this is a purely ideological construction, but one with a long historical lineage (Tucker 1990, pp. 66-75). It is, however, currently being challenged.

The model presupposes that OHS regimes do not operate apart from or independently of the social context in which they are located, and are shaped by and, to a lesser extent, shape that context. The work of Paul Shrivastava (1987) on Bhopal is relevant here for its insistence that technological and organizational systems must be located in their broader social context in order to appreciate both their risks and the possibility of averting future industrial crises. Here, too, the relation between the OHS regime and its social context is vital to our model because it permits a better understanding of why the regime operated in the manner that it did prior to the disaster and of the regime's vulnerability to de-legitimation in the disaster's aftermath. It is hypothesized that when an OHS regime enjoys near hegemonic status or faces opponents who are poorly positioned to challenge it, the crisis potential of disasters is less likely to materialize in significant and effective pressure for change.

The next locus of inquiry is the characteristics of disaster itself, including the number of workers killed or injured, whether the harm is confined to the workplace or spreads to members of the broader community, and its time frame (e.g., a traumatic event inflicting immediate harm as opposed to the slow onset of harm from long-term exposures or the accumulation of single instances of harm). These characteristics, however, are only meaningful because they are imbued with significance through social and institutional processes and must be understood in the broader social context in which they occur. For example, to the extent that workplace deaths have been naturalized, even when they involve single incidents that kill many workers at once, the crisis-producing potential of the incident—which may not even be socially construed as a disaster—will be diminished. But it is also hypothesized in this model that there is an interactive relationship between the disaster and the social context, such that a disaster may produce shifts in the balance of power, alter perceptions of the legitimacy of the existing regimes of regulation or governance, and generate different organizational and strategic responses. These interactions will vitally influence the impact of the disaster on the institutional mechanisms for redress (including legislatures, courts, commissions of inquiry, administrative agencies, and legislatures). This is because the identification of objectives and the ability of social actors to achieve them will depend on a variety of social forces and processes. The work of Renn (1992) using the social arena metaphor is helpful here. Renn argues that to be successful groups must mobilize social resources, including money, power, social influence, value commitment, and evidence. His emphasis on the scope for political action and the plurality of social resources helps avoid reductionist tendencies present in more structural accounts of policy processes. However, while Renn recognizes that resources are unequally distributed and that arenas operate under certain constraints, his focus on environmental harms and their more broadly dispersed effects, in conjunction with a generally liberal-pluralist perspective, leaves untheorized the structural basis for unequal resource distribution or the nature of the constraints operating within policy arenas. These lacunae in Renn's approach become major omissions in the context of OHS where class and class conflict are often central. Therefore, a political economy approach will be used to deepen the analysis of the operation of social arenas (Nichols 1999; Pearce and Tombs 1999).

From this perspective, it is absolutely essential to recognize that the overwhelming majority of the immediate victims and their families are working-class. Writers such as Michael Reich (1991) have demonstrated that, in the aftermath of disaster, victims and their families are drawn out of their private worlds and become involved "in another world of problems, conflicts identities and institutions" as they seek redress (Reich 1994, p. 181). They will frequently form associations to represent and advance their common interests before the institutions of redress. Often, they will be joined and supported by trade unions, especially when the victims were trade-union members themselves. However, the goals of victims' groups and trade unions may not be identical, as the former may be more immediately concerned with individual and organization accountability for the deaths and compensation while the latter may be more strongly focused on system accountability and reform of the OHS regime to better protect health and safety in the future. In the aftermath of a disaster, both groups are likely to be better positioned than at other times to mobilize political and ideological resources that will shift the balance of power in favor of redress and regime reform.

It is important, however, to recognize that working-class actors are likely to face significant opposition unless their demands stay within narrow and accepted channels. The disaster-employer in particular and employer organizations in general also can be expected to mobilize. They will do so to defend themselves against legal liabilities, adverse ideological and political effects, and unwanted legal and institutional changes. However, in the immediate aftermath of a disaster, their ability to mobilize social resources may be weakened, especially if there is *prima facie* evidence that the disaster-employer's failure to meet its legal obligations to its victim-workers was an operative cause of the disaster. Notwithstanding such disruptions of normal politics, we must keep in mind that any resulting power re-balancing will take place within a larger political economy that is unlikely to have been fundamentally altered by the disaster. The structural power imbalances between labor and capital will still be operative and exert a continuing influence over efforts to re-negotiate the OHS health and safety regime and its underlying assumptions.

Disaster politics are often conducted in a number of distinct institutional settings or policy arenas, each of which has its own particular possibilities and constraints. Criminal trials, civil actions, administrative decision-making, public inquiries, and legislatures use different procedures and are bound by different decision-making rules. For example, the rules of evidence and those defining the burden of proof are different in criminal trials than in tort actions and public inquiries. These systems also place different limits on the chains of causality that can be pursued. As well, some social resources are formally permitted to operate in some institutions but not others. For instance—at least in theory—the outcome of a criminal trial is not to be influenced by money or social influence, but only by evidence of a certain kind. Judges are meant to be neutral and a number of formal safeguards are in place to immunize them from outside influences. Decision-making is to be guided by prescribed rules. In contrast, decisions of legislatures are formally open to lobbying, petitions, and other kinds of political influence.

Lastly, the model's analysis must be attentive to the different forms of redress that actors might be seeking and that institutional processes can produce. Thus, it will often be the case that efforts are being made to seek compensation, punish the offenders, and reform the OHS regime, all at the same time. Not only are some of these goals more achievable than others, but we must also be cognizant of the formal and informal interactions between these goals and the institutions invoked to achieve them. While it is not necessarily the case that the pursuit of one goal comes at the expense of another, we cannot ignore the fact that actors have finite amounts of energy and resources and, for a variety of legal reasons, efforts in one arena may limit those in others. However, it may also be the case that the outcome in one arena may influence outcomes in others and, in particular, that the failure to hold individuals and organizations accountable for egregious wrongdoing may reinforce demands for legal reforms that address the accountability gap.

REDRESS IN THE AFTERMATH OF
THE WESTRAY DISASTER

The Pre-Disaster OHS Regime and
Its Social Context

Nova Scotia, like all other Canadian jurisdictions, adopted an OHS regime of mandated partial self-regulation (Rees 1988; Tucker 1995a). An essential characteristic of this regime is that it requires employers and employees to self-manage their health and safety according to certain legally prescribed processes and standards (the so-called internal responsibility system or IRS) while also maintaining a system of direct state regulation (the so called external responsibility system or ERS). In Canada, the IRS provides a role for worker participation through the right to know, the right to participate in mandatory bipartite local health and safety committees, and the right to refuse unsafe work. The ERS imposes duties on employers and employees through statutes and regulations that are enforceable by inspectors and through prosecutions.

Within these broad parameters, mandated partial self-regulation can assume many different forms. Two crucial variables are the strength of worker participation rights and the balance between internal and external responsibility systems. The Nova Scotia variant, adopted in 1985, took a particularly restrictive approach to the right to refuse. It provided that workers could not refuse because of dangers that were "inherent" in the job and that work refusals could not continue after a unanimous joint committee had determined that the work was safe or labor department officials had advised the employee to return to work. Confusion about the right to be paid during a work refusal further reduced the willingness of workers to exercise it (Nova Scotia 1985).[1] The external responsibility system in Nova Scotia was also a weak one. Neither old mine safety statutes, nor industrial and construction safety regulations were updated. In addition, the maximum fine under the Act was on the low end of the spectrum ($10,000). More importantly, the government adopted an enforcement policy that depended almost exclusively on persuasion. Between 1985 and 1990, a total of 14 prosecutions were undertaken for violations of health and safety laws and the largest fine imposed was $2,500. Not a single mining company was prosecuted, notwithstanding the fact that 1037 formal directives were issued to mine operators to correct violations of health and safety laws between 1987-88 and 1991-92 (Glasbeek and Tucker 1993, p. 25).

The weak powers granted to workers in the IRS and the lacks of enforcement in the ERS are justified on the assumption that employers and workers have a common interest in respect of OHS. It is posited that, to employers, "reasonable" safety pays and that "reasonable" employees should be satisfied with that level of safety. As a result, social relations between employers and workers should be cooperative and the parties should be able to self-regulate without significant external intervention. The emergence of conflict is constructed as a sign of deviance, either on the part of an employer who fails to understand that the expected level of safety pays, or on the part of employees who are irrational in their demands for safety or who may be using OHS to achieve other (e.g., collective bargaining) objectives.

These institutional arrangements and ideological assumptions are rooted in a local political economy that is best characterized by its underdevelopment (Brym and Sacouman 1979). The Nova Scotia economy has been heavily dependent on the export of staples into volatile and increasingly unfavorable world markets. As a result, governments have been particularly anxious to attract would-be investors to provide much needed jobs. Moreover, these conditions have adversely affected the Nova Scotia labor movement, which has gone from being one of the strongest and most militant in the country to being much less effective and influential (Earle 1989). As a result, organized labor in Nova Scotia has not been particularly aggressive on OHS issues and has not challenged the assumptions and practices embedded in the regime. As well, the Conservative Party had dominated provincial politics, holding office continuously from 1956 to 1993, leaving the labor movement with little political leverage.

These conditions set the stage for the Westray mine disaster. Not only were the developers of the mine able to extract very sizeable government loan guarantees and favorable contract commitments to purchase its coal, but during the approval process their mining plans were not scrutinized by officials to determine if they could be executed safely. The top priority of politicians was to secure funding for and approval of the project, and regulatory officials implicitly understood these priorities. The mine developer's main concern was coal production, but it continually encountered setbacks in meeting its goals. As a result, pressure was placed on local managers to get the coal out, fostering a culture of risk-taking and a cavalier attitude toward safety (Cooke 2003). Regulatory officials responsible for monitoring mine safety and adherence to approved plans consistently failed to ensure that detected breaches of regulatory requirements were rectified (Glasbeek and Tucker 1993; Jobb 1994; Richard 1997). As hazardous conditions became manifest, experienced miners quit when they saw that their concerns were not going to be addressed by management and that the inspectors were not going to take effective action to force the company to operate safely. The growing fears of the remaining inexperienced and non-unionized Westray miners remained "private trouble" (Comish 1993; Mills 1959, p. 8)—until it was too late.

Mobilizing the Institutions of Redress

In the immediate aftermath of the explosion on May 9, 1992 it was not known whether there were any survivors. As rescue teams rushed into action, intensive media attention focused on the unfolding drama. Although from the outset, the company devised a media strategy that aimed to deflect blame from itself, it could not contain the flow of information about the miners' prior expressions of concern, the issuance of orders by the mine inspectors, and the failure of the company to comply with those orders (Richards 1998). As it became clear that no miners survived and that human agency rather than ineluctable natural forces caused the explosion, there was widespread questioning of the efficacy and legitimacy of the existing regime of OHS regulation and a demand that responsible individuals and institutions be held to account. And so a multitude of institutions of redress were mobilized in response to demands for accountability and reform. One of the immediate influences of the disaster on the balance of social forces was that it gave rise to a new and important voice: the victims' families. Many of them formed the Westray Families Group to pursue their demands for justice. In so doing, they were drawn out of their private worlds into the public sphere, taking on an unfamiliar and uncomfortable role that they felt compelled to assume if only to vindicate the reputations of their loved ones against suggestions that the men were responsible for what had happened (Dodd 1998, 2001). The labor movement, particularly the United Steelworkers of America (USWA), which was in the midst of an organizing drive at the Westray mine at the time of the explosion,[2] also assumed an active role in demanding redress.

Against this background, Donald Cameron, the Conservative Premier of the province at the time, promised a public inquiry. Within days after the suspension of the rescue effort, Cameron appointed Mr. Justice Richard to head up an inquiry under the *Public Inquiries Act* and the *Coal Mine Regulation Act*. The provincial auditor commissioned a private consultant (Coopers Lybrand) to conduct a review of management practices at the Department of Labor, and the Nova Scotia Occupational Health and Safety Advisory Council, representing both labor and management, was commissioned to review the *Occupational Health and Safety Act* (*OHSA*) and its regulations and to make recommendations for reform. A police investigation was commenced as well and the Royal Canadian Mounted Police (RCMP) took control of the mine site 12 days after the explosion. That fall, charges were laid against the employer under the provincial *OHSA* but were subsequently dropped in April 1993 after the employer (Curragh Corporation) and two local managers, Gerald Philips and Roger Parry, were charged with manslaughter and criminal negligence causing death. The entitlement of the surviving family members under the province's workers' compensation law was never in question and so that aspect of compensation was handled routinely and without much controversy. Workers' compensation, however, is a no-fault system, so no findings of blame or responsibility were made. The level of compensation is set by legislation, and it neither fully reimburses victims and their families for their economic loss, nor awards punitive or other non-economic damages. As a result, the surviving families launched a civil action against Curragh, its board of directors, Clifford Frame (Curragh's chief executive officer), the manufacturers of machinery used in the mine, and the governments of Nova Scotia and Canada.

It is beyond the scope of this chapter to provide a detailed account of the conduct and fate of each mechanism of redress (Jobb 1999; Tucker 1995b). Rather, the focus here is on the broader question of their outcome and the social and institutional forces that shaped these results. Although it is somewhat artificial to draw a sharp line between accountability and reform, since mechanisms for holding individuals and organizations accountable (e.g., the civil and criminal law) may also be seen to have systemic effects on the OHS regime, and since some responses, like inquiries combine these functions (often uneasily), it is nevertheless useful for our purposes to draw this distinction.

Accountability

Partial Compensation, but No Fault—A prominent demand of victims in the aftermath of a disaster is that they be compensated for their losses, both economic (e.g., lost income) and non-economic (e.g., pain and suffering). Redress of this sort is typically obtained through the workers' compensation and/or the tort system.[3] Victims may also look to the tort system as a means of holding individuals and organizations publicly accountable for their actions because the court must determine that there was intentional or negligent conduct before it can award damages. Some also believe that the tort system can promote systemic change by deterring potential wrongdoers who will wish to avoid being named and blamed, and to pay damages to the victims. This section examines the ability of the Westray families to mobilize these systems and achieve their objectives of obtaining compensation, holding individuals and organizations accountable for their wrongdoing, and deterring such behavior in the future. Their experience will be related to broader debates about the responsiveness of these institutions to workers' concerns in the aftermath of a disaster and their potential effectiveness as an element of the OHS regime.

Workers' compensation in most Canadian jurisdictions compensates surviving family members for their economic losses reasonably well. Compensation is payable without the need to prove that death was the fault of the employer and, where the work-relatedness of the death is obvious as in the Westray case, administrative officials make entitlement determinations quickly so that compensation payments start shortly after the loss occurs. Payment is made out of a state-administered insurance fund paid for by employer premiums. Payment is secure, even in the face of large claims in the aftermath of disaster, and lawyers are rarely involved in the claims process, so none of the compensation payments are lost to legal costs.

Under Nova Scotia law as it stood at the time of the Westray explosion, widows were entitled to a life pension calculated at 75% of pre-accident gross earnings up to a maximum of $36,000. Because the percentage is based on gross rather than net earnings, the widows' pension will replace nearly all of the lost income, provided the deceased worker made no more than the maximum. In the case of the Westray miners, most were earning more than the maximum, and as a result the widows are not being fully compensated for the loss of their partners' income. However, these benefits are indexed to ensure that they keep pace with the cost of living and the level of the pension will increase as the maximum earnings cut-off is increased in the future. Survivors also get an additional monthly payment for each child that continues until age 18 or, if the child remains in school, to 25. In addition, the families of the deceased miners received a lump sum death benefit of $15,000 and $4,000 for funeral expenses. A spokesperson for the NS workers' compensation board estimated that it would pay out $15 million in benefits, but that this could increase to $25 or $26 million, depending on inflation and future increases to the maximum pension level (COHSN, 8 Feb. 1993).

Although the workers' compensation did not fully replace the families' economic losses, its performance in response to the Westray disaster did not attract significant criticism,[4] despite the widespread discontent of Nova Scotia workers with the system's treatment of workers with permanent disabilities and appeal backlogs. Indeed, neither the Westray families nor the labor movement mobilized in pursuit of legislative or administrative reforms in response to the Board's handling of the Westray claims.[5] These groups also recognized, and implicitly accepted, that the design of the system does not provide for assignment of blame or the award of exemplary damages, that it pays very little compensation for non-economic losses, and that it has little deterrent effect.[6]

Because of these limitations, disaster victims often find the tort system attractive, as did a number of Westray families. They commenced a $30 million damage action against the employer (Curragh Corporation), out-of-province manufacturers of equipment used at the mine, the Governments of Canada and Nova Scotia, and the mines' inspectors. However, this lawsuit faced a formidable legal barrier. In Nova Scotia and other Canadian jurisdictions, workers' compensation laws severely limit the right of injured workers and their survivors to sue. The statutory bar precludes actions against the worker's employer and any other employer covered by the province's workers' compensation legislation. It also forecloses actions against employees of covered employers.

The action against Curragh was subsequently dropped, both because it stood no chance of being allowed to go ahead and because Curragh was bankrupt. The lawsuit against out-of-province equipment manufacturers was also dropped, not because it was barred by statute, but because the families were advised that it would take years to resolve and would be very costly to pursue (*Bell v. Canada (Attorney General)* 2001). This left the governments of Nova Scotia and Canada as defendants.

In 1998, following the report of the Westray Inquiry, the Westray families initiated settlement talks with the Nova Scotia government, lowering their damage claim $12.6 million. After much delay, the government announced in December of that year that it would not offer an out-of-court settlement. This was consistent with its position that it did not accept legal liability for the disaster. The government subsequently moved to have the action against it dismissed on the grounds that it was an employer under the statute and, therefore, protected by the statutory bar.

The status of the government as a protected employer under workers' compensation statutes had recently been before the Supreme Court of Canada in *Pasiechnyk v. Saskatchewan (Workers' Compensation Board)* (1997) where the court held that it was reasonable for the WCB to conclude that the government was protected by the statutory bar, notwithstanding that it was being sued in its capacity as regulator and not employer. While this left open the possibility that different conclusions might be reached by workers' compensation boards in other jurisdictions, the court's holding undoubtedly strengthened the Nova Scotia government's position that the statutory bar protected it.

In dismissing the families' action, Mr. Justice Davison began his analysis with a quote from the dissenting judgment of Justice L'Heureux-Dubé in *Pasiechnyk*:

> The tragic factual circumstances that have led to these proceedings are irrelevant to the . . . legal question at issue. (1997, p. 920)

Having established the requisite emotional distance, Davison J. then dryly parsed the applicable statutory language and rules of interpretation, concluding that the government is an employer for the purpose of the statute and is thus protected against tort claims by injured employees. The effect of this judgment also precluded an action against the provincial inspectors, because the bar also protects employees of covered employers from civil liability. The Nova Scotia Court of Appeal upheld Davison J.'s judgment and the Supreme Court of Canada denied leave to appeal. Although the families vowed to fight on (Brooks 2002), they have no real prospect of advancing their suit and so it is extremely unlikely that tort litigation will help achieve their goals of obtaining a formal assignment of blame and additional compensation, or deterring future employers and governments from creating and/or tolerating unsafe working conditions.

Clearly, even in the face of what a court might characterize as gross negligence by the employer and the mines inspectors, the victims were unable to convince the government that it should voluntarily pay additional compensation or to persuade the judiciary to open the door to tort litigation. Moreover, they were unable to mobilize broader support for their demands, so that neither the government nor the court (nor for that matter, the law it was interpreting) has faced much criticism, suggesting that in Canada, unlike the United States, civil actions against employers and governments are not widely viewed as an avenue of redress that victims of workplace disasters should be entitled to pursue.[7]

Given this outcome, the Westray experience adds little to debates over the tort system's efficacy in delivering the kinds of redress that it is, at least in principle, institutionally capable of providing to disaster victims. However, a few brief comments are still in order.[8] First, the goals of denunciation, compensation, and deterrence are only advanced if the appropriate defendant is found to be at fault. Although the onus of proof is on the plaintiff, unlike in a criminal proceeding, it is enough to prove liability on a balance of probabilities. As well, corporate defendants will be held vicariously responsible for the negligent acts of their officers and employees. Finally, the discovery process assists the plaintiff in getting information from the defendant. Still, plaintiffs face serious hurdles, including the fact that, in the first instance, they bear the cost of gathering and presenting the evidence. Moreover, well-off or well-insured defendants who have a significant stake in the litigation will take advantage of the tort system to delay proceedings and increase the plaintiff's costs. In short, there are significant obstacles to holding individuals and organizations accountable through the tort system.

Second, it is not clear that success in litigation would produce more compensation for victims. The workers' compensation board would have been subrogated to the action and entitled to reimbursement for its expenses out of the proceeds. Thus, the plaintiffs would only be better off to the extent that the tort damages exceeded the workers' compensation award and, according to one recent assessment, that outcome is unlikely (Hyatt and Law 2000, pp. 338-351).

Third, the deterrent effect of tort is premised on the desire of potential torfeasors to avoid the shame attached to civil blame, as well as its financial cost. How strong are these effects? If the case is successful, a finding against the defendant is one that attaches blame and, while it does not have the same significance as a guilty verdict in a criminal trial, it can still cause embarrassment, especially when the court finds there has been reckless disregard for human life in the pursuit of profit. However, just as in a criminal trial, it is likely that the case will be presented in such a way as to emphasize the deviance of the defendants, rather than the systemic nature of hazardous working conditions (see Johnstone, ch. 8 this volume). So, contrary to the claims of Bale (1989), successful tort actions are unlikely to undermine the legitimacy of the systems that encourage the creation of hazardous work environments. Moreover, because the defendant is most likely a corporation, individual officers and managers will escape personal blame.

Perhaps even more than shame, the deterrent effect of the tort system rests on its supposed ability to impose significant financial costs on wrongdoers, thus creating an incentive for persons engaging in potentially hazardous activities to take greater care to avoid causing harm to others. The empirical support for this hypothesis, however, is thin. First, as Ison argued, the tort system is a "forensic lottery" that delivers compensation to only a fraction of those who have valid claims (Ison 1967). Second, although exemplary and punitive damages are becoming more common in Canada, they are still rare and usually modest (Feldthusen 2000, *Whiten v. Pilot Insurance* 2002), and damages for pain and suffering have been capped. Third, most defendants are likely to be insured, so that they will probably not have to bear directly the cost of the damage award

(Atiyah 1997). Fourth, even if the award exceeds the insurance coverage, defendants facing large damage awards have developed an array of strategies, including bankruptcy protection, to reduce their financial exposure.

In sum, if the Westray families had been able to sue successfully for damages, they would have gained whatever satisfaction comes from having a formal determination of fault made by a court. However, it is unlikely that they would have been that much further ahead financially or that the deterrent effect of a successful lawsuit would have been very significant (Dewees, Duff, and Trebilcock 1996, ch. 6). It is even less likely that the litigation would have challenged the underlying ideological assumptions and institutional arrangements that contribute to the problem of unhealthy and unsafe work.

Crime Without Punishment—Criminal prosecutions are first and foremost a way of holding individuals and, to a lesser extent, organizations such as corporations accountable. The choice of wrongs that are deemed to be of such a serious nature that they warrant criminal sanctions as opposed to private remedies through civil actions is a deeply political and ideological one. Historically, the criminal law has not been applied against employers whose actions have caused death and injury to their workers. In part, this is because employment relations are viewed as a realm of voluntarism in which workers assume some risk of injury in exchange for wages. Because this consensus view informs much of contemporary OHS regulation, it has been argued that the use of criminal sanctions against employers becomes a means of challenging the conventional wisdom and promoting system reform (Glasbeek 1988).

The Westray criminal prosecutions were a legal disaster from start to finish (Jobb 1999). The Nova Scotia government initially refused to assign a full-time crown attorney to the case, despite a plea from the RCMP to do so. The two prosecutors finally appointed in September 1992, three-and-a-half months after the disaster, complained that they were not provided with the most basic resources needed to do their job properly, leading them to resign in February 1993. This contributed to a slip-up whereby the prosecution failed to obtain a court order needed to retain evidence seized from Curragh pursuant to a search warrant. In response to an application from Curragh's lawyers, the prosecution was given one month to lay charges or hand over the evidence. So, on April 20, 1993, the RCMP announced that Curragh Corporation and two of its onsite managers, Gerald Phillips and Roger Parry, were being charged with manslaughter and criminal negligence causing death. However, those charges were subsequently quashed in July 1993 by a provincial judge who found them too vaguely worded *R v. Curragh Inc.* 1993). New charges were filed shortly thereafter and these survived legal challenge *R v. Curragh Inc.* 1994).

By then, a new legal team had been put in charge of the prosecution and had been given a budget to enable it to manage the mass of evidence that was involved in this complex case. The trial began in February 1995. The defense repeatedly claimed that it had not been given adequate disclosure of Crown evidence as required by Canadian law. The case was dragging ahead slowly when the presiding judge, Robert Anderson, phoned the head of the prosecution service to demand the removal of the lead prosecutor. The Crown demanded a mistrial but was refused by Justice Anderson. The Crown secured an emergency hearing before the Supreme Court of Canada on April 5 but this Court determined that it had no jurisdiction to intervene in the midst of a trial (*R. v. Curragh Inc.* 1995a). The trial resumed before Justice Anderson and continued until June, when he granted a defense motion to stay the charges because of the failure of the Crown to disclose key evidence about methane sensors and coal dust samples (*R. v. Curragh Inc.* 1995b).

The Crown appealed Anderson's ruling to the Nova Scotia Court of Appeal. In its judgment, issued in December 1995, the court ruled that Anderson's behavior gave rise to a reasonable apprehension of bias and ordered a new trial (*R. v. Curragh Inc.* 1995c). A new prosecution team was assigned to the case and given additional resources, much of which were devoted to cataloguing the mass of documents in the Crown's possession in order to avoid future disclosure problems. The defense challenged the Court of Appeal's decision before the Supreme Court of Canada. Its judgment was issued in March 1997. A 7-2 majority upheld the Court of Appeal's order for a new trial, agreeing that the trial judge's conduct had created an apprehension of bias (*R. v. Curragh Inc.* 1997). The majority did not comment directly on the Crown's failure to disclose, but it did order the Crown to pay the defendants' reasonable legal costs.[9]

The Director of Public Prosecutions in Nova Scotia, however, was losing his enthusiasm for a case that was already absorbing a significant portion of his office's budget and that threatened to become even more costly. Moreover, by then the commission of inquiry (see *infra.*, p. 295) had issued its report which attributed the explosion to a persistent pattern of disregard for basic mine safety and a breakdown of regulatory systems. Guilt was pervasive. Following the commission's report, one of the prosecutors, Jack Hagell was asked to prepare a report assessing the strength of the Crown's case. His recommendation, given in October 1997, was that the charges be withdrawn because it would be "fundamentally unfair" to prosecute only Phillips and Parry when many others, including miners, foremen, and government inspectors, shared responsibility for the explosion. Hagell was also critical of the investigation and the early handling of the case. While Hagell withdrew from further involvement with the case, his colleagues labored on. A further internal assessment estimated that the prosecution would cost in the vicinity of $10 million, that there was no consensus on the likelihood of conviction, and that a jail sentence was unlikely even if there was a conviction (McCormick 1999b, p. 21). In July 1998 the Nova Scotia Justice Minister announced that the criminal charges were being stayed and would not be revived. A prosecution could not be pursued under provincial OHS laws either because the Crown had previously stayed charges in order to clear the way for the criminal prosecution.

While the immediate causes of the failure of the Westray prosecution were a combination of incompetence and lack of political and fiscal support for the effort, it would be wrong to assume that successful criminal prosecutions are usual in the aftermath of a health and safety disaster in Canada or elsewhere (Hopkins 1989; Slapper 1999). For example, in twentieth century Canada, research to date has uncovered only 10 instances in which employers were charged with criminal offences in relation to dangerous working conditions, and only one conviction that withstood appeal (Law Reform Commission of Canada 1986; Tucker 1995b). In 1943, Brazeau Collieries Ltd. was convicted of criminal negligence after 29 coal miners died in a methane gas explosion. Chief Justice Ives imposed a fine of $5,000. He justified this small penalty because of the "close and friendly association between mine officials and miners" (*Calgary Herald* 19 January 1943; *Rex v. Brazeau Mines* 1942).

Why has the criminal law been so marginal to OHS regulation and why is it so hard for it to be deployed as mechanism to denounce and punish employer wrongdoing in the aftermath of a disaster?

There are at least two levels of explanation for criminal law's separation from the OHS regime: the sociological and the legal-institutional. According to many radical criminologists, the criminal law does not stand in an external relation to society, but rather is a product of and an instrument for maintaining unequal social relations. As a result, there has been enormous resistance in capitalist societies to categorizing wrongdoing by the economically powerful as criminal activity (Chambliss and Seidman 1971; Pearce 1976; Pearce and Tombs 1999; Slapper 1993; Taylor, Walton, and Young 1973). Resistance is particularly high when it is alleged that an employer has committed a crime in the course of profit-making workplace activity. This is because of the underlying assumptions that employment relations are consensual and that employees accept some level of risk. This, after all, is one of the justifications for the IRS. A criminal charge represents a social judgment about the unacceptability of certain risks and does not permit individual consent to them. As such, its use in the employment context is anomalous.

This closure, however, is never complete in liberal societies that also embrace the ideal of equality before the law and some commitment, however thin, to minimum standards of social welfare for all citizens. So while the deep-seated assumption that capitalist production gone wrong is to be treated differently than analogous behavior occurring in other contexts that are not similarly valued is rarely questioned during normal times, workplace and other disasters often produce a popular demand for justice that, in the Anglo-American context, is increasingly fulfilled through the prosecution and punishment of wrongdoers under the criminal law (Wells 1995, ch. 7).[10] This was certainly the case in the aftermath of the Westray disaster. Although trade unions and the Westray Families Group took the lead in making this demand, they gained popular support as knowledge of the employer's reckless behavior became widespread through media reports. Thus, the very act of charging an employer or its agents with a criminal offense challenges the normative order, throwing into question assumptions about common interests between workers and employers and challenging the legitimacy of profit-maximizing behavior (Glasbeek 1984).

The symbolic importance of criminalizing employer misconduct, however, virtually ensures that attempts to do this will encounter institutional resistance and that powerful actors will mobilize to limit the threat. This points toward the second level of explanation that focuses on legal and institutional impediments to successful prosecutions of corporate/capital crime. The large body of literature on this subject can only be touched upon lightly here. One problem that commentators have identified is that of assigning criminal responsibility to individuals who act within a corporate structure that is designed to shield individuals from legal liability. Connecting high-level corporate officers and directors to the crime can be a difficult task in an organization in which responsibility is diffuse and in which operational decisions are taken by lower-level officials in the corporate hierarchy (Tombs 1995). Collecting evidence from the boardroom and weaving together a coherent and compelling story for the jury that will implicate senior corporate actors is likely to be such a time-consuming and daunting task that police and prosecutors are hesitant to proceed. Of course, it is also possible to prosecute the lower-level corporate officials, such as the on-site managers, for their personal wrongdoing (as was done in the case of Westray), but this may be resisted by prosecutors and judges who feel that it is unfair to let the small fry take the blame when the big fish have gotten away.

It is often assumed that it is easier to prosecute the corporation itself rather than particular corporate officials. This has been facilitated by developments in the criminal law that, for example, allow corporations to be prosecuted for *mens rea* offenses such as manslaughter. However, the complexity of such cases still is great. According to the headnote in the leading Ontario case on the subject, "[a] corporation is responsible for the criminal acts of its servant only if the servant has authority, express or implied to do the act, or if the servant is virtually its directing mind in the sphere of duty assigned to him so that his actions and intent are the very actions and intent of the corporation itself, provided that in performing the acts in question the agent was acting within the scope of his authority, either express or implied" (*R. v. McNamara et al. (No. 1)* 1981). However, as in the case of prosecuting individuals, the cost and difficulty of gathering evidence necessary to prove all elements of the offense beyond a reasonable doubt is likely to be great. Corporations and senior company officials have the resources to mount a vigorous defense, ensuring that their rights are scrupulously respected and using the complexity of the corporate organization to undermine the prosecution's case. This means that the prosecution will have to be prepared to devote considerable resources to the case, often when it is operating under fiscal restraints. Resource allocation decisions are also likely to be influenced by underlying attitudes about the appropriateness of prosecuting corporate actors in the first place, by direct political considerations, and by doubts about whether the game is worth the candle when a conviction will be difficult to obtain and, if the corporation is the accused, there is literally no body to punish (Benson 2001; Coffee 1981; Geis & DiMento 1995; Slapper 1999). Often, as in the case of Curragh, the corporation will have ceased to exist or other creditors will have seized its assets, making any fine impossible to collect.

Finally, the theory of criminal liability in these cases is likely to be that the employer behaved in a reckless manner. To increase the probability of success, the prosecution is likely to adopt a strategy of decontextualization and individualization. Rather than emphasizing the broader context that promotes the behavior in question, or drawing attention to the frequency of unlawful employer conduct, both the prosecution and the media will tend to focus on the particular facts of the case and to characterize corporate defendants as bad apples in what is a generally good barrel (Johnstone, ch. 8 this volume; McMullan and Hinze 1998). Thus, even in those rare cases where the popular demand for justice overcomes the deeply ingrained resistance to seeing respectable members of the employing classes condemned as pariahs for their undisciplined pursuit of profits resulting in death and destruction, there is a danger that a conviction will be interpreted as an affirmation, rather than a critique, of the normative order.

So while the problems encountered in the Westray prosecution initially look idiosyncratic, upon closer examination the failure of the criminal prosecution in that case appears typical of the criminal law's response to corporate/capital wrongdoing. The public outcry in the immediate aftermath of the disaster pushed a reluctant government to pursue a criminal investigation and to file charges, but the initial failure to provide the necessary resources resulted in legal missteps that nearly saw the charges dismissed and produced substantial delay. By the time those problems were resolved—nearly five years after the explosion—a differently constituted government, under marginally less public pressure, was not prepared to commit substantial resources to a prosecution whose outcome was uncertain and that targeted two low-level managers of a now bankrupt corporate employer. This failure of accountability produced a demand for criminal law reform, which will be examined in the next section of the chapter.

Reform

Public Inquiry: Naming, Blaming, and Recommending More of the Same— Inherent in criminal trials and tort actions is a focus on the actions of particular defendants. Thus, any broader impact of a successful prosecution or law suit will be indirect, either by contributing to a shift in the way people view health and safety in the workplace, or through general deterrence. Public inquiries, however, usually have a broader mandate. While they too search for accountability, they make no legal determinations of wrongdoing. Rather, they typically look for systemic problems and make recommendations aimed at preventing their recurrence. Because of their different mandate, inquiries are not conducted according the rules that govern trials: they are not restricted by rules of evidence; participation in the proceedings is relatively open; and it is not up to those who are seeking particular recommendations to prove its factual predicate on a balance of probabilities. For these reasons, public inquiries can be an important institution through which to raise issues of organizational and social accountability for events, and to influence the public thinking and the future direction of state policy (Roach 1995).

Almost inevitably, inquiries of one sort or another are established in the aftermath of a mining death, so there is little difficulty in activating this institution of redress. Legal impediments, however, still may arise. There has been recent concern that provincial inquiries aimed at alleged wrongdoing of specific individuals are invalid because they are tantamount to criminal proceedings, a matter within federal jurisdiction. As well, the power of inquiries to compel individuals to testify has been challenged in respect of persons facing criminal charges on the ground that it would violate their right to remain silent. Both of these issues were raised in respect of the Westray inquiry. Ultimately, the Nova Scotia Court of Appeal upheld the authority of the province to call the inquiry on the ground that its dominant purpose was to make findings in respect of a coal-mine disaster rather than to investigate whether a criminal offence had been committed (*Phillips v. Nova Scotia (Commission of Inquiry)* 1993), and the Supreme Court of Canada upheld the right of the commissioner to compel testimony from persons facing criminal charges because of the importance of the public interest at stake and because they were protected against having that testimony or derivative evidence used in a subsequent trial (*Phillips v. Nova Scotia (Commission of Inquiry)* 1995). This litigation delayed the start of the inquiry's public proceedings until November 1995, three-and-a-half years after it was established. Although the inquiry ultimately did not hear from senior Curragh officials and Phillips or Parry, the two local officials still facing criminal charges at the time,[11] 71 witnesses testified in 76 days of well-publicized hearings, including the former Premier, the mine inspectors, former Westray miners, and families of the deceased miners. It also received numerous written submissions, including ones from the Westray families, the USW, and other labor organizations.

Its report, released in November 1997, was scathing in its criticism of the operators of the Westray mine and of the government for failing to properly regulate and stop their dangerous and unlawful mining practices. In respect of Curragh, the commission found that "it created a workplace that fostered a disregard for worker safety. . . . [M]anagement's drive for production, together with its disdain for safety, played a key role in the devastation of the Westray mine" (Richard 1997, p. 135). The commission's condemnation of the government's failures started at the top with Donald Cameron, the premier at the time, who in his testimony had blamed the miners for the explosion. Cameron's explanation was characterized as "self-serving, cynical and simplistic" (1997, p. 222) and his aggressive pursuit of the project was seen to have sent a signal to the bureaucracy that Westray was to be given special treatment. The departments of Natural Resources and Labor, which had direct oversight of the mining, were both found to be derelict in meeting their statutory responsibilities. The commission made 73 recommendations to the Nova Scotia government, which accepted them all within days of the inquiry's report (Nova Scotia 1997).

The Westray families, trade unions, and the media welcomed the report's findings (e.g., *Halifax Daily News* 7 December 1997). For the families, the exoneration of the men from blame in their own deaths and the condemnation of Curragh and Cameron was particularly satisfying (Dodd 2001), while the unions, particularly the USW, were pleased with the recommendations to increase corporate accountability (King 1998). However, despite its angry condemnation of employer misbehavior and government inaction, the report failed to confront many of the underlying structural conditions and ideological assumptions that make the production of unsafe conditions and government non-enforcement so common (Tucker 1999).

Almost totally missing from the report was any discussion of the relation between safety and profit. Of course, the pursuit of both safety and profits is not necessarily inconsistent: safe production methods will sometimes enhance profitability. But the potential for conflict is always there, especially in a situation where those immediately responsible for production are under pressure to show a profit in the short run. Instead of addressing this problem, the report makes it magically disappear:

> Once a mine is open, there begins the process of trade-off between production and safety. From the chief executive officer to the miner at the working face, the objective must be to operate the mine in a manner that ensures the personal safety of the worker over the economic imperatives of increased production. The two seemingly competing concepts—safety and production—must be so harmonized that they can co-exist without doing harm to each other. (Richard 1997, p. viii)

But how are they to co-exist? The answer is given on the next page. The Westray management "through either incompetence or ignorance, lost sight of the basic tenet of coal mining: the safe mining of coal is good business" (Richard 1997, p. ix). So, after all, there is no need for a trade off. But if safe production is always good business, then, given the tragic history of coal mining disasters and the high frequency of work-related death and disease in the industry, one is at a loss to explain why mine operators have tended to be such ignorant or incompetent business people.

This understanding of the production of OHS hazards contributes to the report's faulty analysis of the failure of the government inspectors to enforce the law. Richard claimed that it was an erroneous understanding of the IRS that "was a major deterrent to effective enforcement of the safety regulations" (Richard 1997, p. 455). The error lay in ascribing to inspectors the role of being persuaders and facilitators whose mandate was to promote the capacity of the workplace parties to assume primary responsibility for OHS in the workplace. The problem with this analysis, however, is that Richard failed to recognize that this approach to enforcement is not a corruption of the IRS model but rather is a manifestation of its ordinary operation. Even in Ontario, which has the most OHS prosecutions in Canada, the emphasis is on the promotion of self-reliance and inspectors almost never launch a prosecution until after a worker has been killed or seriously injured as a result of a violation of OHS laws and regulations. The reason for taking this approach is the core belief that workers and employers share a common interest in OHS and therefore should, with a little gentle persuasion and advice from the inspector, be able to self-regulate. Thus, despite Richard's denunciation of the failure to enforce in this particular case, the report embraces a model wherein the very behavior he criticizes is the norm. It is telling that Richard makes no specific recommendation in his report that the inspectors should use their coercive powers more frequently against employers who are found to be in violation of the law. Instead, the Inquiry recommended that an independent consultant should be retained to evaluate the inspectorate and its personnel (Richard 1997, rec. 56).

Ironically, the Westray Inquiry proved to be more effective at holding individuals and organizations accountable (even though it could not impose sanctions) than it was at interrogating critically the system of OHS regulation that arguably fostered the unacceptable behavior it condemned so strongly. Indeed, the thrust of its report was that the existing OHS system was fundamentally sound, if badly managed. The Westray Inquiry is not unique in this regard. For example, Susan Dodd's study of mine disaster inquiries in Nova Scotia found that mine inquiries have tended to reflect the conventional wisdom of their time (Dodd, ch. 9 this volume). Why does this happen?

As our model suggests, an important reason is that, as with other state and legal institutions, public inquiries do not stand in an external relation to society. While they are, in legal principle, both independent of government and civil society, and therefore free to challenge conventional wisdom and to recommend major system reform, they also face institutional and social constraints that shape their outcomes. Liora Salter notes in her study of public inquiries that there is a contradiction between their radical potential and their often disappoint-ingly limited results (Salter 1990). She points to the widespread practice by governments of appointing commissioners who they see as "sound." Often, as in the case of the Westray Inquiry, they are judges who, as a group, are likely to be fairly conservative in their outlook. Moreover, Salter argues, there is an implicit understanding by the commissioners that their mandate is to produce a report that the government of the day will find acceptable and act upon. These appointment practices and understandings promote self-censorship and the dominance of narrow pragmatism. These tendencies are further reinforced by the appointment of researchers and other commission staff members whose views are well within the mainstream and, therefore, will be unlikely to promote critical perspectives. It is notable, for example, that the Westray Inquiry hired Ian Plummer, Ontario's former Chief Mines Inspector, who espouses a view of the IRS that minimizes the importance of worker participation and empowerment (Plummer, Strahlendorf, and Holliday 1999), to advise it on the IRS model.

The overall result is that public inquiries often function as schemes of legitimation (Ashforth 1990; Sheriff, 1983). They listen to society and speak to the state, but the vision of the common good that they advance has been filtered through a conservative understanding of proper social relations and the role of government. Legitimation, however, cannot simply be produced in a top-down manner, divorced from social reality. Rather, the inquiry process is part of a two-way conversation between state and society, albeit one that is mediated in the ways we have described. Still, the very legitimacy of the public inquiry itself derives, in part, from its public hearings at which interested groups are given the opportunity to express their views, as well as from its responsiveness to expressed concerns. Indeed, the utility of public inquiries to government is not limited to their pacification effect, but also comes from their ability to communicate to government the boundaries of what is politically acceptable in the aftermath of a disruptive event like a disaster. So, from time to time, the conservative institutional tendencies of inquiries are overcome, systems are held accountable, and more wide-sweeping recommendations are made (McEvoy 1995). The likelihood of this happening may partially be a function of the idiosyncrasies of individual commissioners, but a more important influence is the ability of victims' groups and their supporters to use the disaster to articulate a critical perspective and to translate the heightened moral authority they enjoy into popular support for system changes.

Neither was done very successfully in the aftermath of the Westray disaster. In part this was because the Westray Families and the labor movement were understandably focused on the need to hold individuals and organizations accountable (and to rebut assertions by the Premier, Donald Cameron, that the miners themselves were at fault). Of course, that was not their exclusive concern, but it was the one that tended to take precedence and for which public support was highest. Also significant was the fact that the labor movement does not have a unified position on OHS regulation. While many OHS activists were sharply critical of the current regime, a significant number of trade union leaders have embraced it, seeing it both pragmatically as the best deal they can cut politically, and as a means of providing workers with a voice in the workplace and in government, even if only as junior partners. As a result, the labor movement has tended to support modest modifications to, rather than radical critique of, the current regime. Indeed, even before the Westray Inquiry reported, the province's OHS law had been amended, pursuant to a series of recommendations produced by a bipartite advisory council (see below).

In sum, as in the Aberfan disaster (McLean and Johnes 2000), existing corporatist arrangements undercut the potential of the disaster to call into question the legitimacy of the OHS regime. Instead, public attention was focused on the personal and organizational failures of the mine operator and the government regulators. Under these conditions, the normal institutional tendencies of public inquiries to reflect, repair, and reproduce dominant understandings operated with little opposition.

Changing the OHS Law and Its Administration: More of the Same?—Not only does government set in motion institutions of redress like public inquiries; it provides redress directly through its own actions, whether through legislation or administrative action in response to recommendations from other bodies or on its own initiative. As we already noted, the Nova Scotia government immediately accepted all the recommendations that were within its authority to implement, including the appointment of a consultant to review the inspectors' actions. But even before the inquiry had started, in December 1992, the government initiated a review of the province's health and safety laws by the Nova Scotia Occupational Health and Safety Advisory Council (NSOHSAC), a bipartite labor-management body. They issued their consensus report, entitled *Taking Responsibility* (NSOHSAC 1995), a little over two years later.

The report largely endorsed the underlying principles and practices of the existing IRS. Employer and worker cooperation was expected to be the norm and the role of the government was to clarify the responsibilities of the workplace parties and support their efforts, resorting to enforcement only when necessary. The recommendations aimed to better institutionalize this system by, for example, providing better access to information and improving training for joint health and safety committee members. The issue of worker empowerment, however, was not touched upon, except in the call for greater clarity about the right of workers refusing unsafe work to be paid. Some recommendations were made in respect of enforcement, including an increase in the level of fines, but nothing was said about the level and intensity of enforcement activity. These recommendations were embodied in Bill 13, passed without dissent in 1996 by the then-Liberal government.

In the world of OHS regulation, however, administrative practice is at least as important as formal legislation. While the inspectors directly involved with Westray were terminated, it is questionable whether the division has adopted a fundamentally different approach to enforcement. Data from the annual reports of the OHS Division of the Department of Environment and Labor (Nova Scotia, various years) indicate that since 1996-97 (the first year for which systematic data are available) the annual number of inspections and stop work orders has fluctuated, but the number of orders has more than doubled (see Table 1). As

Table 1. Nova Scotia, Department of Labor, Occupational Health and
Safety Division Enforcement Activity, 1996-97–2000-04

	1996-97	1997-98	1998-99	1999-2000	2000-01	2001-02	2002-03	2003-04
General inspections	1368	1288	1022	1563	1897	1287	1039	1460
Orders issued	2684	3754	4276	6976	8610	5860	6692	7034
Stop work orders	126	80	167	202	144	137	141	123
Prosecutions	12	8	14	32	14	24	28	45
Work refusals	10	19	24	18	8	?	?	?

Source: Nova Scotia, Department of Environment and Labor, *OHS Division, 2003-04.*

well, in the past few years there has been an increase in the number of prosecutions. These data suggest some improvement in the enforcement effort, but there is need for caution in their interpretation.

For example, the 2001 report of the Nova Scotia Auditor General raised numerous concerns about the department's enforcement practices: the department only had a little more than one-third of the businesses in the province in its tracking system; at the current rate of inspections it would take ten years to complete a full cycle of inspections; the department lacked a rigorous approach to targeting higher-risk workplaces; there was inadequate follow-up of compliance orders issued; resource limitations could result in suspected offenders not being prosecuted; finally, there were not adequate procedures in place to monitor the work activity of inspectors (NS Auditor General 2001, ch. 9). In 2003-04 the department reported that there was still an ongoing problem of achieving timely compliance with orders. As well, it reported that nearly two-thirds of prosecutions were in the construction industry. Fines for convictions are generally low; the average was less than $10,000, while the highest was a fine of $45,000 levied against the province's Ministry of Transport and Public Works. The largest fine against a private sector employer was $28,000. As well, the department also reported that there is still significant non-compliance with the requirements of the IRS. Although the situation has improved in recent years, in 2003-04 one-third of employers with 20 or more employees failed to meet each of five measures of IRS compliance.

In short, while the Westray mine disaster forced the government to acknowledge that its practice of OHS regulation was deficient, the underlying assumptions that supported those practices were not seriously called into question. The few groups that raised concerns about unequal power relations in the workplace and the need to recognize that employers and workers will frequently have conflicting interests in OHS regulation were easily marginalized in a political climate where the labor movement not only lacks clout, but also has bought into the weak form of corporatism that OHS bipartism represents. The result is that, while personnel changes have been made, the ideology and practice of OHS regulation has largely been reconstructed in its pre-Westray form.

Criminal Law Reform—The impediments to and ultimate failure of the Westray prosecutions fueled popular support criminal law reforms that would overcome at least some of the technical difficulties that have shielded employers from being held criminally responsible for reckless conduct that caused death and injury to workers. The efforts of trade unions (particularly the USWA) and the Westray Families Group to have the *Criminal Code* amended received a substantial boost when the Westray inquiry accepted their submission on this point and recommended that the federal government should amend the criminal law as necessary to ensure that corporate executives and directors are held accountable for workplace safety (Richard 1997, rec. 73). As well, the fact that England and a number of jurisdictions in Australia have either enacted or are considering similar kinds of changes to their criminal laws both reflects a widespread crisis of legitimacy over the criminal law's lack of even-handedness and makes such changes appear less radical than might otherwise be the case (Glasbeek 2004a). But still, the process of reforming the criminal law was painfully slow and difficult.

Following the commission recommendation, Alexa McDonough, then the leader of the Federal NDP and herself a Nova Scotian, introduced a private member's bill in February 1998 aimed to increase the exposure of corporations, directors, and officers to criminal liability. Peter McKay, then the Progressive-Conservative Member of Parliament whose riding includes the Westray mine, also introduced a motion calling on the government to implement that recommendation. Neither the bill nor the motion proceeded in that session, but both were reintroduced in the next where, by a margin of 216 to 15, the House of Commons voted to refer McKay's motion to the Standing Committee on Justice and Human Rights. In preparation for that meeting, the Steelworkers commissioned a national poll in which 85% supported a law that "would establish fines and jail terms for corporate executives and directors found to be criminally responsible for harm or injury to employees or members of the public." Thirty-seven percent felt that the best way to prevent future Westrays was to make corporate directors criminally accountable, while another 31% supported more government inspectors (MacKinnon 2000). As well, the Steelworkers conducted an intensive four-day lobby involving members brought to Ottawa from around the country.

At the Committee, members from every political party, including from the most conservative, spoke in favor of the motion and a report issued endorsing an amendment to the *Criminal Code* that would ensure that "corporate executives and directors are held properly accountable for workplace safety" (Canada 2000). It also recommended to the Minister of Justice that legislation be brought forward in accordance with the motion and the principles underlying McDonough's private member's bill. Later that fall, the House of Commons concurred in the report, but shortly thereafter elections were called and Parliament was dissolved.

Another large Liberal majority government was returned and the private member's bill was reintroduced in February 2001. The House of Commons once again voted to send the matter to the Standing Committee, which, held hearings in 2002, and issued a report in November calling for legislation dealing with the criminal liability of corporations, officers and directors. The government accepted this recommendation and on June 12, 2003 introduced a bill (Bill 45 2003) that according to the Department of Justice (2003) "sends a clear message to employers: those who fail to provide safe workplaces will be dealt with severely through the criminal law." The bill passed and received Royal Assent on November 7, 2003. It came into force on 31 March 2004, nearly 12 years after the disaster.[12]

The two most pertinent changes made by the Westray Bill are that it establishes a new set of legal duties in the *Criminal Code* and that it makes it easier to hold an organization responsible for the acts of its senior officials. The new s. 217.1 provides:

> Every one who undertakes, or has authority, to direct how another person does work or performs a task is under a legal duty to take reasonable steps to prevent bodily harm to that person, or any other person, arising from that work or harm.

The effect of the section is to impose individual criminal responsibility quite broadly. Anyone with authority to direct work, not just managerial employees, is under a duty to take reasonable steps to prevent harm. This could include, for example, the lowest level supervisory employees, a matter that concerns unions based on their experience with provincial health and safety prosecutions of co-workers, perhaps as a means of demonstrating the regulators' neutrality when also charging employers. As well, the law will impose liability for harm done to people outside the workplace, a responsibility that is not covered by most provincial health and safety laws (Nova Scotia is an exception). To successfully prosecute an individual under this section, it will not be enough to establish a breach of the relevant provincial health and safety law subject to the defense of due diligence; rather, it will be necessary to prove beyond a reasonable doubt that the individual breached her or his s. 217.1 duty recklessly or with intent.

To get at employing organizations, the *Code* was amended to make them parties to offences in a broader range of circumstances than in the past. First, the law does not just apply to corporations, but to organizations, including corporations, partnerships, and trade unions. Second, under the pre-existing law, corporations could only be held responsible for criminal conduct committed by a directing mind with *policy* responsibility. Under Bill C-45 organizational liability has been broadened to include criminal conduct committed at an *operational* level. Third, organizational responsibility has been extended deeper into the organization. In the past, corporations were only parties if criminality was found at its highest levels. Under the current law, it can be held criminally responsible if one of its representatives (which could include employees, agents, and contractors as well as directors and partners) is a party to an offense, and if a senior officer responsible for a relevant aspect of the organization's activities "departs markedly from the standard of care that, in the circumstances, could reasonably be expected to prevent a representative of the organization from being a party."[13] Thus, under the new law organizations are responsible not only for monitoring the activities of their own officers and employees, but for their agents and contractors, and corporate directors cannot insulate the organization from liability by sloughing off responsibility to senior operating officials lower in the hierarchy. Finally, the new law addresses the problem of diffusion of responsibility within the organization by allowing the prosecution to prove that senior officers collectively departed markedly from the standard of care expected of them. However, it is important to note that it will not be sufficient to show that the senior officers were negligent in their oversight. The crown will have to prove criminal recklessness to establish a marked departure from the standard of care.[14]

It is too early to tell whether the Westray Bill will bring the criminal law more fully into OHS regime, by making it an effective weapon in the arsenal of OHS regulators and law enforcement officials. The first and, so far, only charge under Bill C-45 is against an Ontario man supervising a trench excavation performed without proper shoring. The walls collapsed and a worker was killed (Keith 2004). The charge has since been dropped. For those who hoped Bill C-45 would be used to impose criminal sanctions on corporations, this is an inauspicious beginning. Prosecutions aside, the immediate impact of the passage of Bill C-45 has been to generate business for professional risk managers (Fraser 2004; Keith 2004; McGillivray 2004) and, undoubtedly, large employers will take some measures to reduce their exposure. While this could include instituting better health and safety measures in the workplace, they may also adopt legal strategies, such as invoking their right to counsel and their right to remain silent in the aftermath of a workplace death or serious injury, that do nothing to reduce *worker* risk exposure. In the longer term, the impact will depend, in part, on the extent to which the amendments overcome the technical difficulties crown prosecutors faced in the past. In turn, this will depend on how the courts interpret a number of ambiguous terms in the law. The more important determinant, however, will be the extent to which crown prosecutors attempt to use the law. This brings us back to the sociological analysis discussed earlier. As long as the assumption is made that the workplace is a realm of voluntarism in which respectable employers are engaged in the respectable pursuit of profit, then it will remain difficult to convince enforcement officials to resort to criminal prosecutions. Indeed, recall that presently they rarely prosecute for violations of provincial health and safety laws. However, the enactment of this legislation, and the efforts in other jurisdictions to make employers criminally responsible for workplace deaths and injuries show that this assumption is being challenged. Westray has become a potent cultural and political symbol of unpunished employer criminality and the need for legal, institutional and, perhaps ultimately, social change to redress this situation.

CONCLUSION

The Westray disaster disrupted the pre-existing OHS regime that had, in effect, made private the troubles experienced by the miners and their families. It gave them and their supporters a greater public voice and opportunities to mobilize institutions of redress in pursuit of accountability for the loss of 26 lives and reform to prevent future disasters. But in the end, they met with limited success in achieving their objectives.

Monetary compensation was the least problematic because the province's workers' compensation system makes the payment of survivors' benefits a routine matter, not requiring any assignment of fault. But as a result, the workers' compensation system did not address the demands for individual, organizational, and systemic accountability. Tort law provides a mechanism for holding individuals and organizations accountable, but in Canada the statutory bar in workers' compensation statutes has virtually eliminated this form of redress, even in the aftermath of a disaster caused by serious wrongdoing. The strongest form of public accountability is through the criminal law, but though a combination of bungling, lack of government support, and technical obstacles, the Westray prosecution failed miserably. However, public outrage over employers getting away with criminal disregard for the lives of their workers, in conjunction with a broader crisis of corporate legitimacy fueled by recent scandals, created a political environment in which politicians of all political stripes felt the need to demonstrate their commitment to equality before the law, by removing at least some of the technical barriers to the successful prosecution of individuals and their employing organizations when they grossly neglect their duty to insure that work is performed safely. But in the long run, the success of the Westray Bill will depend on whether the underlying assumptions about the consensual nature of work relations that have informed health and safety regulation since the nineteenth century are changed. Ironically, the Richard commission of inquiry, which provided much needed support for criminal law reform, endorsed the very assumptions that have undermined all previous efforts to strengthen the enforcement of health and safety laws, including the incorporation of the criminal law into the OHS regime.

Thus, while the legacy of Westray remains uncertain in terms of its impact on the OHS regime, it continues to be a potent reminder of the dangers that workers face in a world in which there is systemic pressure on employers to maximize profits, even if that means putting production ahead of safety, and on governments to provide business-friendly regulatory climates.

ENDNOTES

1. Interview with Robert Wells, CUPE Health and Safety Representative, 11 November 2000.
2. Twenty days after the explosion the surviving miners voted in favor of the union.
3. There may also be economic losses to persons who do not suffer injury. In the case of Westray, surviving employees were laid off because of the mine's closure. The Labor Standards Board, a provincial tribunal, held that 117 miners were entitled to 12 weeks of severance pay. However, because the employer is bankrupt, the employees, who turned to Nova Scotia government for payment, were promised that they will be paid out of the proceeds of the sale of the remaining company assets.
4. There was a problem with compensation for at least one Westray miner who suffered psychological trauma arising out of his experiences in the mine rescue and recovery operations, but he recently won an appeal that awarded him $101,000 in back payments and a monthly pension of $675 (Naiberg 2004, pp. 20-21).
5. Quite independently of the Westray explosion, employers were already pressing the government to amend the workers' compensation legislation to address their concerns about rising costs and unfunded liabilities. Amendments enacted in 1995 responded to the employers' cost-cutting agenda, but did not adversely affect the Westray families. On the general pattern of North American workers' compensation "reforms," see McCluskey (1998).
6. Workers' compensation boards in Canada have increasingly asserted that prevention is an important part of their mandate and have pursued this goal through education and the use of economic incentives, principally experience rating. This is not the place to engage with the literature on the efficacy of experience rating except to note that it also creates incentives to engage in claims management. Claims management was pursued with a vengeance at the Westray mine. Indeed, Curragh was awarded a prestigious safety award just prior to the explosion on the basis of its fraudulently low claims experience. The award, which had been accepted by one of the miners killed in the explosion, was subsequently withdrawn (Comish 1993).
7. Part of the reason for this difference is that workers' compensation in the United States is usually less generous than in Canada and involves lawyers to a far greater extent.
8. For a somewhat longer discussion with fuller references, see Tucker (1995b).
9. The dissenting judges would have refused to order a new trial because the conduct of the Crown had brought the administration of justice into disrepute by its failures to disclose evidence and its attempts to cover this up and mislead the court.
10. It is still far more common for employers to be prosecuted under regulatory statutes, but these do not have the same normative purchase as criminal prosecutions.
11. Clifford Frame and Marvin Pelley, two senior Curragh executives, fiercely resisted efforts to subpoena them. Eventually, the commission decided to issue its report without waiting for their testimony.

12. *An Act to amend the Criminal Code (criminal liability of organizations)*, S.C. 2003, c. 21.
13. S. 22.1(b).
14. For a fuller discussion of the *Criminal Code* amendments and a critical assessment, see Archibald, Jull, and Roach (2004) and Glasbeek (2004b).

REFERENCES

Archibald, T., Jull, K., and Roach, K. (2004) The Changed Face of Corporate Criminal Liability. *Criminal Law Quarterly, 48*: 367-396.

Ashforth, A. (1990) Reckoning Schemes of Legitimation: On Commissions of Inquiry as Power/Knowledge Forms. *Journal of Historical Sociology, 3*: 1-22.

Atiyah, P. S. (1997) *The Damages Lottery*. Oxford: Hart.

Bale, A. (1989) America's First Compensation Crisis: Conflict over the Value and Meaning of Workplace Injuries under the Employers' Liability System. In D. Rosner and G. Markowitz (eds.), *Dying for Work* (pp. 34-52). Bloomington: Indiana University Press.

Bill C-45. (2003) *An Act to amend the Criminal Code (criminal liability of organizations)*. House of Commons of Canada, Second Session, Thirty-seventh Parliament. (Now S.C. 2003, c. 21).

Bell v. Canada (Attorney General) (2001), 204 D.L.R. (4th) 486 (NSSC), aff'd. (2002), 208 D.L.R. (4th) 654 (N.S.C.A.), leave to appeal denied [2002] S.C.C.A. No. 135, online QL.

Benson, M. L. (2001) Prosecuting Corporate Crime: Problems and Constraints. In N. Shover and J. P. Wright (eds.), *Crimes of Privilege* (pp. 381-391). New York: Oxford.

Brooks, P. (2002) Westray Appeal Rejected. *Halifax Herald*. 16 August 2002.

Brym, R. J., and Sacouman, R. J. (eds.). (1979) *Underdevelopment and Social Movements in Atlantic Canada*. Toronto: New Hogtown Press.

Canada. (2000) House of Commons. Standing Committee on Justice and Human Rights. Fifth Report (6 June).

Calgary Herald (18 January 1943) Nasdegg Mine is Fined $5,000.

Chambliss, W., and Seidman, B. (1971) *Law, Order and Power*. London: Addison-Wesley.

Coffee, J. Jr. (1981) "No Soul to Damn: No Body to Kick": An Unscandalized Inquiry into the Problem of Corporate Punishment. *Michigan Law Review, 79*: 386-459.

COHSN (8 Feb. 1993) NS WCB to pay Westray survivors about $15 million in pensions, one-time costs.

Comish, S. (1993) *The Westray Tragedy: A Miner's Story*. Halifax: Fernwood.

Cooke, D. L. (2003) A System Dynamics Analysis of the Westray Mine Disaster. *System Dynamics Review, 19*: 139-166.

Department of Justice (2003) *New Measures to Address Capital Markets Fraud, Promote Workplace Safety and Modernize the Laws Regarding Corporate Criminal Liability.* Press Release, 12 June 2003, available online at http://canada.justice.gc.ca/en/news/sp/2003/doc_30930.html.

Dewees, D., Duff, D., and Trebilcock, M. (1996) *Exploring the Domain of Accident Law*. New York: Oxford University Press.

Dodd, S. (1998) Unsettled Accounts after Westray. In C. McCormick (1999a). pp. 218-249.

Dodd, S. (2001) *The Writing of the Westray Story: An Discursive Analysis of the After-math of the Westray Coal Mine Explosion*. Ph.D. Dissertation. York University.

Earle, M. J. (ed.). (1989) *Workers and the State in Twentieth Century Nova Scotia*. Fredericton: Acadiensis Press.

Feldthusen, B. (2000) Punitive Damages: Hard Choices and High Stakes. In J. M. Flaherty and K. A. Carpenter-Gunn (eds.), *Personal Injury* (pp. 583-624). Ottawa: Law Society of Upper Canada.

Fraser, J. L. (2004, May) Legislating Safety—A Contentious Claim. *CMA Management, 78*(3): 30-32.

Geis, G., and DiMento J. (1995) Should We Prosecute Corporations and/or Individuals. In F. Pearce and L. Snider (eds.), *Corporate Crimes: Contemporary Debates* (pp. 72-86). Toronto: University of Toronto Press.

Glasbeek, H. (1984) Why Corporate Deviance Is Not Treated as a Crime—The Need to Make Profits a Dirty Word. *Osgoode Hall Law Journal, 22*: 393-439.

Glasbeek, H. (1988) A Role for Criminal Sanctions in Occupational Health and Safety. In Meredith Memorial Lectures: New Developments in Employment Law (pp. 125-149). Cowansville, Que.: Editions Yvon Blais.

Glasbeek, H. (2004a) Crime, Health and Safety and Corporations: Meanings of the Failed Crimes (*Workplace Deaths and Serious Injuries*) Bill. University of Melbourne, Faculty of Law Legal Studies Research Paper No. 62, Online at http://papers.ssrn.com/sol2/papers.cfm?abstract_id=521662.

Glasbeek, H. (2004b) *More Criminalization in Canada: More of the Same?* Paper presented at the Industrial and Corporate Manslaughter Seminar, Flinders Law School and GREWC, University of South Australia, Adelaide (March 12).

Glasbeek, H., and Tucker, E. (1993) Death by Consensus: The Westray Story. *New Solutions, 3*(4): 14-41.

Halifax Daily News (7 December 1997) Westray Exposed Governments' Shortcomings, p. 2.

Hopkins, A. (1989) Crime Without Punishment: The Appin Mine Disaster. In P. Grabosky and A. Sutton (eds.), *Stains on a White Collar* (pp. 160-174). Annandale, NSW: Federation Press.

Hyatt, D., and Law, D. K. (2000) Should Work-Injury Compensation Continue to Imbibe at the Tort Bar? In M. Gunderson and D. Hyatt (eds.), *Workers' Compensation: Foundations for Reform* (pp. 327-360). Toronto: University of Toronto Press.

Ison, T. G. (1967) *The Forensic Lottery*. London: Staples.

Jobb, D. (1994) *Calculated Greed: Greed, Politics and the Westray Tragedy*. Halifax: Nimbus.

Jobb, D. (1999) Legal Disaster: Westray and the Justice System. In C. McCormick (ed.), *The Westray Chronicles* (pp. 163-182). Halifax: Fernwood.

Keith, N. (2004) Letting Loose on Supervisors. *OHS Canada* October/November: 54.

King, A. (1998) The Price of Coal. *Our Times,* May/June: 37-40.

MacKinnon, M. (2000) Canadians Want Executives to Pay for Fatal Mistakes in Workplace. *Globe and Mail,* (6 June), A2.

McCluskey, M. T. (1998) The Illusion of Efficiency in Workers' Compensation Reform. *Rutgers Law Review, 50*: 657-941.

McCormick, C. (ed.). (1999a) *The Westray Chronicles*. Halifax: Fernwood.

McCormick, C. (1999b) Preface to Disaster. In C. McCormick (ed.). (1999a). 12-39.

McEvoy, A. F. (1995) The Triangle Shirtwaist Factory Fire of 1911: Social Change, Industrial Accidents, and the Evolution of Common-Sense Causality. *Law & Social Inquiry, 20*: 621-651.

McGillivray, G. (2004, March) The Dawn of Corporate Responsibility. *Canadian Underwriter, 71*(3): 38-43.

McLean, I., and Johnes, M. (2000) *Aberfan[:] Government and Disasters.* Cardiff: Welsh Academic Press.

McMullan, J., and Hinze, S. (1999) Westray: The Press, Ideology, and Corporate Crime. In C. McCormick (ed.). (1999a).

Mills, C. W. (1959) *The Sociological Imagination.* New York: Oxford University Press.

Naiberg, D. (2004) Miner Wins Benefits Decade After Westray. *OHS Canada,* (April/June): 20-21.

Nichols, T. (1999) *The Sociology of Industrial Injury.* London: Mansell.

Nova Scotia (1985) *Occupational Health and Safety Act,* S.N.S. 1985, c. 3.

Nova Scotia (1997) *Westray* [:] *A Plan of Action.*

Nova Scotia (various years) *Department of Environment and Labor, OHS Division, Annual Report.*

NS Auditor General (2001) *Annual Report, 2001.*

NSOHSAC (1995) *Taking Responsibility.* Halifax: NSOHSAC.

Pasiechnyk v. Saskatchewan (Workers' Compensation Board) (1997) [1997] 2 S.C.R. 890.

Pearce, F. (1976) *Crimes of the Powerful.* London: Pluto.

Pearce F., and Snider, L. (eds.). (1995) *Corporate Crime: Contemporary Debates.* Toronto: University of Toronto Press.

Pearce F., and Tombs, S. (1999) *Toxic Capitalism: Corporate Crime and the Chemical Industry.* Toronto: Canadian Scholars' Press.

Phillips v. Nova Scotia (Commission of Inquiry) (1993) 100 D.L.R. 79 (NSCA).

Phillips v. Nova Scotia (Commission of Inquiry) (1995) [1995] 2 S.C.R. 97.

Plummer I., Strahlendorf, P. S., and Holliday, M. G. (1999) *The Internal Responsibility System in Ontario Mines* (Interim Report #1: Description of the IRS).

R. v. Curragh Inc. (1993) 124 N.S.R. (2d) 59 (Prov. Ct.).

R. v. Curragh Inc. (1994) 125 N.S.R. (2d) 185 (Prov. Ct.).

R. v. Curragh Inc. (1995a) [1995] S.C.C.A. No. 138 (S.C.C.).

R. v. Curragh Inc. (1995b) [1995] N.S.J. No. 275. (Prov. Ct.).

R. v. Curragh Inc. (1995c) 146 N.S.R. (2d) 161 (C.A.).

R. v. Curragh Inc. (1997) [1997] 1 S.C.R. 537 (S.C.C.).

R. v. McNamara et al. (No. 1) (1981) 56 C.C.C. (2d) 193 (Ont. C.A.), 198.

Rex.v. Brazeau Collieries (1942) 3 W.W.R. 570.

Reich, M. R. (1991) *Toxic Politics: Responding to Chemical Disasters.* Ithaca, NY: Cornell University Press.

Reich, M. R. (1994) Toxic Politics and Victims in the Third World. In S. Jasanoff (ed.), *Learning from Disaster* (pp. 180-203). Philadelphia, PA: University of Pennsylvania Press.

Rees, J. V. (1988) *Reforming the Workplace: A Study of Self-Regulation in Occupational Safety.* Philadelphia: University of Pennsylvania Press.

Renn, O. (1992) The Social Arena Concept of Risk Debates. In S. Krimsky and D. Golding (eds.), *Social Theories of Risk* (pp. 179-196). Westport, CT: Praeger.

Richard, K. P. (1997) *The Westray Story[:] A Predictable Path to Disaster*. Report of the Westray Mine Public Inquiry. Halifax.

Richards, T. (1998) Public Relations and the Westray Mine Explosion. In C. McCormick (1998). pp. 136-162.

Roach, K. (1995) Canadian Public Inquiries and Accountability. In P. Stenning (ed.), *Accountability for Criminal Justice* (pp. 268-293). Toronto: University of Toronto Press.

Salter, L. (1990) The Two Contradictions in Public Inquiries. In A. P. Ross et al. (eds.), *Commissions of Inquiry* (pp. 173-195). Toronto: Carswell.

Sheriff, P. E. (1983) State Theory, Social Science, and Government Commissions. *American Behavioral Scientist, 26*: 669-680.

Shrivastava, P. (1987) *Bhopal: Anatomy of a Crisis*. Cambridge, MA: Ballinger.

Slapper, G. (1993) Corporate Manslaughter: An Examination of the Determinants of Prosecutorial Policy. *Social and Legal Studies, 2*: 423-443.

Slapper, G. (1999) *Blood in the Bank: Social and Legal Aspects of Death at Work*. Aldershot: Ashgate.

Taylor, I., Walton, P., and Young, J. (eds.). (1973) *Critical Criminology*. London: Routledge & Kegan Paul.

Tombs, S. (1995) Corporate Crimes and New Organizational Forms. In F. Pearce and L. Snider (eds.). (pp. 132-146).

Tucker, E. (1990) *Administering Danger in the Workplace: The Law and Politics of Occupational Health and Safety Regulation in Ontario*. Toronto: University of Toronto Press.

Tucker, E. (1995a) And Defeat Goes On: An Assessment of Third Wave Health and Safety Regulation. In F. Pearce and L. Snider (eds.). (1995). pp. 245-267.

Tucker, E. (1995b) The Westray Mine Disaster and its Aftermath: The Politics of Causation. *Canadian Journal of Law and Society, 10*: 91-123.

Tucker, E. (1999) The Road from Westray: A Predictable Path to Disaster? *Acadiensis, 28*: 132-139.

Wells, C. (1995) *Negotiating Tragedy: Law and Disasters*. London: Sweet & Maxwell.

Whiten v. Pilot Insurance [2002] 1 S.C.R 595.

Contributors

SUSAN DODD, B.A. (King's), M.A. (Political Science, York University), Ph.D. (Sociology, York University). Susan Dodd is a Senior Fellow in the Foundation Year Programme at the University of King's College, Halifax, Nova Scotia. Her doctoral dissertation, in Sociology at York University, is a study of the ideological effects of *The Westray Story,* the report of the Public Inquiry into the Westray coal mine disaster. This study combines text analysis with ethnographic interviews and archival research to explore the implications, for family members, of the release of the report. She has published articles also on the aftermath of the *Ocean Ranger* oil rig disaster of 1982.

ANDREW HOPKINS, Reader in Sociology, Australian National University in Canberra. He has written extensively on occupational injury and on the regulation and management of workplace safety. Among his publications are: *Lessons from Longford: The Esso Gas Pant Explosion* (CCH Australia 2000), *Managing Major Hazards: the Lessons of the Moura Mine Disaster* (Allen & Unwin 1999), and *Making Safety Work: Getting Management Commitment to Occupational Health and Safety* (Allen & Unwin 1998).

RICHARD JOHNSTONE, Professor of Law and Director of the Socio-Legal Research Centre, Griffith University, Australia, and Adjunct Professor, National Research Centre for Occupational Health and Safety Regulation, in the Regulatory Institutions Network, in the Research School of Social Sciences at the Australian National University. His books include *Occupational Health and Safety Law and Policy* (2nd ed.) (LBC 2004), *Occupational Health and Safety, Courts and Crime* (Federation Press 2003); with Neil Gunningham, *Regulating Workplace Safety: Systems and Sanctions* (Oxford University Press 1999); and with Liz Bluff and Neil Gunningham, *OHS Regulation for a Changing World of Work* (Federation Press 2004).

CLAIRE MAYHEW, Senior Research Scientist, National Occupational Health and Safety Commission, Australia. She is the co-editor (with Chris Peterson) of *Occupational Health and Safety in Australia: Industry, Public Sector and Small Business* (Allen & Unwin 1999) and has authored numerous articles and chapters in books on occupational health and safety.

MICHAEL QUINLAN, B.Ec. (hons), Ph.D. (Syd) is a professor in the School of Industrial Relations and Organisational Behaviour at the University of New South Wales, Sydney, Australia, and adjunct associate professor, Middlesex University, United Kingdom. The main focus of his research has been industrial relations policy/history and occupational health and safety (OHS). He is the co-author or editor/co-editor of several books, including *A Divided Working Class* (Routledge 1998), *Managing Occupational Health and Safety* (Macmillan 1991 and 2nd edition 2000), *Work and Health* (Macmillan 1993) and *Systematic OHS Management* (Elsevier 2000). A particular focus of his research has been the effects of institutions, regulation and employment status on OHS. In 2000-01 he undertook an inquiry into safety in the long-haul trucking industry for the Motor Accidents Authority of New South Wales and the NSW government.

PATRICIA REEVE is a doctoral candidate at Boston College, Massachusetts, where she is completing a study of the evolving law of industrial accidents in the United States and its effects on wage earners' civic and social status. Reeve is the former Director of the Labor Resource Center at the University of Massachusetts, Boston. She has worked in and with the labor movement since 1979 as a member, staff person, and university-based labor educator.

RICHARD RENNIE grew up in St. Lawrence, Newfoundland, and his father was one of the many victims of the industrial disaster described here. He holds a Ph.D. in history from Memorial University of Newfoundland, and his doctoral dissertation was awarded the 2003 Eugene Forsey Prize in Canadian Labor and Working-Class History. Rennie has worked as an academic and in the labor movement. He currently lives in Winnipeg, Manitoba, where he works for the provincial government and teaches in the Department of Labor and Workplace Studies at the University of Manitoba.

ANNETTE THÖRNQUIST, Ph.D., is an Associate professor of History at the National Institute for Working Life in Sweden (Department for Labor Market and Work Organization). Her main research field concerns Labor History, Industrial Relations and OHS. Among her recent publications are: "The Silicosis Problem in the Swedish Iron and Steel Industry during the 20th Century." In A. Thörnquist (ed.), *Work Life, Work Environment and Work Safety in Transition. Historical and Sociological Perspectives on the Development in Sweden during the 20th Century* (National Institute for Working Life 2001) and "From Centralized Self-Regulation to Organized Decentralization: Occupational Health and Safety (OHS) in Sweden 1940-2002." In D. Fleming and C. Thörnquist (eds.), *Nordic Management-Labor Relations and Internationalization. Converging and Diverging Tendencies* (Nordic Council of Ministers 2003).

ERIC TUCKER, Professor, Osgoode Hall Law School, York University. Professor Tucker is the author of *Administering Danger in the Workplace: The Law and Politics of Occupational Health and Safety Regulation in Ontario 1850-1914* (University of Toronto Press 1990) and co-author of *Labor Before the Law: The Legal Regulation of Workers' Collective Action 1900-1948*

(Oxford University Press 2001) (with Judy Fudge) and *Self Employed Workers Organize: Law, Politics, and Unions* (McGill-Queen's University Press 2005) (with Cynthia Cranford, Judy Fudge, and Leah Vosko). He has also published numerous articles on contemporary occupational health and safety regulation.

DAVID WHYTE is Lecturer in Criminology at the University of Stirling where he specializes in regulation and corporate crime. His publications include *Unmasking the Crimes of the Powerful* (Peter Lang 2003) (with Steve Tombs).

Index